Integrated Holistic Yoga Psychology

Volume 1 in Therapeutic Yoga Teaching, Clinical Service, and Practice

ALSO BY CHRISTIANE BREMS, PhD, ABPP, ERYT500, C-IAYT

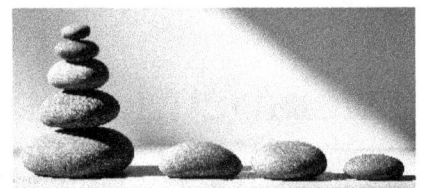

Therapeutic Breathwork: Clinical Research and Practice in Healthcare and Yoga

Comprehensive Guide to Child Psychotherapy and Counseling (4th edition)

Basic Skills in Psychotherapy and Counseling

Instructor's Manual for "Basic Skills in Psychotherapy and Counseling"

Dealing with Challenges in Psychotherapy and Counseling

Psychotherapy: Processes and Techniques

The Child Therapist: Personal Traits and Markers of Effectiveness

Between Two People: Exercises Toward Intimacy (with Johnson & Fortman)

Integrated Holistic Yoga Psychology

Volume 1 in THERAPEUTIC YOGA TEACHING, CLINICAL SERVICE, AND PRACTICE

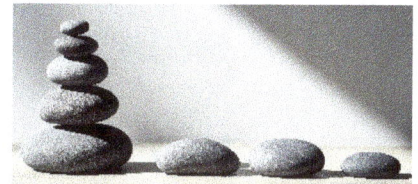

Christiane Brems, PhD, ABPP, ERYT500, C-IAYT

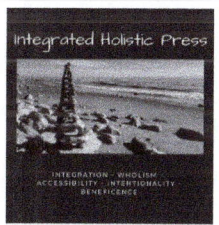

**Integrated Holistic Yoga Psychology:
Volume 1 in Therapeutic Yoga Teaching, Clinical Service, and Practice**

Copyright © 2025 by Christiane Brems, PhD, ABPP, ERYT500, C-IAYT
Integrated Holistic Press
Santa Barbara, California

All rights reserved. No part of this publication may be reproduced, stored in a retrieval system, or transmitted in any form or by any means, electronic, mechanical, photocopying, recording, or otherwise, without the prior written permission of the publisher and copyright holder.

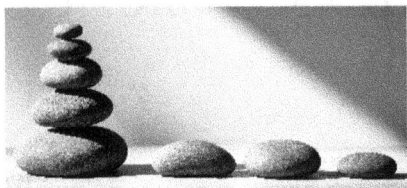

US Library of Congress Cataloging-in-Publication Data:

Title:	*Integrated Holistic Yoga Psychology: Volume 1 in Therapeutic Yoga Teaching, Clinical Service, and Practice*
Author:	Christiane Brems, PhD, ABPP, ERYT500, C-IAYT
Format:	Softcover
ISBN:	979-8-9928567-1-2
Publication Date:	2025
Disclaimers:	The information provided in this book is not intended to substitute for medical, movement, breathing, or other practice advice of qualified healthcare providers. This book is not intended to diagnose or treat any medical or mental health conditions, but rather serves to describe an approach to integrated holistic movement, breathing, and inner yoga practices. Readers are advised to consult with their qualified healthcare providers if they have questions about the appropriateness of any of the strategies offered in this book for themselves or their students or clients. The publisher and the author is not liable for any injuries, damages, or negative consequences allegedly arising from any actions, movements, applications, or preparations by anyone reading or otherwise perusing the information in this book.
	References and websites provided throughout this book are strictly for informational purposes and do not constitute an endorsement of any websites or other named sources. Readers should also be aware that website addresses listed in this book may change. The information and references included in this book were up to date at the time of its writing but given that medical evidence progresses quickly, they may not be up to date by the time of reading.
Cover Image:	Rock Cairns by Victor Gladkov (Data source: istock.com)

Dedication

This book is dedicated to all yoga practitioners everywhere.

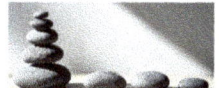

May your practice serve your health and wellbeing
and provide you a sense of agency and personal empowerment.

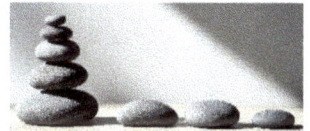

May your practice invite compassion, lovingkindness,
appreciative and altruistic joy, and equanimity.

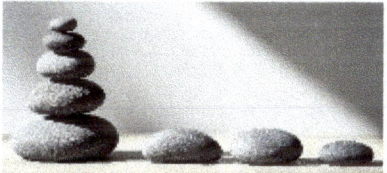

May your practice reverberate into your communities,
creating wholesome collectives that serve
the greater good for all human and sentient beings,
as well as this planet.

Foreword

"A human being is a part of the whole, called by us 'Universe', a part limited in time and space. He (sic) experiences himself, ... thoughts and feelings as something separated from the rest – a kind of optical delusion of ... consciousness. This delusion is a kind or prison for us, restricting us to our personal desires and to affection for a few persons nearest to us. Our task must be to free ourselves from this prison by widening our circle of compassion to embrace all living creatures and the whole of nature in its beauty."
Albert Einstein

> *"Most [humans] lead lives of quiet desperation and go to the grave with the song still in them."*
> *Henry David Thoreau*

The quest to know who we are and to express this true essence guides our day-to-day lives and major decisions. Yet, the ideas we form about our self-definition are often distorted, outdated, rooted in habit, or determined by others. Not surprisingly, we often live an unquestioned life, lacking a sense of meaning or purpose and being caught up in habits or ruts. We go about our lives as if they were a preparation for something else – simply a rehearsal for a better future. Yet occasionally we wake up and realize that this is it – this life is the one to live in a way that counts, that improves the world, that gives something back, that makes a difference. In those moments, we begin our existential search for a better way to be and we turn to ancient traditions and modern science for guideposts and advice on how to accomplish this task. One such practice, combining ancient wisdom and current-day research, is yoga.

Ancient yogis, dating back as far as 500 BCE, and modern yoginis have defined paths toward more meaningful existence and have provided guidance for purposeful lives. They have given us a framework for day-to-day living that explores the many aspects of self that flow into each action we take and every decision we make. They have discovered that by becoming more mindfully aware of how we make choices, gain insight into the truth of human life, and become more compassionate with ourselves and the entire web of life, we can improve ourselves and our impact on our world. We can free the song in our heart and let it brighten our individual and collective existence.

Yoga training in general, and this series of three books in particular, is offered as a way to begin the journey home to ourselves and to set free the song in our hearts. It is an invitation to become curious, interested, patient, mindful, open-minded, open-hearted, grateful, joyful, equanimous, and compassionate. The journey begins with this volume that explores how yoga as an art and science invites us to explore ourselves, guide our students and clients, and enlighten our communities from a place of awareness, insight, and compassion. It offers a deep exploration of yoga psychology from a developmental perspective. It hones a deep understanding of human physicality, vitality, mind, emotions, behaviors, and relationships as profound expressions of our humanity and power to create change not only for ourselves but our greater communities.

Enjoy the journey. With love,

Chris Brems

Content Overview of the Series
Therapeutic Yoga Teaching, Clinical Service, and Practice

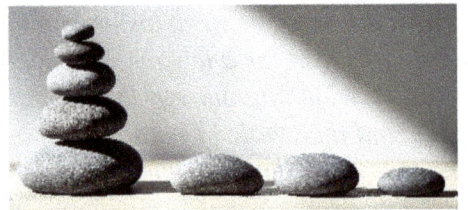

Volume 1 – Integrated Holistic Yoga Psychology

Section 1: Integrated Holistic Yoga History and Psychology

Section 2: Integrated Holistic Yoga Pedagogy and Practice Principles

Volume 2 – Integrated Holistic Yoga Movement

Section 1: Integrated Holistic Yoga Anatomy and Physiology

Section 2: Integrated Holistic Yoga Approaches to Asana

Volume 3 – Integrated Holistic Introspective Yoga Practices

Section 1: Integrated Holistic Yoga Approaches to Pranayama

Section 2: Integrated Holistic Yoga Approaches to Inner Practices

Introduction to the Series
Therapeutic Yoga Teaching, Clinical Service, and Practice

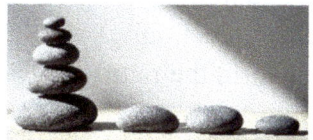

The three-volume series *"Therapeutic Yoga Teaching, Clinical Service, and Practice"* offers an integrated holistic approach to the teaching, clinical service provision, and practice of therapeutic yoga. Integrated holistic yoga is defined by its focus on intentionality, beneficence, accessibility, wholism, and integration. It carefully reviews, weaves together, and scientifically and practically grounds therapeutic yoga practices and lifestyles in the traditional eight limbs of yoga. It simultaneously contextualizes all offered yoga principles and practices within the wholism of the five layers of human experience postulated by ancient wisdom and supported by modern science. It explores and honors interrelationships among body, vitality (energy and affect), mind (emotions and thoughts), wisdom and self-discovery, and relationships within families and communities, in support of personal and collective healing and thriving.

Therapeutic Yoga Contents Covered in the Series

In three comprehensive volumes, the series *"Therapeutic Yoga Teaching, Clinical Service, and Practice"* elucidates the principles of therapeutic yoga guided by a strong commitment to wholism and integration.

- Volume 1, *Integrated Holistic Yoga Psychology*, explores neurophysiological and psychological mechanisms underlying physical, energetic, emotional, cognitive, and relational patterns and habits, combining ancient wisdom about human nature with modern scientific findings. Relying on yoga psychology – ancient and modern, it dives deeply into mind and emotion, exploring the development and transformation of physical, mental, and emotional habits, based on the cultivation of compassion, awareness, and insight to serve personal and collective healing and thriving.
- Volume 2, *Integrated Holistic Yoga Movement*, reviews anatomical and physiological science as relevant to the teaching of yoga movements and forms, integrating ancient wisdom with modern anatomical and kinesiological research. A multitude of movement teaching principles and practice strategies are offered for supporting enhanced health and wellbeing through therapeutic yoga classes, yoga-therapeutically informed healthcare, and individually-tailored personal practices.
- Volume 3, *Integrated Holistic Introspective Yoga Practices,* offers scientifically-based and ancient yogic approaches to breathwork, sense-guarding, concentration, and meditation practices. It offers scientific insights that guide applied inner practices (including mindfulness). Offered practices lead practitioners toward the cultivation of compassion, awareness, and wisdom, with deliberate implications for personal and collective wellbeing.

Therapeutic Yoga Audiences for the Series

The series *"Therapeutic Yoga Teaching, Clinical Service, and Practice"* is written for
- yoga teacher and therapeutic yoga training programs
- individuals seeking yoga teacher credentials,
- yoga teachers who seek to transform their current teaching to become more therapeutic and person-centered,
- dedicated yoga practitioners who want to deepen and tailor their personal practice, and
- healthcare providers seeking to integrate yoga therapeutics into their clinical practice.

The series is an excellent resource for yoga teacher training programs, carefully designed to exceed educational contents and standards required by Yoga Alliance, the association that registers yoga schools, programs, and teachers internationally. It augment current yoga teachers' training by offering a unique therapeutic lens that allows yoga professionals to broaden their yoga teaching skills and understanding to serve populations of students and clients in community health settings and healthcare systems. The volumes in the series are an invaluable resource for healthcare practitioners who hope to integrate therapeutic yoga strategies into their extant clinical practice. They provide an in-depth exploration of how therapeutic yoga can serve patients in healthcare and mental health care and how it can be infused in clinical service delivery. The series is also appropriate for advanced yoga practitioners who seek to refine their yoga practice to be more person-centered, relevant to their unique biopsychosociocultural context, and tailored to their specific physical, vital, emotional, mental, behavioral, and relational needs.

Therapeutic Yoga Approach and Lineage of the Series

The series *"Therapeutic Yoga Teaching, Clinical Service, and Practice"* offers historically-respectful, science-informed guidance for therapeutic yoga practices and interventions development across all limbs of yoga – from *asana*; *pranayama*; mindfulness, concentration, and meditation; to ethical and committed lifestyle practices – emerging from a respectful context of tradition and science. The series focuses on yoga therapeutics, highlighting yoga as a transformative lifestyle and healing practice that is available to and appropriate for all humans.

The series is unique due to its embrace of the integrated holistic yoga (IHY) paradigm that is defined by accessibility, intentionality, beneficence, wholism, and integration. This unique approach to the teaching, clinical offering, and personal practice of yoga was developed by the author to create a system of yoga therapeutics that offer yoga to the very populations who can most benefit from, but often have limited access to, the practice.

The integrated holistic yoga approach offers a vision that honors the deep cultural traditions of transformative practices, such as yoga and Buddhism, that date back thousands of years. It integrates modern neuroscience with ancient psychologies and practices; it demonstrates the profound wisdoms from the original teachings that we are relearning and rediscovering every day, with research increasingly supporting their usefulness. The integrated holistic framework underlying all practices offered in the series embraces inclusiveness, access, diversity, health, wellbeing, and resilience for everyone. It is a practice of and for community; it honors interdependence and co-regulation. Integrated holistic work embraces an honoring of traditional yogic practices – practices (grounded in the eight limbs of yoga) that are physical only to prepare practitioners for more important interior practices (such as concentration and meditation) and interpersonal applications of a thoughtful and deliberate code of ethics, lifestyle, and discipline.

The integrated holistic approach combines body, emotion, mind, spirit, and community through a comprehensive lifestyle with implications for individual and collective wellbeing. It promotes self-compassion, introspection, and community that lead to insights that alter human physiology and anatomy and – perhaps more importantly – emotions, cognitions, behaviors, and relationships. Integrated holistic practices are accessible to anyone who can breathe without assistance, almost anywhere, for little to no cost. They motivate practitioners to adhere to a complete practice that honors all human needs and experiences, more so than a unidimensional posture practice and freed from Western stereotypes that tend to limit who engages with yoga or other types of transformative work. The following central principles of IHY are interwoven throughout all volumes in the series and guide all teachings and practices.

- *Integrated Holistic Yoga is a practice of intentionality* – commitment to making the world a better place; to living and practicing with intention, purpose, and meaning; to helping all beings develop meaningful goals and life purpose
- *Integrated Holistic Yoga is a practice of beneficence* – commitment to facilitating mechanisms of change that do no harm and lead to positive health and mental health outcomes
- *Integrated Holistic Yoga is a practice of accessibility* – commitment to creating communities of healing that honor and practice diversity, inclusion, equity, advocacy, engaged action, and personal as well collective empowerment
- *Integrated Holistic Yoga is a practice of wholeness* – commitment to honor human complexity, biopsychosociocultural contexts, interconnection, and community
- *Integrated Holistic Yoga is a practice of integration* – commitment to offering a diversity of integrated practices, carefully tailored to individual and collective needs of all humans, interweaving science and soul, as well as interdependence and coregulation

In sum, the three-volume series "*Therapeutic Yoga Teaching, Clinical Service, and Practice*"
- uses an integrated holistic model that covers a multitude of yoga practices for body, breath, mind, and relationships;
- focuses on preparing yoga professionals who offer therapeutic applications of yoga, especially in healthcare settings; and
- is a perfect and unique accompaniment for therapeutic yoga teacher training, personal yoga practice, and self-study to adapt clinical services or standard yoga teaching to become therapeutic, person-centered, and individually tailored.

Please enjoy the three volumes in this series and the journey into self-discovery and thriving that may result. I wish you and your students, clients, and patients the wisdom, awareness, compassion, and joy that is inherent in an integrated holistic practice of yoga. May you and yours discover a practice that leads to coping, healing, and thriving – individually and collectively.

Gratefully,

Chris Brems

Acknowledgements

No book is ever a solitary effort. All books arise out of a particular context and set of experiences, causes, and conditions This book is no exception – I am forever grateful to all the individuals and collectives that have contributed to the emergence of this book during the many decades of my life.

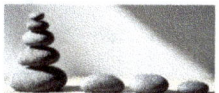

Deep appreciation and ever-lasting gratitude also goes to my many teachers and guides on the path to self-discovery. Your collective depth of knowledge and commitment left indelible marks on my work and my life. All of you remain in my heart always. You have shaped me as a human being, teacher, clinician, colleague, and partner. I am filled with gratitude to each and every one of you.

Klaus, my very first yoga teacher when I was just a wide-eyed youth – you started me on this journey and I cannot thank you enough. I may have forgotten your last name (it was after all 50 years ago), but your impact on my life is as palpable today as it was back then. Lynne Minton – you are an eye-opening inspiration, a yogi in the truest sense of the word, and a wonderful mentor as I started my journey into teaching yoga. Monica Devine, Sarahjoy Marsh, Judith Hansen Lasater, and Christopher Wallis – you inspired me and guided me in the most meaningful ways.

Marty Rossman – you gave me the gift of guided imagery; Patrick McKeown – you shared your profound wisdom and belief in the Buteyko method; Stephen Porges – you imparted your insights into polyvagal theory; Yongey Mingyur Rinpoche, Joseph Goldstein, and Lama Tillmann Borghardt – your Buddhist teachings have deeply inspired and transformed me although I never met them in person.

My commitment to diversity, equity, and accessibility was shared, shaped, and nourished by two beloved (late) colleagues – indigenous psychologist Robert Morgan and Yupik healer Rita Blumenstein (once an elder on the International Council of 13 Grandmothers).

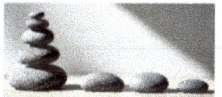

I am forever grateful to you, my students and clients, who may have taught and changed me most of all. I am grateful to you for sharing your wisdom, insights, vulnerabilities, faith, courage, hearts, and experiences. Nothing in life taught me more than being a part of your journeys and witnessing your resilience, joy, and learning. I have learned more from you than I could have ever hoped for. I am filled with the deepest gratitude and love for all of you. You have enriched my life in endless ways that will be with me always.

To my *Breast Cancer Resource Center* 'students' (well, you are really my teachers as much as I am yours) who have shared the journey through cancer – my weekly time with you has been nothing short of miraculous. You have shown the strongest spirit, deep capacity for mutual compassion and caring, and enormous resilience in the wake of intense suffering.

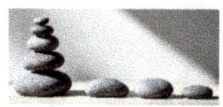

I am filled with gratitude and love for all of my German family, especially my father Bernard Brems, my sister Gabriele Strubel, and brother-in-law Floh Strubel. You are my roots. We may be thousands of miles apart; yet whenever we meet, whenever we talk, whenever we are in one another's thoughts, the distance is gone. We are connected in spirit – always. I am deeply thankful for your presence in my life –
Ich danke Euch allen von ganzem Herzen.

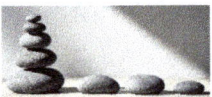

Finally, I am most profoundly and eternally grateful for my intrepid, compassionate, patient (beyond belief), supportive, loving, funny (thanks for the strong core muscles), and unwavering partner, Mark Johnson. You are the love of my life, my best friend, my most trusted human being, and my inspiration. You have helped shape my way of being in the world more than anyone. You constantly rekindle my faith and my joy; you help me feel whole. The greatest miracle in my life was crossing paths with you nearly 40 years ago and having shared a road ever since.

Thank you all!
Chris

Integrated Holistic Yoga Psychology
Volume 1 in Therapeutic Yoga Teaching, Clinical Service, and Practice

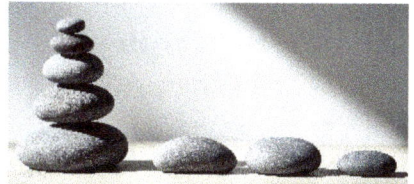

Table of Contents

Section 1: Integrated Holistic Yoga History and Psychology 1

Section 1 Introduction 3
    Yoga History and Psychology Overview 3
    Yoga History and Psychology Learning Objectives 5
    Yoga History and Psychology Recommended Readings 6

Chapter 1: History of Integrated Holistic Yoga 7

Defining Integrated Holistic Yoga 7
    Integrated Holistic Yoga: A Commitment to Wholism 9
        Wholism Avoids Reductionism and Embraces Complexity 10
        Wholism Honors all Human Layers of Consciousness or Experience 10
        Wholism Recognizes Interdependence and Embeddedness in Community 11
        BioPsychoSocioCultural (BPSC) Paradigm 12
    Integrated Holistic Yoga: A Commitment to Integration 15
    Integrated Holistic Yoga: A Commitment to Accessibility, Equity, and Belonging 16
    Integrated Holistic Yoga: A Commitment to Intentionality 18
    Integrated Holistic Yoga: Beneficence and Doing No Harm 20
        Changes that Emerge from an Integrated Yoga Practice 21

A Brief History of Yoga 25
    The Yoga Sutras of Patanjali 28
    Bhagavad Gita 31
    Hatha Yoga Pradipika 33

Chapter 2: Eight Limbs of Yoga 35

Overview of Limbs 1 and 2: A Yoga of Safety and Intention 37
    Limb 1: Yama or Life Choices for Ethical Living 37
        Five Aspirations of Limb 1 38
    Limb 2: Niyamas or Life Choices for Purposeful Living 43
        The Five Commitments of Limb 2 43

Limb 3: Asana or Healing through Form and Movement 47
    Central Principles of Asana 49

Limb 4: Pranayama or Healing through Freeing the Breath 50
    Central Principles of Pranayama 51
        Breath Observation and Awareness 52
        Optimally Functional Breathing 52
        Breathing as Informed by Polyvagal Theory and the Gunas 53

Overview of Limbs 5 to 7: Interior Practices or Healing by Drawing Inward 54
    Limb 5: Pratyahara or Guarding the Senses 54
        Central Principles of Pratyahara 55
    Limb 6: Dharana or Finding Single-Pointed Focus 56
        Central Principles of Dharana 57
    Limb 7: Dhyana or Meditative Awareness 58
        Central Principles of Dhyana 58

Limb 8: Samadhi or Accessing Enlightenment 59

Summary of the Eight Limbs of Yoga 60

Chapter 3: Koshas or Layers of Experience 63

Koshas as Co-Arising and Interdependent Systems 63

Health and Wellness and Their Relationship to the Koshas 66

A Contextual Model of the Koshas 66

The Developmental Perspective of the Koshas 68
    Transcendence and Integration of the Koshas 68
    Feedback and Feedforward across the Interconnected Koshas 70

Annamaya Kosha or Embodied Self or Somatic Consciousness 72
    Some Characteristics of Annamaya Kosha 73
    Annamaya Kosha's Primary Neural Signatures 75

Pranamaya Kosha or Affective or Vital Self or Affective Consciousness 76
    Some Characteristics of Pranamaya Kosha 77
    Pranamaya Kosha's Primary Neural Signatures 78

Manomaya Kosha → Verbal and Social Self or Mental and Emotional Consciousness .. 80
    Some Characteristics of Manomaya Kosha 80
    Developmental Layers within Manomaya Kosha 81
    Manomaya Kosha's Primary Neural Signatures 82

Vijnanamaya Kosha → Wise, Reflective, Decentered Self or Wisdom Consciousness ... 85
    Some Characteristics of Vijnanamaya Kosha 86
    Vijnanamaya Kosha's Primary Neural Signatures 87

Anandamaya Kosha → Joyful and Connected Self; Union or Unity 88

Habitual Identification with a Particular Kosha 89

Chapter 4: Connecting to the Deeper Dimensions of Being 91

Gunas or Fundamental Qualities of Nature 92
- Rajas in Yoga Psychology 94
- Tamas in Yoga Psychology 95
- Sattva in Yoga Psychology 95
- Gunas Interacting with Koshas 96
- Gunas in Nature and the Environment 98
- Gunas in the Context of Polyvagal Theory 103
  - Neuroception of Safety 105
  - Neuroception of Danger 106
  - Neuroception of Life Threat 107
  - Mixed Polyvagal States and Gunas 108

Kleshas or the Roots of Suffering 113
- Raga or Craving, Clinging, Grasping, Wanting 116
- Dvesha or Aversion, Anger, Hatred 116
- Asmita or Clinging to Ego, Rigid Role Identities for Self and Others 117
- Abhinivesha or Fear of Change, Fear of Loss of Life, Fear of Loss of Self 118
- Avidya or Non-Seeing 118
  - Confusing the Impermanent with the Permanent 119
  - Confusing the Story with the Truth 120
  - Confusing Pleasure with Pain 120
  - Confusing Roles and Superficial Identities with Who We Really Are 120
- Collective Expressions of the Kleshas 122
- A Modern Psychology Perspective on Avidya 123

Chapter 5: Moving Toward Transformation 125

Vrittis or the Yogic Expressions of Mind 126
- Development of the Vrittis 126
- Stickiness of Identifying with Our Mind Contents 127
- Pramana or Right Perception 129
- Viparyaya or Misperception 130
  - Modern Science Perspective on Perception and Misperception 131
- Smriti or Memory 134
  - Modern Science Perspective on Memory 134
- Vikalpa or Creativity 137
  - Modern Science Perspective on Imagination 137
- Nidra or Deep Dreamless Sleep 138
  - Modern Science Perspective on Sleep 139

Mind States 147
- Kshipta or Disturbed Mind 147
- Mudha or Dull Mind 147
- Vikshipta or Distracted Mind 148
- Ekagra or Pointer Dog or Bird Dog Mind, Bear Mind; One-Pointed Mind 148
- Niruddha or Luminous Mind 148
- The Path Toward Transforming the Vrittis 149

***Samskaras* or Habits, Patterns, and Reactivities** 150
    Development of Samskaras 150
    Samskaras as Pattern Locks 152
    Opening Heart and Mind To Transforming Pattern Locks 155
        RAIN Framework of Honest and Ethical Inquiry 157
        Awareness-Based Framework of Honest and Ethical Inquiry 157

Karma or The Law of Cause and Effect 158
    Tools for Auspicious Choices in Each Moment 161
        Concentration and Awareness 161
        Discernment and Wisdom 162
        Virtue and Positive Intention 162
        Generosity 163

Brahma Viharas 163
    Upekṣā or Equanimity 164
    Maitri or Lovingkindness 165
    Karuna or Compassion 166
    Mudita or Altruistic and Appreciative Joy 167

Application of Yoga Psychology to Yoga Services 168

Section 2: Integrated Holistic Yoga Pedagogy and Practice Principles 169

Section 2 Introduction 171
    Yoga Pedagogy and Practice Principles Overview 171
    Yoga Pedagogy and Practice Principles Learning Objectives 173
    Yoga Pedagogy and Practice Principles Recommended Readings 174

Chapter 6: Yoga Services Based in Integrated Holistic Yoga Psychology 175

Yoga Pedagogy as Rooted in Integrated Holistic Yoga Psychology 175

Environments of Safety, Accessibility, and Ongoing Consent 178
    Clarity and Consistency in Logistical Procedures, Structure, and Rules 178
        Safety- and Respect-Related Etiquette 178
        Class Structures and Logistics 179
        Time Management Commitments 179
    Clarity in Personal Boundaries and Priorities 179

Provider Qualities for Client Empowerment and Safety 182
    Personal Alignment with Yogic Principles 183
    Cultural Skillfulness and Sensitivity 183
    Interpersonally Relevant Traits for Relationship-Building 184
    Qualities with Impact on Teaching Style, Management Style, and Optimizing Safety ... 184
    Additional Aspects of Creating Safety in Healthcare, Clinical, and Residential Settings .. 185

Teaching or Yoga Service Delivery Styles 185
    Styles and Types 185
    Preparedness 187

Prioritizing Accessibility, Diversity, Equity, and Social Justice 187
    Optimization and Embrace of Accessibility, Diversity, Equity, and Inclusion 188

    Optimization of Safety via Conducive Environmental Features 188
    Creation of Procedural Clarity and Embrace of a Strong Code of Conduct 189
    Marketing, Social Media, and Public Relations 190

Stages of Learning 190
    Stage 1: Unconscious Incompetence 191
    Stage 2: Conscious Incompetence 191
    Stage 3: Conscious Competence 191
    Stage 4: Unconscious Competence 191

Chapter 7: Principles of Sequencing and Teaching with Intention 193

Teaching with Intention 193
    Elements of the Sankalpa Teaching Spiderweb 194
        Student or Client Variables 196
        Aim or Intention 196
        New Learning 196
        Koshas 197
        Applied Psychology 197
        Limbs of Yoga 198
        Pedagogy 198
        Affiliation and Safety 198

Sequencing for Safety and Meaning 200
    Auspicious Session Sequencing 200
    Sequence-Planning with Intention 202
        Considerations in Choosing a Class Intention or Theme 202
        Considerations in Choosing Peak Practices 204
        Considerations in Planning Session Opening 204
        Considerations in Planning Breathwork 205
        Considerations in Planning Warm-Up and Preparation Poses 205
        Considerations in Planning and Offering Counter- and Recovery Procedures ... 206
        Considerations in Planning Cool-Down and Release 207
        Considerations in Planning Inner Practice, Meditation, and Savasana 207
        Considerations for Planning Practice Closure 208

Chapter 8: Principles for Teaching with Integration and Wholism 209

Principles that Create Opportunities for Safety and Self-Agency 209
    Honoring Yoga Ethics, Commitments, and Intentions 209
    Healthful Physical, Vital, and Cognitive/Emotional Boundaries in all Koshas 211

Scaffolding across the Koshas 212

Balancing Effort and Ease 213
    Sthiram – Commitment to Working the Path 214
    Sukham – Commitment to Staying Playful and Serene 214
    Balancing Sthira and Sukha 214
    Abhyasa (Practice) and Vairagyam (Non-Attachment) 217

Cultivating Grounding, Expansion, and Stability 218
    Rootedness of Grounding 218

    Openness of Expansion 220
    Courage of Stability 222

Working with Lines of Energy 226
    Physical Lines of Energy 226
    Life Energy or Pranic Lines of Energy 226
    Emotional and Mental Energies 228

Cuing Mindfulness, Attention/Attunement, and Awareness 228
    Attention and Awareness: Presence with Focus or Spaciousness 228
        Cuing Attention 230
        Cuing Awareness 230
    Befriending the Present Moment 230
    The Four '-Ceptions' – Our Portal into Experience and Being 232
    LET Be 235

Embracing Trauma-Informed Yoga Principles 236
    Types of Traumata 236
    Beneficial TIY Principles and Practices to Cultivate 237
    Contraindicated Practices in TIY To Avoid 239

Chapter 9: Cuing, Demonstration, and Observation *241*

Choices for Successful Cuing, Speech, Action and Class Leadership 241
    Thinking Before Speaking and Doing 242
    Perspective-Taking in How Cuing, Speech, and Action May Land 243
        Statements versus Questions 244
        Phrasing and Language 244
        Possible Connotations and Meanings of Questions, Cues, and Statements 244
    Observation of the Impact of Cuing, Speech, and Actions on Students' Experience 244
        Being Open to Experience: Coming Into the Present Moment 245
        Maintaining Beginner's Mind: Inviting Openness for Something New 246

Considered Use of Specific Language Constructions 246
    Grammatical Constructions 246
    Efficiency, Poignancy, and Student-Centeredness 247
    Attention to Language Connotations 248
    Types of Language 249

Wisdom of Intentional Demonstration 250

Wisdom of Observation: Holistic Seeing and Integrated Understanding 251
    Seeing and Understanding People as an Integrated Whole 251
    Basic Principles of Seeing and Understanding Students 253
        Annamaya Kosha Observations 254
        Pranamaya Kosha Observations 254
        Annamaya and Pranamaya Kosha Observations 254
        Manomaya Kosha Observations 255
        Vijnanamaya and Anandamaya Kosha Observations 255
    Basic Aspects of Nonverbal Communication 256
    Seeing and Understanding Collapsing, Contracting, and Yielding in All Koshas 258

    Collapsing or Buckling 260
    Contracting or Bracing 261
    Resilience or Yielding 263

Chapter 10: Skillfulness in Providing Tailored Therapeutic Yoga 267

Wise Choices about Yoga Props 267
    Creating or Impairing Accessibility Through the Use of Props 268
    Potentially Helpful Yoga Props 268

Planning for Variations, Adaptations, and Alternatives 272
    Offering Variations to Meet People Where They Are 272
    Recognizing and Drawing on Students Resources and Strengths 272
    Preplanning and Revising on the Fly 273

A Few Additional Considerations 274
    Importance of Variations 274
    Importance of Adaptations and Propping 274
    Knowledgeability about Alternatives 275

Guiding via Cuing, Assisting, Adjusting, and Adapting 276
    Cuing 276
    Adjusting 276
    Assisting 277
    Intervening 277

Applications of Cuing, Assisting, Adjusting, and Adapting 277
    Types of Demonstration, Cuing, Adjustment, Assisting, and Intervening 278
    Developmental and Respectful Approaches to Guiding Clients 279
    Safety Considerations in Choices for Supporting or Guiding Clients 279

Supportive Guidelines Related to Physical or Tactile Assists and Use of Touch 279
    Explicit and Ongoing Informed Consent 280
    Clear Intention with Explicit Verbalization of Purpose and Planned Action 281
        Verbalize a Clear Intention 281
        Provide Specifics 282
        Be Patient and Take Enough Time 282
    Continuous Yielding of Power and Agency to the Student 283
        Ensuring Privacy 283
        Choosing Least Restrictive and Least Intrusive Interventions 283
        Recognizing the Personal Impact 284
    Protections for the Yoga Professional While Using Tactile Assists 285
    Types of Tactile Contact Defined With Examples 286
        Student-Initiated Touch 286
        Guiding Touch 287
        Directional Touch 287
        Supportive Touch 288
        Stabilizing Touch 289
        Auspicious Alignment Touch 291

Chapter 11: Foundational Ethics and Commitments.. 293
Ethics Aspects of Being a Yoga Professional.. 293
Ethics in Relationship 293
Ethics in the Yoga Room – Preparation, Teaching, Debriefing, and More 295
Relevant Ethical and Professional Resources 297
Yoga Alliance 297
Ethical Commitments and Professionalism in the Context of Yoga Services 298
Legal Commitments in the Context of Yoga Services 299
A Few Final Notes 299

Professional Development Aspects of Being a Yoga Professional 300
Credentialing and Commitment to Ethics and Professionalism 300
Scope of Practice Definitions.. 300
Yoga Classes.. 302
Therapeutic Yoga Classes.. 302
Yoga Therapeutics in Healthcare 303
Yoga Therapy.. 303
Details about Yoga Teaching and Yoga Therapy Credentialing 304
Yoga Teaching – Certification Preparation and Credentials 304
Yoga Teaching – Registration Preparation and Credentials 304
Therapeutic Yoga Preparation and Credentials 305
Yoga Therapy Preparation and Credentials 306

Concluding Thoughts.. 308
Bibliography and Citations.. 309
Index.. 317

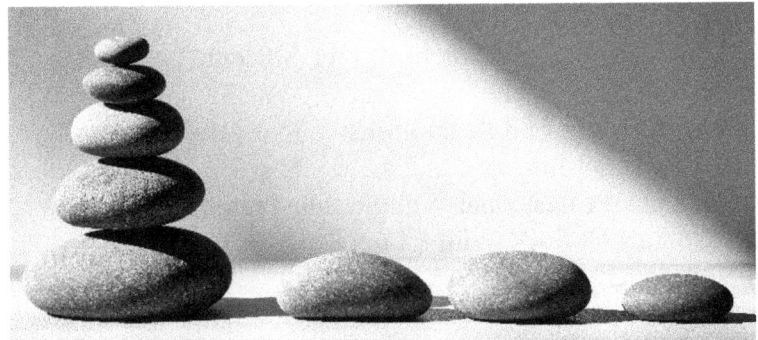

Section 1: Integrated Holistic Yoga History and Psychology

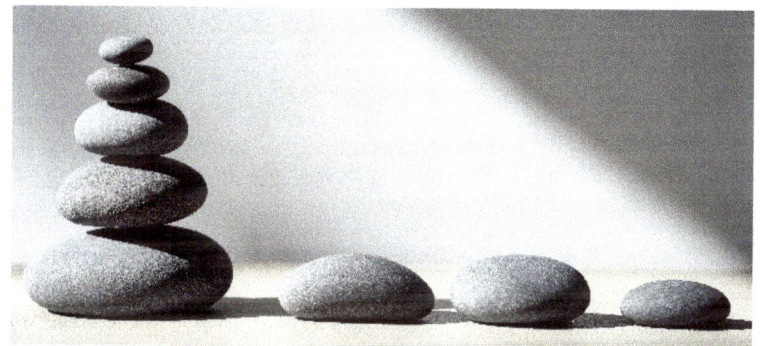

Section 1 Introduction

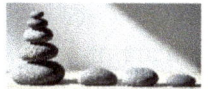

Yoga History and Psychology Overview

Given that competent yoga teachers understand the deep historical and scientific foundations of yoga, this chapter provides an immersion into important historical, philosophical, and psychological contexts, including the eight limbs of yoga, Yoga Sutras of Patanjali, and other important texts. The perspective in this section is one of yoga as a psychology, focusing on the essence of the conceptual and practical (or applied) aspects of yoga. It introduces a lineage of yoga called Integrated Holistic Yoga that is dedicated to integration, wholism, intention, beneficence, and accessibility. *Integration* refers to the interwoven and complete practice of yoga as consisting of at least eight aspects of practice – from lifestyle and ethics, to physical practices of movement and breathing, to inner practice reaching from sense guarding to concentration and meditation, ultimately inviting a joyful and connected experience of being human. *Wholism* refers to the honoring of all five layers of human experience, from the physical to the vital, the mental and emotional, the wise and altruistic, to the joyful and connected. *Accessibility* focuses on creating a path into the practice for all humans – regardless of context, background, abilities, preferences, or other aspects of being human in all its diversity and complexity. *Beneficence* means that all that is offered in a yoga practice (whether on the mat or as a lifestyle) has positive ripples for the individual practitioner and the communities and systems in which they are embedded. Therefore, every action in the context of a yoga practice is engaged in with *intention* and clarity of purpose.

Honoring *integration*, yoga is understood as a practice of eight sets of ancient practices called *limbs of yoga*, grouped into four categories based on modern research. *Values and Lifestyle Practices* of yoga (yamas, niyamas) help yoga practitioners and teachers develop and ethical and intentional living informed by purposeful values and meaningful life goals. *Physical Practices* (asanas) transform practitioners' anatomy and physiology, support accurate sensory perception of the body from the inside out and of the environment from the outside in. *Breathing Practices* (pranayama) stimulate the parasympathetic nervous system, allowing access to a calm, relaxed state from which to become adaptively responsive to inner and outer life demands, achieving systemic homeostasis in body and mind. *Interior Practices* (pratyahara, dharana, dhyana, and samadhi) draw the practitioner and teacher into self-exploration, personal insight, and interpersonal transformation, shedding maladaptive habits, reactivity, and stereotypes while opening space for new choices, adaptive responsiveness, and resilience in body, emotions, mind, and relationships.

The yoga sutras are presented as the essential philosophical text that elucidates the *intention*, purpose, meaning and importance of the eight limbs of yoga. The yoga sutras are highlighted as a treatise that has reemerged in significance across the centuries, inspiring reinterpretation and modernization as life has evolved and yoga has been introduced in different contexts, cultures, and societies. The sutras are presented as a "thread" – as the science of yoga – that links teachings, teachers, students, and communities together, in line with the meaning of the word yoga, *to yoke or unite*. The sutras are introduced as a practical guide and manual of concise aphorisms of evolving, individual, and cultural meanings and interpretations. They are used to highlight the multitude of approaches to the practice and teaching of yoga, and to reinforce the idea that both practice and teaching of yoga are most auspiciously grounded in a greater intention and purpose that reaches beyond the mat into daily life.

Wholism clarifies the importance of seeing, feeling, hearing, and experiencing the entirety of each human being regardless of how or what they present when they seek out yoga, healthcare, or education. Wholism places each individual in their individual biopsychosociocultural context and seeks to understand their past and current circumstances, life, and embeddedness. As this approach highlights, it is helpful to see ourselves, our students, our clients – everyone we encounter – in all their layers, trying to understand, honor, respect, and value their *embodied* self (i.e., their physical development and experience), their *vital* self (i.e., their energetic and affective development and experience), their *verbal and social* self (i.e., their emotional and mental experience), their *wise decentered* self (i.e., their development and experience in relationships and ways of expressing what is in their hearts), and their *joyfully connected* self (i.e., their capacity to feel deeply grounded in a particular biopsychosociocultural context and interpersonal matrix). In yogic language, we recognize all *koshas* – or layers of human experience – and honor these layers in our practice, in our teachings. and interactions with students, clients, and patients, and ourselves.

Intention, beneficence, and accessibility are honored through the deep exploration of central psychological yoga principles and practices that create deepening insights into personal lifestyle choices, habits, and decisions. Internal inquiry is encouraged to help readers, practitioners, and teachers apply yoga psychology to their personal life, teaching, and personal and professional transformation. There is an interweaving of the limbs and koshas in the context of human development across the lifespan. Concepts such as the yogic expressions of nature (i.e., gunas) are integrated with the modern science of polyvagal theory. Concepts such as the emotional afflictions (or kleshas) are linked to modern science of the development and transformation of emotion, mood, and affect. Mind states, mental fluctuations and preoccupations (i.e., yogic vrittis) are placed into scientific contexts of perception and misperception, memory and imagination, and the importance of sleep and calm abiding. Pattern locks (or samskaras) are juxtaposed with principles of transforming reactivity into responsiveness and into choices that serve the greater good. All practices and psychological principles are explored as transformative forces and deeper dimensions of yoga that move practitioners and teachers toward self-discovery, self-inquiry, and conscious decision-making while living and teaching with intention and purpose. The wish is for all to access compassion, lovingkindness, altruistic and appreciative joy, experienced with equanimity and deep contentment in every moment of daily life.

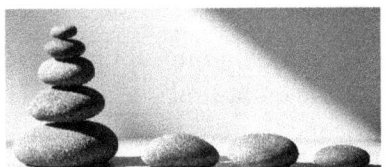

Yoga History and Psychology Learning Objectives

1. Know, understand, and be able to explain and operationalize the eight limbs of yoga, providing for each basic definition, central intention, central principles, and central practices
   a. yamas and niyamas
   b. asana and pranayama
   c. pratyahara, dharana, and dhyana
   d. samadhi

2. Be knowledgeable and versed in yoga psychology, as well as able to use philosophical principles in teaching and planning class content and flow
   a. read, understand, explain, and translate into action the yoga sutras, with special emphasis on the first four sutras and padas 1 and 2
   b. read, understand, explain, and translate into action the Bhagavad Gita, with special emphasis on the importance of a teacher and the four paths of yoga (karma, raja, jnana, and bhakti)

3. Be able to define, explain, and incorporate into yoga teachings several of the primary yoga philosophies relevant to the interior practices of yoga; minimally, be able to cover
   a. koshas
   b. gunas
   c. kleshas
   d. vrittis, samskara, and mind states
   e. karma and transcendence

4. Understand and operationalize integrated holistic yoga psychology in participant-provider, provider-mentor, and participant-participant relationships, weighing and making ethical, lifestyle, teaching, and relationship decisions about issues such as
   a. integration of yoga practices with scientific wisdom
   b. wholism that honors all layers of human experience in its biopsychosociocultural context
   c. purpose and clear intentionality for all actions and teachings
   d. beneficence in intention, thought, action, behavior, and relationships
   e. accessibility through awareness of individual and collective needs of students and creating environments of kindness, compassion, joy, and contentment

5. Become intentional and proactive with regard to understanding and taking responsibility for increasing equity, inclusion, and accessibility of yoga for all by committing to providing yoga teachings and services that are
   a. inclusive in didactics, language, approach, settings, and psychology
   b. based on practice accessibility accomplished via multiple modalities, ranging from creating safe and accessible spaces to using trauma-informed and accessible language to offering accessible variations in asana and pranayama
   c. actively geared toward creating equity, in the yoga classroom, as well as in the greater community, and social network

Yoga History and Psychology Recommended Readings

Yoga Sutras of Patanjali. Many translations exist and you can choose one. Several are available for free online (http://www.swamij.com/yoga-sutras.htm and http://www.arlingtoncenter.org/Sanskrit-English.pdf).

Barkataki, S. (2020). *Embrace yoga's roots: Courageous ways to deepen your yoga practice*. Ignite Yoga and Wellness Institute.

Porges, S. W., & Dana, D. (2018). *Clinical applications of the polyvagal theory: The emergence of polyvagal-informed therapies*. W.W. Norton.

Feuerstein, G. (2013). *The psychology of yoga: Integrating eastern and western approaches for understanding the mind*. Shambala.

Johnson, M. C. (2021). *Skill in action: Radicalizing your yoga practice to create a just world*. Shambhala.

Stone, M. (2008). *The inner tradition of yoga*. Shambhala.

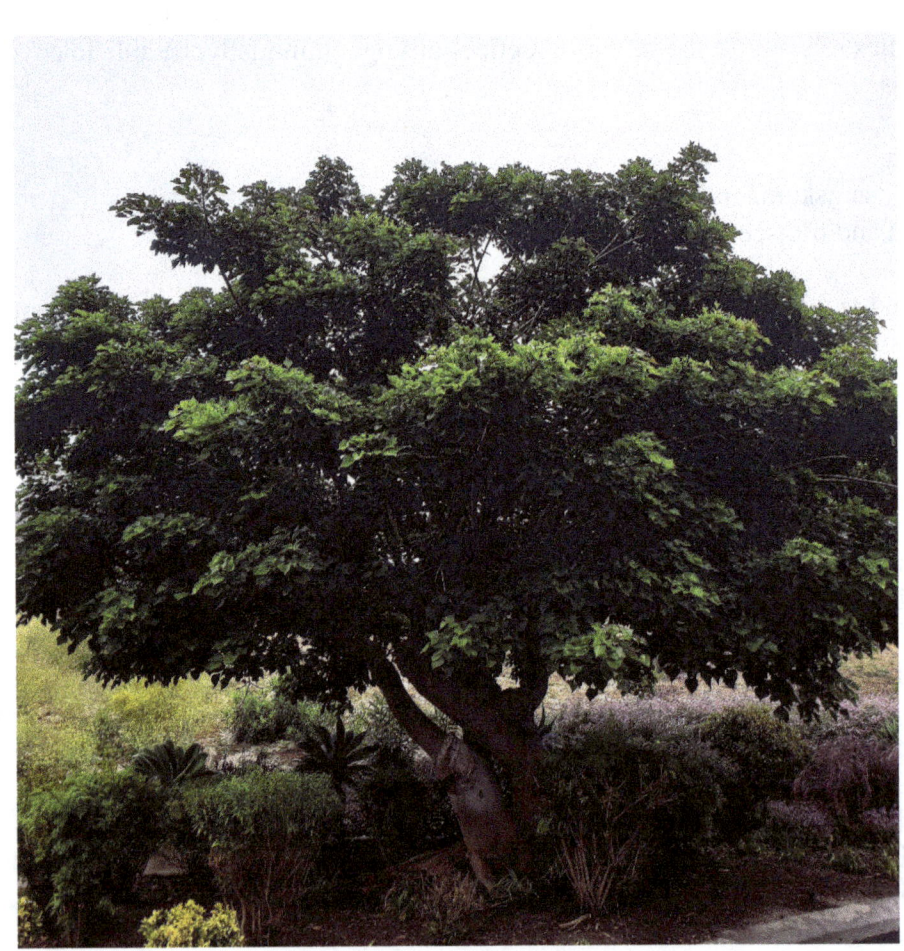

Chapter 1: History of Integrated Holistic Yoga

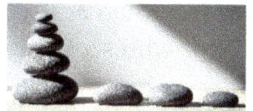

The practice of yoga in the U.S. has seen a tremendous increase in numbers of practitioners (IPSOS Public Affairs, 2016) and has been identified as among the top ten alternative and integrative practices sought out by patients in physical and mental healthcare settings (Barnes et al., 2007; Barnett et al., 2014). Yoga's increase in popularity has been largely due to the strong interest in posture practice as a form of exercise. Posture practice has become a point of focus in gyms, schools, and even workplaces and is touted as a way of combatting stress, increasing mindfulness, and staying physically healthy. Yoga from the postural practice perspective is a physical or exercise-based system that helps promote physical health, strength, and balance. Many yoga classes – especially in conventional venues such as typical yoga studios and gyms – offer strenuous physical practices proven to enhance the physical wellbeing of practitioner.

The postural practice of modern Western yoga has brought keen media attention to the practice along with a certain amount of notoriety. In fact, yoga has become a bit of a loaded word these days. Modern postural yoga elicits visions of sweaty bodies in large rooms, full of people who are working hard to build a healthy physique. It may also bring up images of young, healthy people – often well-to-do and often female – who are able to move their body in ways that most humans cannot and who wear tight clothes and fancy accessories. However, yoga as an integrated holistic practice or life philosophy goes far beyond posture (or physical) practice alone. Integrated holistic yoga brings us a different vision – a vision focused on physical, behavioral, mental, emotional, and relational health; on centeredness in mind, breath, emotions, and body; and on a psychology of wellness and resilience.

Defining Integrated Holistic Yoga

Integrated holistic yoga offers a vision that honors the deep cultural tradition that dates yoga back thousands of years. It integrates modern neuroscience with ancient practices to demonstrate the profound wisdoms in the original teachings that we are relearning and rediscovering every day. Integrated holistic yoga embraces inclusiveness, access, diversity, health, wellbeing, and resilience for all. It is a practice of and for community; it honors interdependence and co-regulation. Integrated holistic yoga represents a return to yoga as it was traditionally practiced. Ancient yoga was physical only to prepare practitioners for the more important interior practices (such as concentration and meditation) and interpersonal applications of a thoughtful and deliberate code of life and discipline (Brems et al., 2016; Freeman et al., 2017).

Similarly, modern integrated holistic yoga (as defined by (Brems, 2024a) is a practice that combines body, emotion, mind, spirit, and community through a comprehensive lifestyle with implications for individual and collective wellbeing (Feuerstein, 2013; Iyengar, 2006; White, 2007). It promotes self-compassion, introspection, and community that lead to insights that alter human physiology and anatomy, and – perhaps more importantly – emotions, cognitions, behaviors, and relationships. Integrated holistic yoga can be practiced by anyone who can breathe without assistance, almost anywhere, for little to no cost (Dittman & Freedman, 2009; Ross et al., 2013). Integrated holistic yoga motivates practitioners to adhere to the practice more so than a unidimensional posture practice (Dittman & Freedman, 2009) and is freed from Western media stereotypes that tend to limit who seeks access to yoga.

Ancient or traditional yoga consists of eight sets of ancient practices called limbs of yoga (Hartranft, 2003; Iyengar, 2006), grouped into four categories based on modern research (Gard et al., 2014; Ward et al., 2014). *Values and Lifestyle Practices* of yoga direct practitioners toward ethical (yama) and intentional (niyama) living informed by purposeful values and meaningful life goals. *Physical Practices* (asana) transform the practitioner's anatomy and physiology, and support accurate sensory perception of the body from the inside out and of the environment from the outside in. *Breathing Practices* (pranayama) stimulate the parasympathetic nervous system, allowing access to a calm, relaxed state from which to become adaptively responsive to inner and outer life demands, achieving systemic homeostasis in body and mind. *Interior Practices* (pratyahara, dharana, and dhyana) draw the practitioner into self-exploration, personal insight, and interpersonal transformation, leading to the shedding of maladaptive habits, reactivity, and stereotypes while opening space for new choices, adaptive responsiveness, and resilience in body, emotions, mind, and relationships. These practices are enormously beneficial to the practitioner – and have been so for millennia. Modern sciences are finally catching up to this recognition that yoga – as an integrated practice, not a single-minded postural practice – has profound impacts on human wellbeing, as explored in detail below.

Integrated holistic yoga (Brems, 2015, 2022) provides access to the many benefits of yoga by:
- Inviting practitioners to begin to understand their own complexity as well as their deep grounding in relationships and communities;
- Blending ancient wisdoms and modern science, integrating a multitude of practices;
- Inviting everyone into the practice, creating accessibility, equity, and engagement; and
- Inviting practitioners to make a whole-hearted and open-minded commitment to a practice that reflects intentional lifestyle choices.

Integrated Holistic Yoga – A Definition and Commitment

- A practice for accessibility – creating affiliation, solidarity, and belonging; promoting social justice, engaged action, and personal as well collective empowerment
- A practice of intentionality – promising to making the world a better place; living with intention; committing to basic ethical values and practices
- A practice of beneficence – creating access to the health and mental health benefits of yoga via several mechanisms of change; pledging first to do no harm
- A practice of wholeness – addressing the layered experiences of consciousness, biopsychosociocultural context, interconnection, and community in all their complexity
- A practice of integration – embracing the eight traditional practices (aka limbs) of yoga, four ways to glean a deeper understanding of our students or clients, interweaving of science and soul, and interdependence and coregulation

Integrated Holistic Yoga: A Commitment to Wholism

Integrated holistic yoga – the type of yoga that facilitates maximum physical and mental benefits – is a yoga of wholism that honors mind as much as body, breath as much as calming of the nervous system, individuals as much as the collective, stillness as much as movement, and effort as much as ease. It looks at and addresses the needs and resources of *whole people in all of their layers* (or koshas, in Sanskrit): body, breath, mind, heart, and spirit – grounded in community and a complex interpersonal setting (or matrix) of biological, psychological, social, and cultural influences. It is particularly well-suited to applications in healthcare settings.

Integrated holistic yoga teachers always remember that the physical posture is only the tiniest tip of the iceberg – the real work happens energetically, emotionally, and mentally. We understand and are in the physical world first and hence we grow and evolve from there. Yoga teaches us to understand, acknowledge and inhabit our bodies – not deny, repress, or dissociate from them. We learn to understand the physical and how to rest in equanimity regardless of what happens in the body. Alongside the work with the body, we work with breath and energy, mind and emotions, and ultimately, we move toward samadhi or enlightenment (awakening to a new level of consciousness).

> **Holistic systems consider the interaction of all living beings to create an environment for the maximum benefit of all. They do not focus on specific components or features, instead being dedicated to the understanding, wellbeing, and support of the entire system in all its multidimensional complexities. Nothing is ignored; nothing is left out.**
>
> **Teaching and learning approaches that embrace holism integrate all human traits, attending to the physical, energetic, mental, emotional, behavioral, relational, and psychological aspects of all who are coming together for the purpose of learning.**
>
> **Holistic approaches to healthcare, education, politics, environmental policy, gardening, and so on encourage personal and collective responsibility, accountability, duty, wellbeing, welfare, security, health, and happiness.**

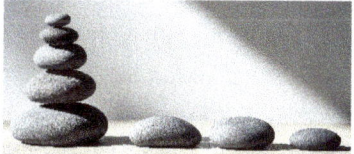

Wholism Avoids Reductionism and Embraces Complexity

Working from an integrated holistic paradigm of teaching yoga allows us to avoid reductionism and invites us to embrace *wholism*. It embraces the complexity of human life and growth while resting in the simplicity of a well-designed practice. Just like a spiderweb, a yoga class is the weaving together of many intricate strands with great attention and purpose. The result is a complex structure that is beautiful to behold in its seeming simplicity and genuine clarity.

What does reductionism look like? Reductionism hones in on a single or a couple of aspects of the individual who is coming to the practice of yoga without honoring their full history, experience, and complexity. It may hone in on the physical aspect of the individual or the practice, treating a single symptom or using a single intervention. It may hone in on perceptions of people as unidimensional or as stereotypes and fails to acknowledge each person's unique expressions, needs, or contexts. Likewise, yoga practices (or other interventions, such as healthcare, educational approaches, recommended physical activities, endorsed nutritional styles, and more) may be prescribed for individuals but are based on generalizations that do not actually apply to their unique circumstances. This 'standard of care' or universal approach may not serve them because they are based on false assumptions. Reductionism tends to exclude and frighten as opposed to include and invite.

The opposite of reductionism is wholism, the honoring of complexity, critical analysis, and thinking as guides to teaching, education, healthcare, and other human interactions. From a holistic paradigm, teachers or care providers teach and support based on principles applied and tailored to the specific students or clients, as well as their circumstances and context, with deep caring and wisdom, informed by the intention for the work and for each component of the work. A holistic paradigm that avoids reductionism is the perfect approach for yoga in healthcare settings. It can help transform challenges faced in modern healthcare by treating the whole person, rather than symptoms.

Wholism Honors all Human Layers of Consciousness or Experience

Wholism makes a point of seeing the entirety of each individual regardless of presenting concern, context, or relationship. The practitioner or client is seen in all layers or koshas – body, vitality and energy, mind and emotion, heart and relationship, and context and belongingness. Ancient yoga was very clear that humans have multiple ways of being conscious of themselves as they live and interact in the real world of daily life. In modern language, we refer to this complexity as the many layers of human experience and consciousness. Ancient yogis conceived of the self as layered – composed of several aspects or components that make up our experience or consciousness (a consciousness to which we refer as our *self*). In Sanskrit, these layers are called koshas, which can be loosely translated as "sheaths".

The word koshas is used in this text because no English translation can quite capture the complexity of the concept. *Each kosha has a separate and distinct function while also being completely integrated and interdependent with all others.* All layers of consciousness are with us (if only as seeds) from birth to death – yet each takes on particular significance and reaches maturation during different stages of our lives and development. In other words, they develop and become important neurosequentially. The specific meanings and expressions of each kosha depend on the circumstances we face as we move through life and relationships. We will cover the koshas in the next section in great detail. Following is a summary of the five layers of experience as a brief preview of that is to come.

Koshas or Layers of Experience

The word "*kosha*" is translated as *layer* or *sheath* of the self in most western yoga translations. However, they koshas perhaps better understood as layers or stages of consciousness, awareness, or experience. These layers, of course, are simply constructs to help us give labels to experience. Layers of "self" are merely ways of experiencing and communicating about ourselves in the tangible world. In reality, all layers are interconnected, interdependent, and co-regulating. They are a unity of experiences in each moment and across a lifetime, as absorbed in the specifically biopsychosociocultural context in which they develop, transform, and disappear.

Annamaya kosha – embodied self-experiences or physical consciousness ("anna" = food)
Pranamaya kosha – affective or energetic self-experiences or vital consciousness ("prana" = breath; "Prana" = life force)
Manomaya kosha – verbal and social self-experiences or mind consciousness ("mano" = mind)
Vijnanamaya kosha – decentered, wisely intuitive self or wisdom consciousness ("vijnana" = wisdom)
Anandamaya kosha – joyful integrated self-experiences or unity/universal consciousness ("Ananda" = bliss, joy)

Wholism Recognizes Interdependence and Embeddedness in Community

Human development, which can be considered synonymous with development along the lines of the koshas, is profoundly influenced by and dependent upon a multitude of individual, relational, and contextual factors that are utterly interpersonal and interdependent. Human development depends on being solidly and supportively anchored in a greater web of life, especially a web of loving, joyful, kind, and compassionate humans. Human newborns cannot survive outside of a caretaking human matrix of relationships that support their physical survival, emotional needs, and mental growth (Cozolino, 2015, 2024). This interpersonal matrix (Stern, 1985) and its influence has been thoroughly documented in the developmental psychology literature and is unquestioned in the importance of its influence.

In the integrated holistic yoga model (Brems, 2024a), development is viewed as a lifelong process of refinement and emergence, shaped by individuals' experiences in and interactions with their context and environment. Development thus defined resembles evolution (Wilber, 2000) and results in the acquisition of behaviors, useful skills, shaping of new responses, un- and relearning habits, and expansion of awareness (Grant, 2021; Wimbarti & Self, 1992). In this model, development is utterly dependent on the context in which it occurs. How our bodies, energy and vitality, mind and emotions, and ways of being relationship develop, grow, and transform is strongly affected by the context that surrounds us: relationships we experience, environments in which we grow up and grow old, cultural forces that bring us advantages or disadvantages, social and sociopolitical pressures we feel, and educational and career or job opportunities that emerge or fail to emerge. All have profound and long-lasting effects on how we grow, emerge, and evolve in all layers of self, in our relationships, families, and communities.

The integrated holistic yoga model of understanding human development and human existence/experience is premised on continual change, emergence, and evolution that optimizes and integrates learning and experience over time, constantly transcending and improving upon prior learning and conditioning insert (Badenoch, 2011a, 2011b; Cozolino, 2015, 2024; Siegel & Payne Bryson, 2012). The empowering premise that humans are subject to and agents in their own lifelong growth is consistent with findings from modern neuroscience and psychology as well as yogic perspectives on human development.

Ancient traditions and modern sciences recognize that humans change, emerge, and grow in the context of their embeddedness in an interpersonal matrix and need to be understood from the unique developmental and contextual embeddedness at any moment in time. All are equally optimistic and hopeful, by virtue of their developmental focus, that there is an inherent capacity of humans to transcend their current state, to improve with experience and discipline, and to evolve continually, and ultimately to embrace their human interconnection, interrelation, and interdependence – along with the responsibilities that emerge from this recognition of connection. The context in which development and healing happens is relational, collective, and biopsychosociocultural in nature.

BioPsychoSocioCultural (BPSC) Paradigm

The biopsychosociocultural paradigm invites yoga clinicians to gain in-depth understanding of clients' or students' (or their own) webs of life, webs of relationships, and greater connection. It reminds us that sources of challenges, difficulties, and presenting concerns, even overall life experience, are always relational and embedded in a greater context. It leads to recognition of the importance of having an understanding of biopsychosociocultural contexts that have had and continue to have a bearing on the development and experience of human beings. Four dimensions are defined and understood with complexity from a holistic and integrated lens. They are *biological*, *psychological*, *socioeconomic/sociological*, and *cultural/familial* – or **biopsychosociocultural** – in nature (cf., (Brems & Rasmussen, 2019). Biopsychosociocultural context are in and of themselves ever-emerging, always changing, and in flux. This adds complexity, ambiguity, uncertainty, and volatility to our understanding of ourselves and our clients. In other words, our human experience is always grounded in a world that has been said to be marked by volatility, uncertainty, complexity, and ambiguity (VUCA).

Two figures below detail the four biopsychosociocultural factors individually; however, it is important to understand that this is simply for ease of communication. In actuality, these factors co-exist, influence each other, co-arise, and interact deeply and profoundly – they are connected. They weave a complex and whole web of relationships and interactions that deeply shape and affect who we become and how we develop and influence others. Our relationship with our biopsychosociocultural context is entirely reciprocal – our biopsychosociocultural context deeply influences and shapes us; in turn, we can greatly influence and shape it, becoming agents for change and betterment – not just on behalf of ourselves, but for our communities and our world.

The Four Quadrants of the BioPsychoSocioCultural Context	
Biological Factors o genetics o physical disabilities o developmental and health issues o accidents and injuries o illness and disease o nutrition o sleep hygiene o medications and substances o medical family history o physical environment …. and more	**Psychological Factors** o temperament o personality o self-identity o resilience and coping o affect o emotion o cognitive style and learning o intellectual capacity o executive functioning o emotional environment …. and more
BIO	**PSYCHO**
SOCIO	**CULTURAL**
Social, Societal, Socioeconomic Factors o education o employment and career o socioeconomics o social support o sociopolitical circumstances o legal and law enforcement structures o oppression or bias o discrimination o privilege o political climate o access to natural environments …. and more	**Cultural and Familial Factors** o group memberships o values, ethics, and morals o prejudice and stereotypes o choices and options o language and speech o religion and spirituality o family structure o family process/communication o family competence o historical and other trauma o cultural heritage-related environments …. and more

The next figure offers the same content, adding overlapping dimensions between the basic biological, psychological, social and cultural aspects of our environment and experience. The follwing intersections are proposed and outlined:

- Biological and psychological context (behavioral health)
- Biological and social context (public health)
- Psychological and cultural context (family health and functioning) and
- Cultural and social contexts (sociocultural health)

The Expanded Model of the BioPsychoSocioCultural Context

BIO
Biological Factors
- genetics
- physical disabilities
- developmental issues
- health issues
- accidents and injuries
- nutritional status
- sleep quality
- medications
- medical family history

Intersection of Bio-Psycho

Behavioral Health
- nutritional choices
- exercise
- sleep hygiene
- hydration
- addiction
- time in nature

PSYCHO
Psychological Factors
- temperament
- personality
- self-identity
- resilience and coping
- affect and emotion
- cognitive style
- learning styles
- intellectual capacity
- executive functioning

Intersection of Socio-Bio

Public Health
- access to healthcare
- access to health education
- access to insurance
- food insecurity and quality
- air and noise pollution
- access to nature
- environmental safety

Familial Health
- family dynamics
- family structure
- family process
- family communication
- family competence
- family affect
- family values and myths

Intersection of Psycho-Cultural

- affordable, safe housing
- neighborhood safety
- educational access/quality
- educational opportunity
- employment, career, work
- socioeconomic equity
- political systems
- social support networks
- legal structures/equity
- crime exposure/definition

- oppression or bias
- discrimination
- microaggression
- intergenerational trauma
- privilege, supremacy
- gentrification

Sociocultural Health
Intersection of Socio-Cultural

- group memberships
- values, ethics, and morals
- prejudice, stereotypes
- choices and options
- religion and spirituality
- language, speech, symbols
- historical trauma
- customs, rituals, standards
- dress, style, appearance
- expectations and openness

Social and Societal Factors
SOCIO

Cultural Factors
CULTURAL

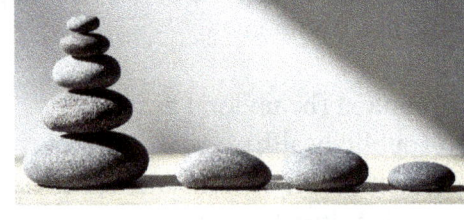

Integrated Holistic Yoga: A Commitment to <u>Integration</u>

Integrated holistic yoga integrates all eight traditional limbs of yoga practice equally, not raising physical performance or practice above the rest. It begins with the understanding that yoga is first and foremost a practice of awareness, compassion, and insight in all the many layers of our modern and ancient conceptions of self (or consciousness). The practice begins with mindfulness of the body, as we tune into personal needs, tailor our physical practice, attune to inner sensation, and develop interoceptive awareness of how our body responds to different demands and actions. Mindfulness also encompasses the breath, to help us find attunement to how we move energy through our body, how the breath enlivens the body, and how affects and arousal arise, are experienced, and dissipate. Mindfulness moves with greater challenge toward cultivating awareness of the fluctuations in the mind to help us transcend and transform mental and emotional habits that impair our psychological growth and transformation, affect our relationships and communities, and flavor our understanding of how life unfolds and interconnects.

From mindfulness of body (sensation), breath (affect), and mind (perceptions, cognition, memory, thoughts, emotions, interpretations, attitudes, opinions, and more), slowly wisdom emerges and guides us toward an appreciation of life as a journey of connection, transformation, growth, and perpetual change. We move toward an understanding that when we find the gap between stimulus and response, we give ourselves the gift of conscious choice, novel ways of being, reshaping our lives and relationships. Of course, we do not practice yoga with a goal in mind – we simply realize its potential and open ourselves to the journey toward perhaps becoming wiser, more equanimous, compassionate, and joyful. We engage in the practice altruistically, for the benefit of our greater community and world.

The integrated journey that is yoga guides us along a varied path of practices that begins with a commitment to and grounding in *ethical practices* (Limb 1: *yama*) that encourage us to strive to live peacefully, truthfully, and with a sense of abundance, joy in moderation, and non-possessiveness. It includes a commitment to purposeful living that embraces simplicity, contentment, impassioned practice, self-reflection, and dedication to a greater purpose. On the foundation of these ethics and *life-choices* (Limb 2: *niyama*), we build a *physical practice* (Limb 3: *asana*) that is mindful, easeful, passionate, and committed to enhancing our capacity to perceive ourselves accurately. Adding mindful *breathing* (Limb 4: *pranayama*) to the physical practice adds feedback mechanisms that calm our nervous systems, help regulate physiological arousal and emotional reactivity, and enhance emotional and psychological resilience.

As we get to know our body and emotions with greater accuracy and honor our physical needs with compassion, we turn our yoga practice inward. We allow time for our mind to become quiet – we settle into the *inner practices* (Limbs 5 [*pratyahara*], 6 [*dharana*], and 7 [*dhyana*]) of yoga. Drawing our senses away from constant (over)stimulation, we develop the capacity to recognize how our mind works, how we can transform its fluctuations, and how we can become more peaceful and rest in stillness. We develop the capacity to become concentrated and achieve a single point of focus, and ultimately we move into a spacious awareness that forges new neural pathways, creating neuroplasticity, increased decisional control, spaciousness, peacefulness, and loving responsiveness to ourselves and others.

What emerges perhaps spontaneously along the path of integration is a sense of being grounded (integrated) in community, a sense of belonging to the earth, a desire to connect and preserve, and a *joyful connection* (Limb 8: *Samadhi*) to something greater, a transformation of suffering. We emerge with a sense of compassion, joy, equanimity, and lovingkindness. We attain a sense of integration and of being whole (again). This practice of yoga is a journey inward so that ultimately we can journey outward – a journey of getting to know ourselves so that we may become a positive force in our communities, in the lives of others. We move inward to move outward. We get to know ourselves to understand all.

Integrated Holistic Yoga: A Commitment to Accessibility, Equity, and Belonging

Yoga is a practice that is meant to be shared; a practice that is for everyone; a practice centered on the practitioner. For this reason, I end up asking almost everyone I know, meet, or run into at some point in our conversations whether they have a yoga, meditation, or mindfulness practice. What I hear from those who say "no" is usually pretty discouraging about how yoga is perceived. I hear things like "yoga is not for guys", "yoga is not for women my age"; "I am too old… too big… too stiff … too lazy … too *whatever* …"; "I am not fit enough"; "I don't fit in"; "yoga conflicts with my religion..."

Some have tried yoga and given up – they stopped going to class when they felt like an outsider, the only one who could not keep up, the only one who did not seem to know what to do, the only one in their demographic. Some gave up because they had pain or physical challenges and did not know how to work within their limitations; some did not know how to move into and out of a pose safely; some were afraid that they would be the only ones left lying on the mat at the end of a pose or class because they could not hear the teacher. Some gave up because they were hurt in class or by a teacher, had strong emotions emerge without support, or were upset about something that was said or done in class.

Among those who do yoga, some have confided that they have encountered teachers whom they perceived as having pushed too hard, made painful adjustments, failed to offer props, been too demanding, had no understanding of their own unique social and cultural circumstances, and had no experience with older people, men, individuals with physical limitations, people with emotional or mental challenges, and on goes the list. Some talk about being bothered by having to look at themselves in a mirror, feeling uncomfortable about their clothes or body, or feeling left out when they cannot access a pose that everyone else in the room seems to do with ease.

As yoga teachers, we need to understand, appreciate, and address these concerns. Most of us are well-intended and thoughtful about prepping classes. That said, we likely all have left students behind in our classes. We can all do better; we can all become more mindful to make yoga more accessible, especially in the settings where people are already served who could benefit from the practice (including in healthcare settings).

As yoga professionals, we can use many tools to make this happen:
- We can accurately label our classes to invite the students who will most benefit from what we have to offer.

- We can offer classes that are focused less on form or posture practice and more on breathing, mindfulness, or meditation.
- We can offer classes that expose students to the psychology and philosophy of yoga, integrating emotional supports and mental coping strategies in a context of physical practice that is easeful and accessible to most, if not all.
- We can offer physical practices that honor varying levels of skill, physicality, emotionality, and psychological needs.
- We can learn to demonstrate multiple expressions of the same pose, giving our students opportunity and permission to choose what is right for their body in any given moment.
- We can adapt, modify, and show variety in all poses, modeling mindful awareness of the range of needs in our classroom.
- We can develop gentler, more accessible physical and breathing practices that are adapted, inviting, and realistic for the average, non-stereotypic practitioner.
- We can use props for every pose – demonstrating all poses with props, encouraging the use of props, and inviting our students to be advanced practitioners by honoring their body and using the proper supports for a safe practice.
- Our language can become clearer, our voice crisper. Our words can be chosen to be more inclusive and inviting.
- We can invite humor and lightness into the practice without making fun of anyone.

As a yoga community, we can remember to work on changing the face of yoga:
- We can develop classes that are specifically geared to non-stereotypic practitioners
  - We can offer appealing and beautiful practices that attract seniors, individuals of all genders, individuals with physical challenges, people who have struggled emotionally, persons who are searching for community, students who want more than exercise, people from all walks of life, all cultures and backgrounds.
  - We can offer classes that are on a sliding fee scale or free to those who cannot afford them (using the honor system – no questions asked).
  - We can offer classes in community centers, museums, classrooms, and libraries – places that are not associated with the "glamor" of yoga.
- We can show more diversity in pictures that demonstrate yoga poses
  - We can show props, modifications, adaptations, restoratives.
  - We can show people – teachers and students – of all ages, shapes, sizes, and more.
- We cannot succumb to the materialism of the practice
  - We can show images of yoga without fancy clothes.
  - We can show fun home-made props.
  - We can offer scholarships and free classes.
  - We cannot make our yoga setting a platform for selling stuff.

All yoga teachers can work on solutions for bringing yoga to everyone. All of us need to collaborate with as many people as possible to transcend current notions about who can practice yoga and who is welcome. We need to create the change that will carry yoga into more lives.

All of us can make efforts to understand and honor the biopsychosociocultural contexts of our students and to offer cues of safety and understanding for all. This may mean that yoga has to get political and has to challenge institutionalized, systemic, and structural racism, White supremacy, and the fantasy that we are all one and the same. All of us need to understand that there is indeed diversity and that there is indeed a huge difference in how all of experience and feel safe (or not) in the world. A yoga of inclusion, accessibility, and equity is a yoga that is political, open-hearted, and open-minded. It is a yoga of values, engaged action, and a commitment to make the world a better place for everyone.

Integrated Holistic Yoga: A Commitment to Intentionality

The basis of any dedicated yoga practice grounded in the eight limbs and five koshas is the setting of an intention for this practice, *sankalpa* in Sanskrit. The Sanskrit word *kalpa* means vow; the Sanskrit root word *san* refers to the highest truth. Setting a sankalpa thus means that we vow to orient our practice to the search for truth; we resolve to search for the deeper meaning of our individual and collective lives; we commit ourselves to a deep search for purpose.

Intentions signal commitment and dedication; they anchor us to a deeper meaning so that we can stay with our practice when it becomes challenging – which it will. Intentions infuse our actions with volition and motivation. They set in motion thought, speech, and action that will infuse the outcomes and impacts of our actions (though intention and impact must not be confused – we can have a positive conscious intention [that may be flavored inauspiciously by other unconscious processes] and yet set off a negative impact).

Intention setting is best woven into yoga practice, psychology, and philosophy from beginning to end. It is a bit like values clarification in that we have to figure out where we want to place our intention, what we truly desire, and to what we want to dedicate ourselves. We can set an intention for an individual practice; we can set an intention for our practice across a lifetime; we can set an intention for a particular timeframe; we can set intentions in many different ways. Intentions are – in a way – a drishti for life – a focal point for our attention and concentration that orients our thoughts, speech, behaviors, and relationships.

Intentions are useful as tools that hone our attention on a particular goal – a goal that we hold loosely while enjoying the journey and what unfolds, rather than clinging to a particular outcome (more about this below). Intentions are not like New Year's resolutions that we set to fix something that is broken or to correct the error of our ways. Intentions are orienting principles that help us stay the course of our practice even when things get tough, when we are tempted to give up, when doubt rears its head.

Intentions are closely linked to motivation, which in turn may help us recognize our primary layer of self or consciousness (i.e., our kosha):
- If intentions are driven by fear (or the avoidance of danger), they may arise from annamaya kosha (our physical body).
- If intentions reflect desire or aversion (wanting or not wanting something), they may arise from pranamaya koshas (our energy, breath, life force).
- If intentions arise from duty or want to do the right or moral thing (to help ensure that we are perceived as a good person), they may arise from manomaya kosha (our mind).
- If intentions reflect love, compassion, kindness, the desire to be of selfless service, they may have arisen from vijnanamaya kosha (our intellect and wisdom).

> *If we want to be serious about our intentions, we may choose to start and end each day with a review of our open-hearted commitment to them.*
>
> - We may *start each day* with one of the following (as examples):
>   - gratitude practice for our life
>   - heart-opening practice
>   - conscious vow to live the day with awareness, compassion, and/or insight
>   - recommitment to our intention as we move into our day
> - We may *end each day* with one of the following (as examples):
>   - review of the day to assess if we were true to our intentions
>   - review of our commitment to awareness, compassion, and insight
>   - recommitment to our intention for the next day
>   - gratitude practice for the gifts of the day

As we will explore shortly, research provides evidence that yoga is an amazingly beneficial practice for physical, emotional, mental, and relational wellbeing and resilience. It would be simple to stop right there. It is certainly enough of an incentive to start a practice. But nothing is ever that simple. It would be reductive to practice yoga because Western research has tested and documented its effectiveness. For one thing, ancient yoga has been known as healthful and transformative for millennia – we did not need Western researchers to tell us this (though it does convey a legitimacy to yoga that now allows us to integrate the practice into modern healthcare and mental healthcare settings – a boon to holistic health).

The view of yoga as being worthy of practice because it is a healthcare strategy is reductive because yoga is so much more. Yoga is a lifestyle; it is a commitment to ourselves, our loved ones, our communities, our world of sentient beings, our environment, and our planet. Yoga brings to our lives clarity of purpose that is larger than our own small world and selfish perspectives. It instills a passion for making the world a better place, for being engaged and feeling responsible for the betterment of society and the earth. Yoga creates growth and change on and off the mat. In fact, yoga is not meant to be limited to the mat (for one thing, there did not even used to be a mat). It is meant to be a lifestyle, a way of reaching clarity and wisdom, a way of living that is of value and about service, a way to move beyond habit into discernment, a way of creating awareness. Yoga based on its ancient roots draws us inside to make us better people on the outside. It is a practice of mindfulness and insight that invites us to transcend narrow and reactive views; that challenges us to take broad and less biased perspectives; that prompts us to be loving, kind, compassionate, joyful, equanimous, and generous; and that reminds us that there is a greater connection and interdependence than we may even be able to fathom.

In Buddhism, intention is the foundational step in cultivating the five strengths or energizing factors that support any type of practice, new routine, or commitment:
- *Determination*: setting an intention and working on or toward it with determination
- *Familiarization*: getting to know ourselves in the midst of the business of life and committing to living with mindfulness to become more familiar with our layers of self and impacts on others

- *Virtue*: living in accordance with values of open-heartedness and open-mindedness as opposed to acting from fear desire or ego; this is the commitment in all layers of self or consciousness (body, breath, mind, wisdom, bliss – the koshas)
- *Reproachment of habit*: letting go of ego, of firmly held habits and patterns in service of freeing ourselves from being locked into some calcified opinions about who, what, how we are - freeing ourselves from habit
- *Aspiration*: aspiring to be of benefit and service of others, even all; awakening our heart and creating connection

---

A Personal Aside: My Reason to Practice

For me, the real reason to practice yoga is that – every single day – it gives me a way to become a better person, to be an agent for change, to fulfill my existential imperative to leave the world better than I entered it, to transcend my shortcomings and grow. If my personal health and resilience improve as a result, that is the icing on the yogic cake. If I am a kinder more loving person in my relationships, that is a relief for my soul. If I am at least able to recognize when I screw up and am hurtful, less than peaceful, or not as generous as I could be, then I have already benefited from the practice. Even the word "benefit", though, can be dangerous. Daily, I remind myself that I do not practice to reap a benefit or achieve a particular outcome. Yoga is not a means to end. Yoga is the end in and of itself; my commitment to the practice – to being present and engaged – is the end in and of itself. Anything that arises from there, is a gift and miracle. And for that I am grateful every day – even if sometimes I forget. ☺

Reflection Exercise:
What is your reason to practice?

Integrated Holistic Yoga: Beneficence and Doing No Harm

The research evidence is clear: any individual with mental or physical health challenges can benefit from a tailored and person-centered yoga practice. Sadly, under-referral to the practice as a healthcare intervention is typical as most healthcare professionals do not understand the wide applicability of yoga (Sulenes et al., 2015). However, given the variety of yoga strategies, almost anyone can benefit from practicing yoga. Lifestyle, breathing, and interior practices are accessible to all bodies; postures come in many forms and can be practiced by nearly everyone, especially with openheartedness about using variations that are individually tailored and compassionate. While Western postural practice is often (and counter to traditional yoga) forceful, energetic, and focused on physical beauty and fitness, yoga's physical practices can be easily modified and adapted to fit the individual practitioner. Widespread stereotypes about yoga postures suggest falsely that yoga is for the fit, the young, the slim, the flexible.

The misleading and stereotypic images of postural yoga create barriers to access to integrated holistic yoga for the very individuals who could benefit most – those with health challenges or who are subjected to chronic stress (Brems et al., 2015; Justice et al., 2016; Sulenes et al., 2015). For the most part, media depictions imply that yoga is only about physical posture and only for those who are already physically adept, slender, White, female, well to-do, educated, flexible, strong, balanced, and healthy (Birdee et al., 2008; Brems et al., 2016; Park et al., 2015; Razmjou et al., 2017). Nothing could be further from the truth. Integrated holistic posture practice is carefully adapted to individual practitioner's needs by being taught holistically with yoga blocks, straps, bolsters, blankets, pillows, and chairs to invite human beings of all shapes, ages, sizes, states of health and mobility, and experiences to participate fully and reap the benefits of mindful self-expression and self-exploration (Vladagina et al., 2016). Properly varied and adapted, nearly all students, clients, or patients, even those with physical challenges and limits, can experience the benefits of yoga.

Integrated yoga practices (Payne et al., 2014) and comprehensive, burgeoning research (Jeter et al., 2015; Khalsa et al., 2016; McCall, 2014) have begun to demonstrate that individuals – if invited into the practice on their own terms (Justice et al., 2016) – can derive substantial benefits. In contrast to Western stereotypes about who practices yoga (Justice et al., 2016; Razmjou et al., 2017), this includes (but is not limited to) individuals with physical, emotional, and mental challenges; with significant life stress and trauma histories (Carter et al., 2013; Justice et al., 2019); with aging bodies; in prisons and jails; in hospitals and other healthcare settings; in schools and universities; and more (Elwy et al., 2014; Freeman et al., 2019; Hayes & Chase, 2010; Khalsa et al., 2016). Positive effects have been documented for a range of physiological, musculoskeletal, and mental health symptoms. Beneficial effects have been demonstrated through clinical trials as well as case studies, surveys, and other means of establishing the utility of interventions for human health and wellbeing.

Changes that Emerge from an Integrated Yoga Practice

Research evidence that yoga, in its many manifestations, is helpful for a variety of challenges and with many types of individuals begs the question how this change is facilitated (McCall, 2013; Riley & Park, 2015) In fact, the synergy of the multitude of practices within yoga has a profound impact on several human systems that greatly affect day-to-day functioning, wellness, and resilience in times of stress, busyness, challenge, and demand (Sullivan et al., 2018b). Yoga optimizes autonomic control, regulates endocrine (e.g., decreases cortisol and increases gamma-aminobutyric acid) and immune function, shapes adaptive emotional and behavioral responses, and lessens reactivity (as evidenced by less widespread arousal, enhanced vagal tone, improved relaxation response, and increased cardiac variability). It facilitates optimal physiological conditions (Taylor et al., 2010), enhances executive functioning and working memory, increases pain tolerance, and enables adaptive emotions and behaviors by facilitating a positive attitude, new ways of dealing with old inputs, and accurate discernments in times of stress and challenge (Schmalzl et al., 2014; Taylor et al., 2010). Yoga increases resilience in body, emotion, and mind and brings about self-regulation that supports adaptive responsiveness to meet the needs of the environment, body, emotions, and mind. These benefits arise because yoga affects and integrates both top-down and bottom-up pathways in the human brain for coping with internal and external demands, while it recalibrates the nervous system and maintains homeostasis in body and mind.

Top-Down Pathways

Top-down mechanisms or pathways are those that arise from the cerebral cortex of the brain and as such are conscious and intentional. They promote self-regulation through a variety of mechanisms, including cognitive appraisal, reframing, goal-setting and follow-through, attention, intentionality, and planning (Sullivan et al., 2018a, 2018b; Taylor et al., 2010). Top-down pathways decrease the level of engagement of the sympathetic nervous system; decrease habitual emotional, mental and behavioral reactivity; enhance working memory and attentional stability; improve executive functioning; and make stress perception more accurate (Field, 2011; Gard et al., 2014, 2015). They can modulate neuroendocrine output, vagal tone, and sympathetic nervous system output. As changes take effect, even immunity and inflammation are improved (Sullivan et al., 2018b).

Yoga integrates many practices that strengthen top-down processing and regulation, not the least of which include the exercising of attention, intention, and mindfulness and the ongoing conscious monitoring of the internal states of body, breath, and mind (Brown et al., 2007). Further, yoga's first and second limbs (i.e., ethical values and lifestyle commitments) as well as other aspects of deeper yoga philosophy (Feuerstein, 2013) help practitioners explore motivations, habits, patterns, and predilections (Sullivan et al., 2018b); engage in metacognition that allows for decentering and perspective-taking to result in less rigid world views and greater behavioral flexibility (Vago & Silbersweig, 2012); and step out of habits to make conscious choices based on clear intentions and deliberate preparatory plans (Payne et al., 2014; Payne & Crane-Godreau, 2015; Vago & Silbersweig, 2012).

Yoga's values clarification practices encourage practitioners to engage in ethical inquiry that supports intentional decision-making and discernment (Sullivan et al., 2018a). Yoga's interior practice of drawing awareness inward supports the development of selective attention and response inhibition, facilitating self-regulation and conscious decision-making (Gard et al., 2015) Concentration practices, as interior or posture practices (via gaze points or mindful attention of a particular part or state of the body), contribute to strengthening downward self-regulatory control and behavioral flexibility. In fact, all interior practices encourage practitioners to reappraise and reframe their lived experience (e.g., reconceptualizing 'discomfort' as 'sensation'; (Schmalzl et al., 2015)). Finally, even posture practices in and of themselves can demonstrate positive effects on top-down pathways through requiring planning, problem-solving, set-shifting, and decision-making skills (Schmalzl et al., 2015).

Bottom-Up Pathways

Bottom-up mechanisms modulate activity in the lower regions of the brain, via ascending pathways that reach from the brain stem, through the limbic system, to the cerebral cortex, including the anterior cingulate and insula (Taylor et al., 2010). Inputs into the bottom-up circuits arise from somatic, sensory, visceral, cardiovascular, and immune receptors in the body and affect immunity, psychological health, and physical wellbeing. Bottom-up inputs also arise from the autonomic nervous system (sympathetic and parasympathetic) and the hypothalamic-pituitary-adrenal axis. Bottom-up mechanisms can contribute to self-regulation; however, they do so not through conscious and intentional cognitive processes (as is the case with top-down processing), but rather through unconscious responsivity to the perceived demand characteristics of a particular input. Symptoms of illness and injury arise from the bottom-up pathways.

Many yoga practices facilitate accurate perception of sensory inputs through careful attention to bodily states, especially as mediated by mindful breath and posture practice (Abel et al., 2013; Sengupta, 2012). Breathing practices induce calmness in the nervous system with subsequent relaxing responses in the neuroendocrine system via release of oxytocin and prolactin (Nivethitha et al., 2016; Schmalzl et al., 2015). Successful autonomic nervous system control and decreased endocrine release in turn results in enhanced social bonding and decreased emotional reactivity (Porges, 2011). Posture practices help practitioners learn to maintain a balanced nervous system in the face of challenge, as physical and sympathetic arousal from movement is effectively managed through careful postural sequencing and processing of exposure, extinction, and adaptive responsiveness (Gard et al., 2014). Finally, while not a limb of yoga, chanting or intoning a mantra such as the word '*om*' are additional yogic practices that assert positive autonomic control (Sullivan et al., 2018a).

Polyvagal System and Top-Down/Bottom-Up Integration

A crucial player in top-down and bottom-up functions is the vagus (10th cranial) nerve or polyvagal system (Porges, 2011). The vagus nerve is the primary conduit for communication to the brain about internal states as perceived through various sensory systems. It relays physical, mental, and environmental sensory input (from the bottom) via the anterior cingulate cortex and the insula to the prefrontal cortex (to the top). It integrates emotion, cognition, and conscious deliberation about sensory input from the top to the bottom, creating a network and integration across brain structures for an integration/collaboration of the top-down and bottom-up pathways. Top-down bottom-up integration facilitates balance in the vagal system, allowing for a calm, integrated, and resilient response (Gard et al., 2014; Schmalzl et al., 2015; Sullivan et al., 2018a, 2018b).

The smooth and adaptive integration of bottom-up and top-down pathways is not ingrained as humans may develop habitual patterns wherein responses are driven reactively by one or the other system (Payne & Crane-Godreau, 2015). The polyvagal system is the human threat detection system that is unconscious and arises at the sensory receptor level via neuroception, a process through which the nervous system detects and interprets cues of safety or danger in the environment or internal state. Neuroception can result in three possible perceptions: safety, danger, or life threat (terror). Neuroception of safety activates the ventral vagal complex (VVC). The VVC supports physiological recovery, emotional processing or interoception, mental regulation, and prosocial behavior (Porges, 2017; Taylor et al., 2010). The VVC facilitates social engagement and connection through release of oxytocin and prolactin, prosocial behavior, engaging voice and facial expressions, and relaxed posture.

Neuroception of danger activates the sympathetic branch of the autonomic nervous system, readying the organism for fight or flight, mobilizing a response that increases the likelihood of survival in light of the perceived threat or peril. It results in increased muscle tone, redirection of blood flow from the periphery to the core, inhibition of the gastrointestinal system, dilation of the bronchi, and increase in heart rate and respiration (among other physiological responses).

Neuroception of life threat activates the dorsal vagal complex and results in behavioral and physiological immobilization, along with emotional and mental collapse. Humans in this situation shut down, freeze, or "play dead". An organism in a state of life threat exhibits decreased muscle tone, decreased cardiac output, and reflexive defecation and urination (among other physiological responses) to reduce life functions to the least amount needed for survival.

Humans tend to have habitual or preferred autonomic nervous system styles (mediated by the vagus) that develop through experience and learning histories over the developmental span (Brems, 2024a; Payne & Crane-Godreau, 2015; Porges, 2011; Porges & Carter, 2017; Sullivan et al., 2018a, 2018b). Some individuals have greater likelihood to perceive safety (living more commonly in their relaxed, engaging and restorative ventral vagal space); others have an autonomic nervous system primed for danger (living in a near-constant state of sympathetic arousal, isolation, and physiological overload or break-down); and some expect life threat and develop a habitual pattern of shrinking back from life, withdrawing – even dissociating – from human experiences. Top-down and bottom-up mechanisms are set in place that perpetuate these nervous system styles and thus can also become the mechanism for change.

Yoga offers many strategies for top-down and bottom-up processing, most of which work in tandem with each other for a natural integration of these pathways through the synergistic combination of the limbs of yoga. Additionally, yoga facilitates changes in habitual autonomic nervous system styles by making practitioners more behaviorally flexible, emotionally resilient, socially available, and cognitively complex to deal responsively with each input in the moment as it unfolds, rather than reactively based on learning history and experience. Through various integrative practices, yoga facilitates top-down bottom-up integration, ushering in greater response flexibility, enhanced impulse inhibition, and decreased reactivity.

Yoga, especially the breathing and interior practices, creates bi-directional feedback and feedforward loops in the brain that result in greater accuracy of input detection and interpretation and in greater resilience and self-regulation in emotional, mental, relational, and behavioral responses (Gard et al., 2014; Sullivan et al., 2018a, 2018b). Yoga stimulates the basal ganglia cortico-thalamic circuits that help humans unlearn maladaptive behaviors and allow for extinction learning. Simultaneously, yoga (especially through mindfulness practices, often using the breath as a mindful focus) creates greater connectivity of the caudate with other (higher and lower) brain regions, facilitating new, goal-directed, flexible learning and behavior (Gard et al., 2015; Schmalzl et al., 2015). Yoga employs breathing strategies that restore balance to the nervous system through supporting autonomic nervous system styles (and, commensurately, unconscious cognitive expectations or predictions) that place the organism into the ventral vagal (i.e., calm, relaxed, interpersonally engaged) space. This effect is important as the polyvagal system regulates allostatic load.

Allostasis and Accurate Sensory Processing

Allostasis is the "ability of an organism to maintain stability/homeostasis through change by actively adjusting to both predictable and unpredictable events" (Schmalzl et al., 2015), p. 13). Yoga offers many tools that decrease allostatic load by offering behavioral choices, emotional flexibility, and cognitive reappraisal and restructuring. Resilience in body, emotion, mind, and behavior facilitates a ventral vagal response and promotes successful, integrated (bottom-up and top-down) self-regulation. Allostasis is dependent on the capacity to take self-regulatory action based on accurate internal (Craig, 2014) and external (Witkiewitz et al., 2017) sensory pathways to bring the organism back into balance. Much of what yoga facilitates is exactly that – it prepares the practitioner to take appropriate and adaptive action in response to accurately perceived demands and needs.

Mindfulness (embedded in all yogic practices and central to many breathing practices) encourages accurate perception of sensory input from internal bodily systems and environmental stimuli through conscious awareness of neuroceptive, interoceptive, exteroceptive, and proprioceptive stimuli. In other words, yoga encourages conscious and accurate processing of sensory input from inside and outside the body to support self-regulation, bidirectional feedback, and adaptive behavior in support of successful allostasis (ongoing change in the service of stability). Yoga facilitates meta-awareness and in-the-moment lived experience of interoceptive, neuroceptive, exteroceptive, and proprioceptive inputs and thus helps integrate information across top-down and bottom-up systems, a process that is largely coordinated by the insula (Gard et al., 2014, 2015; Taylor et al., 2010; Tsakiris et al., 2011).

These inputs and the capacity to recognize their ebbing and flowing (i.e., impermanence) are crucial to psychological wellbeing, via accurate cognitive appraisal of what is perceived (Craig, 2014) and physical health, via supporting physiological homeostasis (Gu et al., 2015) as well as to feeling present, effective, and proactive in the world. They become useful – and are applied in the context of yoga – when they are interwoven with mindful and accurate appraisal of the environment or context to result in adaptive behaviors (Farb et al., 2015) and to break reflexive and reactive cycles of responses. Practitioners of yoga learn to live in a ventral vagal state and to allow for and successfully manage a sympathetic nervous system response during danger. This sense of *preparedness* allows the individual to maintain or re-achieve ease while being ready to take action when environmental demands arise. In moments of terror or life threat, a sense of *surrender* may be triggered, wherein the practitioner moves from the ventral vagal to the dorsal vagal space to allow for momentary submission or freezing if the environmental demand is best met by this response. The resultant level of resilient and adaptive self-regulation reduces allostatic load and brings homeostasis or stability to body, energy and breath, emotion, and mind – equanimity in yoga's language.

A Brief History of Yoga

Yoga dates back to early Indian traditions, possibly as far back as 3000 BCE, based on archaeological evidence from the Indus Valley Civilization. However, scholarly consensus on whether these findings represent actual yoga practices is inconclusive. Yoga began to consolidate as a systematic practice with core principles around the 5th or 6th century BCE, as reflected in the Upanishads and early Buddhist and Jain texts. Yoga traditions have varied widely across Hindu, Buddhist, and Jain contexts, evolving in different ways over time. When studying yoga's history, it is essential to acknowledge the reliance on ancient texts and archaeological evidence that are difficult to date and interpret with certainty. Texts were often transmitted orally for centuries before being written down, leading to multiple interpretations and evolutions over time.

The complexity of these traditions requires an open-minded approach to understanding the context in which yoga emerged, developed, and continues to be practiced.

Central aspects of most yoga traditions include meditation, mindfulness, working with the mind to transcend suffering, cultivating awareness of subtle energies, and recognizing the various layers of self. These common threads appear in Hindu, Buddhist, and Jain traditions, although their interpretations differ. Notably, many ancient texts do not emphasize *asana* (or postural practice) as a central element of yoga; when mentioned, it is primarily as preparation for deeper meditative practices. Shared philosophical concepts across traditions include impermanence, interdependence, and interplay between tangible and subtle aspects of existence. Originally, yoga was a meditative and introspective tradition aimed at achieving inner peace and liberation by transforming cognitive, emotional, and behavioral patterns. The earliest references to yoga-like practices appear in the Vedas (c. 1500–1200 BCE), particularly in the Rig Veda, which includes hymns and mantras that were later incorporated into meditative traditions. The Upanishads, composed between the 8th and 3rd centuries BCE, expanded on these ideas, introducing the concepts of atman (individual soul) and brahman (universal consciousness), as well as the koshas (layers of self). These texts emphasize seated meditation, study with a teacher (guru), and oral transmission of knowledge (*satsang*).

The Bhagavad Gita (composed between 400 BCE and 200 CE), sometimes considered an Upanishadic text, provides one of the first systematic guides to spiritual liberation. It outlines different paths of yoga, namely, *karma* (action), *bhakti* (devotion), *raja* (meditation), and *jnana* (knowledge), each leading toward self-realization and liberation. The Bhagavad Gita incorporates both dualistic and non-dualistic perspectives, presenting a devotional approach to transcendence. The Yoga Sutras of Patanjali (c. 300–500 CE) further refine the philosophical and practical aspects of yoga. The text defines yoga as the calming of mental fluctuations and outlines an eight-limbed path as a means to transcend suffering. Patanjali's philosophy is primarily dualistic, distinguishing between *purusha* (pure consciousness) and *prakriti* (material nature), while also acknowledging *ishvara* (a divine being) as an aid in practice rather than a necessary focus.

Tantric traditions, emerging around the 5th–7th centuries CE, significantly influenced the evolution of yoga. Tantra developed within both Hindu and Buddhist contexts, emphasizing the integration of all aspects of existence – material and spiritual, sacred and profane. It democratized yoga by making practices accessible to householders rather than being limited to ascetics, challenging Brahmanical rules of the time. Tantra's influence can be seen in later forms of yoga, including the mindfulness and subtle energy practices found in Vajrayana Buddhism.

Hatha yoga, which emerged between the 9th and 15th centuries CE, draws heavily from tantric and Nath yogic traditions rather than solely from Buddhist sources. The Hatha Yoga Pradipika (15th century CE) is one of the most influential texts on this tradition. Unlike earlier meditative yoga traditions, Hatha yoga introduced physical postures (*asanas*) and breathwork (*pranayama*) as tools for growth, evolution, and spiritual transformation. However, even in Hatha yoga's early formulations and introductions of *asana,* physical posture was not the central focus of the practice, but a preparatory stage for meditation.

Yoga's introduction to the West occurred through two primary channels: Westerners traveling to India and becoming fascinated with Eastern traditions, and Indian yogis bringing yoga to the West (De Michelis, 2004)De Michelis, 2004). In the late 19th and early 20th centuries, Swami Vivekananda introduced *raja* yoga (via Patanjali's Yoga Sutras) to the West with emphasis on philosophical ponderings and implications and on meditative practices, initially excluding *asana*. Later, postural yoga, as developed in Mysore, India, by teachers such as Krishnamacharya, incorporated colonial influences from Western gymnastics and body-training systems (Singleton, 2010). Krishnamacharya's students, including B.K.S. Iyengar, Pattabhi Jois, and T.K.V. Desikachar, helped spread physically-oriented yoga worldwide, leading to an increased focus in the West on *asana* practice.

Modern transnational yoga movement often emphasized postural (even physical fitness) practice over its meditative and philosophical roots (Lorr, 2012). This shift has been shaped by colonial influences, Western physical culture, and commercial interests. Although contemporary yoga offers many benefits, practitioners need to be aware of yoga's historical context and the ways in which cultural appropriation has shaped its presentation in the modern world (Freeman et al., 2017; Razmjou et al., 2017; Vladagina et al., 2016). Understanding yoga's diverse origins allows for a more respectful and informed engagement with the practice.

A Few Signs of Cultural Appropriation	
General Concept or Definition of Cultural Appropriation	*Examples from the Context of the Cultural Appropriation of Yoga*
• Fail to give credit or acknowledgment to the source of the practice	• Not citing ancient yogic texts, not acknowledging lineage and influences; extracting concepts without giving source attribution
• Apply in ways inconsistent with the original intent of the practice	• Use of asana as a form of exercise; extract a single practice from the eight limbs and present it as the totality of yoga
• Disrespect the original culture, spirituality, or language	• Mispronounce Sanskrit terms; misuse Sanskrit expressions; ignore the cultural or holistic context of yoga
• Use the practice to create or perpetuate structures of oppression or abuse	• Abuse one's power under the guise of being a guru; transgress interpersonal boundaries and abuse students in various ways, including sexually
• Reinforce stereotypes of original practitioners or create new ones, passing them off as ancient	• Perpetuate Western or Eastern stereotypes: yogis as fit White skinny flexible… yogis as ascetic, eccentric, withdrawn from society
• Use the practice for personal gain, profit, or interest	• Monetize yoga by selling merchandise, over-charging, not creating equal financial (and other) access for all
• Give a skewed or altered perspective of the practice, yet pass it off as traditional or ancient	• Present yoga's (more recent) asana practices as ancient; extracting aspects of yoga psychology and failing to contextualize in the entire system of yoga

The Yoga Sutras of Patanjali

The Yoga Sutras, attributed to Patanjali, are a foundational philosophical text dated to approximately 300–500 CE (although some sources claim it came along as early as 4th century BCE). The Yoga Sutras are a practical guide or manual of concise aphorisms or instructions of evolving individual and cultural meanings and interpretations. The Yoga Sutras present a pathway toward psychological wholeness and integration, are at their essence a psychology, and provide students with tools to train the mind, regulate behavior, modulate emotions, refine thoughts, and enhance relationships (De Michelis, 2004; Hartranft, 2003). Patanjali, a deeply mystical figure (likely a conglomeration of many thinkers of the era), is an embodiment of integration as he (or the group of thinkers he represents) was a philosopher/psychologist, ayurvedic physician, and grammarian (or communications specialist) with writing in all three areas. He reminds us again and again that body, breath, mind, spirit, and community are integrated and that we become whole and healthy through integration. The path outlined in the Yoga Sutras is based on comprehensive lifestyle practices that cut across all the layers of self and integrate eight types of practices that take us to ever deepening levels of understanding and awakening. The eight-fold path, referred to as the eight limbs, is considered the royal road of yoga (*raja* yoga).

The meaning of the word 'yoga' is to 'yoke' or 'unite'. The literal translation of the word 'sutra' is 'thread'. As such the yoga sutras are a unitive thread, a science, that links the teachings, teacher, and student. The sutras have reemerged in significance repeatedly across the centuries, inspiring reinterpretation and modernization as life across the centuries has evolved. Yoga is constantly evolving depending on different contexts, cultures, and societies and the interpretations of the Yoga Sutras vary across time and cultures. It is important to read multiple translations to appreciate the breadth and depth of meaning that can be gleaned from the Yoga Sutras, which – by their very writing style – leave a lot of room for interpretation. Each translation tends to reflect the Zeitgeist, beliefs, even consciousness of the translator, and thus interpretations of the Yoga Sutras vary widely and have transformed across the centuries.

The Yoga Sutras consist of four chapters (in Sanskrit called *padas*), summarized here:
- *Samadhi Pada* with 51 sutras – This chapter can be considered the short-cut discourse on how to attain enlightenment through meditative practices and samadhi (absorption). It presents meditation and other advanced states of practice as the speediest way to arrive the essence of yoga, which is the recognition of our true nature. It highlights that if we can collect ourselves fully into the present moment, we can still the fluctuations of the mind and awaken.
- *Sadhana Pada* with 55 sutras – This chapter outlines the eight limbs of yoga as a disciplined way to practice. It is the chapter most relevant for most practitioners as it suggests the eight-limbed path, undergirded by discipline, self-study, and committed purpose (*kriya* yoga), as a way to move toward the readiness to use the inner (concentration and meditation) practice to awaken. It is the yoga for the rest of us – those of us who cannot just get there with the guidance offered in *Samadhi Pada*.
- *Vibhuti Pada* with 56 sutras – This chapter explores more detail about practices of concentration, meditation, and samadhi to help us move into clear seeing – into wisdom and awareness. It also introduces the superpowers (or powers of manifestation) that can

accompany the process of enlightenment. This chapter warns us to not get caught up in attachment to some of these powers as this can become a hindrance on the path.
- *Kaivalya Pada* with 34 sutras – This chapter is dedicated to the attainment of *moksha* (or liberation), which brings us into our true nature, which in Patanjali's vision is consciousness. It frees us from unwholesome karma, as our consciousness has been purified of unwholesome intention, thought, speech, and action.

The following sutras are especially important to beginning yoga professionals as they frame the greater philosophical and psychological context of yoga as a personal practice, service, and teaching. They explain the reason for the practice of yoga and lead us to be curious about how to bring the practice into our lives. For translational details, readers can refer to any English translation of the Yoga Sutras.
- *Atha yoga anushasanam* (1.1): Now is the time for the teachings of yoga.
    - an invitation to directly experience the teachings and undergo the process
    - highlights the importance of presence, attention, and awareness
    - yoga happens in every moment of our life – it is the cultivation of mindfulness
    - yoga is a practice that is most relevant when taken off the mat
- *Yogas chitta vritti nirodhah* (1.2): Yoga is the calming of mental fluctuations (or mental reactivities or thought storms).
    - yoga is presented as a way of freeing ourselves from being trapped into conditioned and habitual tendencies
    - yoga is the removal of the causes of the disturbances of the mind – we cannot calm mental fluctuations without addressing their root causes
    - yoga is a practice that could be based simply on this single sutra that guides us to become aware of and respond deliberately (rather than reactively) to what is happening in the mind
    - yoga creates – over time – increasing awareness of what unfolds in our minds every moment of every day; in that way, it slowly invites us to experience stillness and wellness instead of chaos and disturbance
- *Tadas drasthu svarupe vasthanam (1.3):* Then the practitioner (the one looking within) can rest in their true inner essence.
    - in a way, this is a summary of the whole reason for practicing yoga – to rediscover and rejoice in our self
    - through practice, we remove the obstacles that usually keep us from appreciating who we really are
    - focus on reminding us that we have inherent resilience in all layers of self, including in our communities
    - we have the innate capacity to heal – to be integrated, to be whole (here you see the guiding principle for the lineage of integrated holistic yoga)
- *Vritti sarupyam itaratra (1.4):* Otherwise we stay caught up in misidentification and stay stuck in the dark (in suffering).
    - we mistake reactivity for reality – then we react to circumstances from that place of misunderstanding – that cannot be good ☙
    - not seeing who we really are brings suffering to ourselves and others – it is the precondition for illness and dis-ease
    - not realizing our reactivity keeps us trapped in nonproductive or maladaptive patterns

- o if we identify with our thoughts and emotions (our reactivity), we get stuck in habits or ruts that no longer serve us
  - o leading us to diving into learning about samskaras (habits, repetitive patterns, reactivities, thoughtless actions and more) and karma (action results)
- *Abhyasa vairagyabhyam tan nirodhah (1.12):* Practice (or effort) and non-attachment (or letting go) stops the self-identification with the mind.
  - o we realize that we are not our thoughts and emotions through consistent effort and through letting go
  - o we practice to practice, not to attain a goal - we let go of wanting and striving
  - o through letting go, we find ease with who we are and where we are – we begin to realize our true self
  - o we stay engaged (abhyasa) but without getting insistent or attached (vairagyam)
  - o we find the balance between heroic effort and complete surrender
- *Shraddha virya smrti samadhi prajna purvakah itaresham (1.20):* Freedom from suffering (or wholeness) requires conviction (faith), persistence (energy, passion), mindfulness (remembrance), integration (focus, concentration, alertness), and discernment (wisdom, good judgment).
  - o we meet the practice with faith, not with blind belief – we meet the unknown with openness of heart and mind, not trying to mold reality to our expectations; we open up to the mystery of life with trust and a willingness to jump into the deep end of the pool with wisdom ☙
  - o we commit to the practice with our whole heart and mind
  - o we bring an auspicious attitude to our practice as we realize that how we look at the world is how the world looks back at us
  - o we realize that the journey requires our full passion, commitment, and energy and it needs to be persistent and ongoing
  - o we trust in the worthwhileness of the effort without striving, with wisdom and concentration
- *Heyaṁ duḥkham-anāgatam (2.16):* Any suffering that has not yet come (or been experienced) is to be avoided.
  - o we learn to anticipate more correctly what may bring pain and suffering to ourselves and others and make choices that have a different outcome
  - o we realize that discernment now about how to think, speak, feel, and behave may prevent suffering later
  - o we recognize how we contribute to our own and others' suffering and resolve to make changes that lead to better outcomes
  - o we live more consciously of the consequences of our actions and make discerning choices

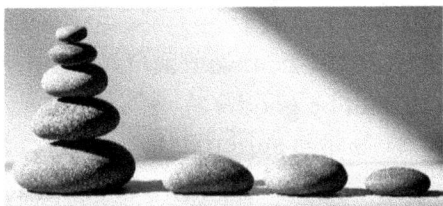

Bhagavad Gita

The Bhagavad Gita or "Divine Song" can be an interesting and controversial springboard for discussion of yoga's ancient meanings – and modern implications (Vyasa, 2020). Some say that the Bhagavad Gita was composed approximately between 400 BCE and 200 CE and is considered by many to be a part of a larger spiritual Hindu epic called the Mahabarata, dating to the end of the era of the Upanishads (though there is some that claim it is a document that emerged much later and faked to seem ancient). Others argue that it was written in 800 CE and attributed to the Mahabarata by its author Shankaracharya to give it the legitimacy of a longer legacy.

It is a philosophical text about a war between two sides of a royal family fighting for power over their kingdom – interpreted as an allegory for good versus evil, right versus wrong, mindful versus thoughtless. Arjuna, the story's hero, guided by Krishna, his mentor, is facing the fact that life is full of struggle and suffering; that we have to face unbelievable horrors and yet need to take action rather than quit in despair. Not each of our actions looks loving on the face of it, some may look downright evil; yet we have to attempt to look beyond the evil to recognize the intention underlying each action and see it in the context of the greater whole and in the context of karma.

The text is often used to teach about the deeper intentions of yoga practice (self-realization) and the many variations of the yogic path. The text points to the heart of some of the greatest human struggles, with a few examples offered below (all pages numbers refer to the source translation by (Easwaran, 2007).

- *Detachment from the outcome of our action*: Passages in the Bhagavad Gita encourage us to be mindful and open-minded as well as openhearted, to be soft and flexible, not set and determined toward a particular end. For example, Krishna advises Arjuna: *"You have the right to work, but never to the fruit of work. You should never engage in action for the sake of reward, nor should you long for inaction. Perform work in this world, Arjuna, as a man established within himself – without selfish attachments, and alike in success and defeat. For yoga is the perfect evenness of mind."* (2:47 and 2:48; (Easwaran, 2007), p. 94).
- *Selfish desire versus selfless action*: Action is our purpose, our dharma, and we have no choice but to engage in it. However, the direction of our action, its underlying intention, is the deciding force about its merits and consequences (or karma). Actions motivated by selfishness or greed may have short-term outcomes that are pleasurable to the self, but their long-term outcomes are negative. Actions motivated by compassion, love, kindness, and understanding and carried out with equanimity will result in positive outcomes. As Krishna points out, *"the spiritually minded, who eat in the spirit of service, are freed from all their sins; but the selfish, who prepare food for their own satisfaction, eat sin."* (3:13; Easwaran, 2007, p. 105) and *"the ignorant work for their own profit, Arjuna; the wise work for the welfare of the world"* (3:25; Easwaran, 2007, p. 107). The ripple effect of positive and selfless action is expressed by Krishna in this passage that gives us (but especially those in leadership positions) pause to think: *"What the outstanding person does, others will try to do. The standards such people create will be followed by the whole world."* (3:21; p. 106).
- *Seeing the deeper ripple effects and dimensions of stillness and mindfulness*: *"The wise see that there is action in the midst of inaction and inaction in the midst of action. Their*

consciousness is unified, and every act is done with complete awareness." (4:18; p. 118.). Much of our lives, especially in the West, are simply about doing. We consistently and constantly confuse action (i.e., meaning or purpose) with activity (i.e., being busy, keeping our time occupied). This passage reminds us that just doing is not the same as being useful or purposeful; in fact, doing can be our undoing. Sometimes taking no action (or doing nothing) is the best action. Being quiet and collecting our thoughts and emotions, not reacting but responding thoughtfully and mindfully, is true action in the sense about which Krishna talks. Wisdom comes not from doing something; it comes from being mindful, thoughtful, compassionate, and clear in our intentions.

The Bhagavad Gita has been interpreted in widely differing ways, sometimes in controversial contexts. Mahatma Gandhi viewed it as a spiritual and ethical guide, emphasizing nonviolent resistance (*ahimsa*) and selfless action (*karma yoga*). He saw the battlefield as an allegory for the internal moral struggle, using the Gita's teachings to inspire his *satyagraha* (truth-force) movement against colonial rule. In stark contrast, Heinrich Himmler, one of the chief architects of Nazi atrocities, misappropriated the Bhagavad Gita to justify his ideology. Fascinated by its discussion of duty (*dharma*), he distorted its message to promote the idea of detached action, using it as a means to rationalize mass violence. However, this was a severe misreading of the text, which frames duty within a broader ethical and spiritual discourse, not as an endorsement of cruelty or genocide. Additionally, Indian rulers and religious authorities have historically cited the Bhagavad Gita in support of the *varna* system (social classification), using it to justify the claim that individuals have innate societal roles. Although the text discusses the fourfold *varna* system, it emphasizes that these roles are based on qualities (*guna*) and actions (*karma*), rather than birth. Over time, however, its teachings have been used to promulgate the rigid, hereditary caste system, perhaps justifying and reflecting later sociopolitical influences rather than the text's original intent.

Despite divergent interpretations, the Bhagavad Gita remains a profound philosophical work that has been adapted to various cultural and ideological contexts, if sometimes in ways that stray from its core message of selfless duty, wisdom, and spiritual liberation. It remains a deeply symbolic and multi-layered text, interpreted in diverse ways across spiritual and philosophical traditions. At its core, the battle described in the text is often seen as an allegory for the internal struggle between humans' highest self and its lesser manifestations – as the conflict between wisdom and ignorance, clarity and confusion, selfless duty and personal desires. Some interpretations present the Bhagavad Gita as a personal instruction manual for navigating the spiritual path, offering guidance tailored to background, disposition, and circumstances. As such, the text serves as a map and guidebook for yogic practice, providing various approaches to self-realization.

The Bhagavad Gita outlines four primary paths of yoga, each suited to different temperaments and inclinations. *Karma* yoga, the path of selfless action, emphasizes performing one's duties without attachment to results. *Raja* yoga, the path of meditation, focuses on disciplining the mind and senses to attain inner stillness and enlightenment. *Jnana* yoga, the path of knowledge or wisdom, involves deep inquiry into the nature of reality and the self. *Bhakti* yoga, the path of devotion, encourages surrender through love and reverence for the divine. While these paths are distinct, they are not mutually exclusive and often overlap in practice.

The Bhagavad Gita also presents profound lessons that have sparked ongoing discussions and debates. One such lesson is the importance of having a teacher (*guru*), a guide on the spiritual path. However, this raises the question of whether this guidance should be seen as an aid to personal discernment or whether it can lead to mindless subservience. Similarly, the text promotes nonattachment, urging practitioners to act without clinging to personal desires. Yet, some question whether this detachment should mean withdrawal from worldly affairs or whether it should be balanced with engaged, ethical action that supports the greater good.

Another significant concept in the Bhagavad Gita is *svadharma*, or personal duty. Traditionally, this has been linked to selfless service, with the idea that each person needs to fulfill their unique role in life without selfish motives. However, this principle has also been debated in the context of ethical autonomy, question whether one's duty should be rigidly determined by social standing versus being defined by the freedom to make empowered choices beyond societal constraints. Similarly, the doctrine of karma and wise action has also been misinterpreted to justify the forced imposition of particular social roles or predetermined life paths and outcomes.

The discussion of *varnas* (social categories) has been one of its most contested aspects of the Bhagavad Gita. It describes *varnas* as a way to define different responsibilities based on inherent qualities and disposition, ideally creating the most fitting opportunity for spiritual progress. However, this concept has been used to reinforce rigid caste structures and interpreted as an endorsement of maintaining fixed social hierarchies rather than a flexible framework for personal and spiritual development. Thus, although the Bhagavad Gita offers a rich and complex philosophy, it is open to multiple interpretations. Its teachings have inspired paths of wisdom, devotion, action, and self-inquiry; however, they have also inspired ideological and historical reinterpretations to justify deviations from a deeper spiritual essence of the yogic past.

Hatha Yoga Pradipika

The Hatha Yoga Pradipika is one of the most foundational and widely referenced texts on hatha yoga. Written in the 15th century by Swatmarama (Svatmarama & Akers, 2002), it serves as a manual for physical and energetic practices aimed at preparing the body and mind for higher states of consciousness. Although it is a later addition to the corpus of classical yoga literature, it remains deeply influential in shaping modern understandings of yoga. Unlike the Yoga Sutras, which emphasize mental discipline and meditative absorption, the Hatha Yoga Pradipika focuses primarily on physical and energetic purification as a means to spiritual transformation. It outlines methods such as *asana* (postures), *pranayama* (breath control), *bandhas* (energy locks), *mudras* (gestures), and *kriyas* (purifications) to awaken and channel *Prana* (life force). These practices are designed to refine human energy systems, readying the human organization for higher states of awareness. Although the text does not explicitly outline ethical precepts like the *yamas* and *niyamas* in the Yoga Sutras, it assumes that the practitioner has already established a strong ethical foundation before engaging in intense physical and energetic practices.

The Hatha Yoga Pradipika teaches that the physical component of yoga is a preparatory step that is essential to attaining a deeper goal of spiritual awakening. The real work of yoga involves awakening and directing *Prana* through the body's subtle channels (*nadis*) and energy centers (*chakras*). Through disciplined practice, the mind becomes more refined, leading the practitioner toward meditative absorption. Importantly, the Hatha Yoga Pradipika does not advocate for dissociation from the body but rather understanding, purifying, and harnessing it as a means to move toward spiritual growth.

A central theme of the Hatha Yoga Pradipika is the distinction between *samadhi* (meditative absorption) and *moksha* (liberation). Samadhi is described as a state where an individual sense of self dissolves, allowing for profound clarity and stillness. However, this is not necessarily equivalent to *moksha*, which is liberation from the cycle of birth and death. The Hatha Yoga Pradipika is primarily concerned with achieving heightened states of awareness through disciplined practice rather than explicitly discussing final liberation. Much like the Yoga Sutras, the Hatha Yoga Pradipika emphasizes discipline, effort, surrender, and inner transformation. However, its approach is deeply rooted in working with the body's energy and breath as a means to transcendence. By refining *prana* and stabilizing the mind, the practitioner moves toward awakening—a process of seeing oneself and the world with greater clarity.

Like the Yoga Sutras, the Hatha Yoga Pradipika has four chapters. The chapters contain 389 shlokas (or verses – similar to the aphorisms in the Yoga Sutras). A more thorough discussion of the Hatha Yoga Pradipika is beyond the scope of this brief historical review (Svatmarama & Akers, 2002).

- Chapter 1 – 67 verses about environment, ethics, and postural practices
- Chapter 2 – 78 verses about breathing, working with energy, and purification
- Chapter 3 – 130 verses about hand gestures and their energetic influences
- Chapter 4 – 114 verses about meditation and union

As you immerse yourself in the yoga, history, psychology, and otherwise,

**'Please work with persistent effort and endurance;
Yet, travel lightly – packing only what you need'.**
Paraphrased from a dharma talk by Western Buddhist Tim Olmstead

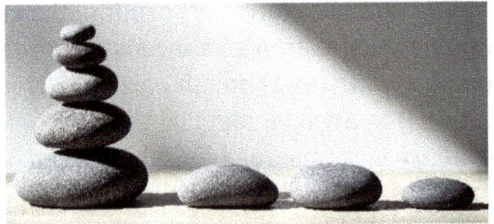

Chapter 2: Eight Limbs of Yoga

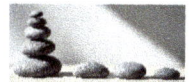

As noted previously, integrated holistic yoga integrates all eight traditional limbs of yoga practice equally, not raising any single limb above or below the others. It is a practice deeply grounded in the ancient traditions of yoga as a lifestyle and as a practice that can support, maintain, enhance, and even recover our physical and mental health and wellbeing. The psychology that undergirds the eight limbs of yoga is closely aligned with the understanding of the koshas. Each limb supports all koshas. Additionally, each limb provides specific access to certain of the koshas to become the primary vehicle that can invite health into that particular experience or consciousness of self. Wellness that arises from the application of a particular limb to a particular kosha, in turn, will penetrate into all other koshas given the profound interconnection and union of all of these layers. This is a true manifestation of the many pathways into health and wellbeing offered by an integrated, all-limbs practice of yoga.

The limbs of yoga interact with the psychology or philosophy of yoga in that they are the application of yoga psychology, the process of bringing the psychology alive in our day-to-day life. Yoga psychology comes alive when understood as a personal and interpersonal practice, informed by yoga psychology. Yoga psychology, history, and psychology are pivotal to understanding and embodying the essence of yoga; they encourage authenticity and deep philosophical grounding in a multi-limbed practice of yoga. The eight limbs of yoga move us from outer lifestyle and ethical commitments toward mindful ways of being in our bodies and with our emotions. These grounding practices then catapult us inward toward exploring our mind, wisdom, and human potential. Ultimately, the practices lead us to a greater purpose to which we devote ourselves with an open heart, an open mind, and no expectations for a particular outcome. The practices allow us to discover – and rediscover – our center, our truth, and our shared humanity (Iyengar, 2006).

Understanding of the eight limbs is most powerful if understood from multiple perspectives, including that of a:
- Yoga student or practitioner
- Teacher integrating the limbs into a lesson plan to frame a class or sequence of classes
- Teacher providing a dharma talk
- Healthcare provider integrating yoga into their extant clinical practice
- Mentor transmitting knowledge to students

Multi-limbs-based yoga is a highly interpersonal, practical, and communal practice. It is a practice for householders, that is, for those individuals who are not interested in a monastic life and yet interested in a spiritual or meaningful life. The most powerful transformations are relational across the layers of the self and across relationships and communities. In other words, the eight limbs are yoga for the rest of us – for those of us who cannot just sit down and gain mastery over the activities of the mind just because we would like to. So, if we are like most people, our yogic path may follow that of the eight limbs. We may start with committing to an ethical and purposefully dedicated life (Limbs 1 [*yamas*] and 2 [*niyamas*]). We may cultivate ease and grace, strength and power, and balance and integration in the body through posture and movement practices (Limb 3 [*asana*]). We may sit and breathe – becoming aware of your breath, observing your breath, and influencing the rhythms and patterns of your breath (Limb 4 [*pranayama*]). We may move inward (Limb 5 [*pratyahara*]) to find single-focused concentration (Limb 6 [*dharana*]) and to access spacious awareness (Limb 7 [*dhyana*]). And if we are patient and dedicated, we may access moments of integration, wholeness, and deep connection to a greater purpose (Limb 8 [*samadhi*]).

As will be explored in detail later, the eight limbs align with the five koshas, that is, the layers of human experience (see Chapter 3), providing practices specific to each layer as well as practices that reverberate through all aspects of experience. As a bit of a preview, here is an outline of this limb-to-kosha alignment:

- *Yamas and niyamas* – Limbs 1 and 2 align with all koshas and profoundly inform the biopsychosociocultural context in which humans grow, develop, interact, and nurture one another
- *Asana* – Limb 3 aligns with the physical layer of self or our somatic consciousness and reverberates through all other koshas
- *Pranayama* – Limb 4 aligns with the energetic layer of self or our affective consciousness and reverberates through all other koshas
- *Pratyahara* – Limb 5 aligns with the layer of cognitive, verbal, and social self or our mind consciousness, especially from the perspective of working with sense perceptions, and then reverberates through all koshas
- *Dharana* – Limb 6 also aligns with the layer of cognitive, verbal, and social self or our mind consciousness, especially as related to becoming aware of self and role consciousness, and then reverberates through all other koshas; it may also align with our wise and intuitive self or wisdom consciousness
- *Dhyana* – Limb 7 still aligns with mind consciousness but really begins to carry us into our wise intuitive self or wisdom consciousness, especially as related to living life with a greater sense of service and purpose that aligns with the greater good
- *Samadhi* – Limb 8 aligns with the layer of joyful self or universal consciousness, attuning us very deeply, wisely, compassionately, and insightfully with our interdependence, the ephemeral nature of all that we are and experience, and the painful state of conditioned states; understanding these truths of human existence allows us to liberate ourselves from suffering and moves us into connection, freedom, and joy

If we are interested in this path, it is most helpful to study with a teacher or a dedicated group of yoga practitioners who follows an integrated 8-limbed path into yoga. Because yoga is an interpersonal practice that relies on community, such a collaboration with a teacher or sangha will add depth and meaning to the journey into yoga, into the eight limbs. Sangha, or a teacher, who provides compassionate presence of others in one's life is a powerful support in maintaining health and resilience, especially in the face of challenge or adversity The big takeaway about the eight limbs is clearly that yoga is neither a solitary nor a singular practice – it is a comprehensive set of lifestyle choices that have a profound impact on how we live our lives, how we understand ourselves and others, and how we choose to be in the world. The eight limbs of yoga are learned, practiced, applied, and integrated into our life as a whole, depending on and reverberating into our interpersonal matrix and biopsychosociocultural context.

Overview of Limbs 1 and 2: A Yoga of Safety and Intention

Limbs 1 and 2 are well conceptualized as the lifestyle limbs of yoga. The practices in these two limbs guide the life choices we make every moment of every day. The principles and practices contained in these two limbs of yoga are considered foundational to all others. They require commitment, ongoing mindfulness, and daily practice. They are the limbs that ground us in community and ethical ways of being, ensuring that as adults we nourish our communities and ourselves with clarity, altruism, and joy. It is through these two limbs that we establish human communities of collaboration that create the biopsychosociocultural backdrop of our lives. The two limbs reflect our collective and individual values and ground us in a way of being with one another that provides the potential for creating safety, connection, opportunity for growth and development, at the individual and collective level.

Limbs 1 and 2 offer pathways toward change and healing applied in the biopsychosociocultural context of student and teacher or client and clinician. They honor the biopsychosociocultural experiences of the practitioner by taking them into account in all cuing and applications of the others limbs, as well as in understanding students' or clients' unique presentations of suffering. The first two limbs can honor the biopsychosociocultural context of by helping teachers or clinicians create relationships and environments that maximize the opportunities for students or clients to move into experiences of feeling heard, supported, and safe.

Through the first two limbs, yoga professionals create a healing context that invites purpose, engaged action, and motivation for change. Firstly, this happens through creating a biopsychosociocultural context and experience in the yoga or therapy room that incorporates environmental cues of safety; a commitment to teacher qualities and traits that invite, honor, and respect autonomy, agency, and empowerment of students; prioritization of creating a practice that is accessible, invites diversity, and honors differences; and clear cultivation of intentions and commitment to the healing journey. Secondly, Limbs 1 and 2 can support healing by helping students and clients to explore how they themselves can find ethical grounding and a committed yogic lifestyle – both of which will ultimately help the individual to find ways to contribute to their biopsychosociocultural context in thoughtful and compassionate ways.

Limb 1: Yama or Life Choices for Ethical Living

The first limb of yoga, *yama*, consists of a set of aspirations that encourage us to engage in values clarification that guides our moment-to-moment choices in thought, speech, actions, and relationships. This limb helps us with decision-making about how to balance the ethical aspirations with one another and within our greater biopsychosociocultural context, weighting in each moment how values and context interact and which principle(s) may need to be prioritized. It inspires us to lean into the behavioral and relational side of wholesomeness versus unwholesomeness. Through adherence to the yamas we aspire to be the best version of ourselves that we can be in the moment and to recognize in that movement how we can become better. It is a lifelong endeavor of refining the wholesomeness with which we show up in the world. In Buddhism, this is called 'ennobling' ourselves. This is the real meaning of the 'noble' truths - they are ways for us to *ennoble* ourselves, improve ourselves, make ourselves better beings who hold a higher truth beyond our own personal wellbeing.

This limb of yoga contains five central aspirations (or principles of ennoblement), each of which has clear and definite applications in day-to-day life for our many layers of the self. Each aspiration applies to each kosha – our body, emotions, mind, and wisdom as applied in relationships and communities. Each aspiration affects our capacity to access joy and a sense of being part of a greater meaningful whole. Each principle reminds us of the interconnectedness of all things – that what we send into the world ripples through everything. Each aspiration underscores the need for each one of us to be ethically and socially responsible and to make choices that cultivate conscious, loving, and compassionate communities. The various ethical aspirations are interdependent and are always applied contextually and interactively. They are applied intrapersonally and interpersonally and can help create balance and integration within ourselves as well as in our relationships.

The set of five aspirational first-person ethics principles outlined in this first limb are neither prescriptions nor proscriptions – they are a lifelong practice of refinement and growth. The emphasis on the word "aspirational" means that this limb offers us guidelines for ethical living to which we aspire and that we know we will *fail t*o heed. Yes, you read that correctly. We know that no matter how hard we try to follow these guidelines, we will not always do so. There will be moments of failure – and that is not only perfectly fine (human), but to be expected. We are human and we are fallible. The best we can do is to set an intention to do our best to bring these principles into our relationship with ourselves and with others.

Another important note about these aspirational principles that will guide our ethics and values is that they interact with each other. As you read their definitions below, you will realize that sometimes these practices and principles may lead us in different directions – following one may result in compromising another. When we encounter such situations, we make conscious choices about which principle to prioritize. For example, if you are struggling with telling someone the truth versus being kind and non-violent, which way will you go? Of course, there is no single answer to this conundrum. Each individual occasion may require a different answer to this question. So, it is important to realize that yogic ethics are not a simple prescription for how to behave. Instead, they are a way of inviting conscious inquiry about how to life our life ethically in each moment. They are a way of teaching us how to weigh the consequences of each intention, thought, decision, action, and relationship. Only once we have weighed the consequences, can we make a fully informed, optimal choice for any given moment in a manner that strengthens relationships and engages communities. We must not misunderstand this considered choice-making as a way to give us permission to let ethics fall to the wayside. That is not at all what weighing these principles suggests. It simply means that when we prioritize one principle over another, we do so consciously and with full willingness to bear the consequences.

Five Aspirations of Limb 1

   Nonharming or Ahimsa

Following the principles of nonviolence and peacefulness toward self, other, and everything, this aspirational ethical guideline invites us to live in a manner that seeks not to cause deliberate pain or harm. It is behaviorally expressed as kindness and compassion toward ourselves – in all koshas – and toward others. It is behaviorally expressed as being kind and peaceful in our intentions, thoughts, speech, actions, and relationships. It reflects the overcoming of hostility, even – or perhaps especially – in our intentions and thoughts. It is the capacity to notice hostility when it is present in our mind and to do what we can to transform and, if we cannot transform it, at least not to express it behaviorally or relationally.

Ahimsa starts with our intentions (though it does not end there) – violent intentions lead to harm even if we try to suppress violent action or aggressive speech. If we start from a place of negativity, hostility, or anger, we will likely do harm to ourselves and ultimately to our communities. Even challenging situations will unfold more auspiciously if we can approach them from a place of peaceful intention, a place of genuine and authentic desire of nonviolence for all. Ahimsa means choosing wise actions that generate and maintain peaceful interactions, relationships (inner and outer), communities, and systems.

<u>Applied collectively</u>, *ahimsa* relates to having compassion, caring, and lovingkindness for *everyone equally*. This means that we support equity – equity in the form of equal human rights and equal access to collective services and goods that support health, wellbeing, food and shelter, and opportunity. Nonharming extends beyond sentient beings to include nonviolence toward nature, the world, our planet, and the universe. Nonviolence is balanced with the other aspirations and always needs to be viewed contextually. Nonviolence does not mean sitting idly by when we witness injustice. Quite the opposite. It means recognizing, truly and consciously and honestly seeing, violence where it is present in our communities and feeling responsible for helping challenge and resolve it. It means speaking up in the face of harm – but not by being harming. Not by swinging an axe against the individual who is violent, but by entering into a dialogue with a heart of peacefulness, inquisitiveness, and openness. It means challenging harm that is being done in a non-violent manner.

> **Yoga Sutra 2.35**
> **Ahimsa pratishthayam tat vaira-tyagah**
> **When we are firmly grounded in nonharming, those we come in contact with naturally lose any feelings of hostility.**
> **→ Ahimsa begets peace**

Truthfulness or Satya

Following the principle of honesty with oneself and in all relationships and befitting to the context creates authenticity and integrity in day-to-day life. This aspirational ethic invites us to live in a manner that is true to our real and ideal self. It is behaviorally expressed as truthfulness, non-defensiveness (i.e., defenselessness), and all-revealing openness with ourselves – in all koshas – and with others. Honesty includes moving into relationship with the entirety of our Self and consciousness, as expressed in present and in the past. It means opening our heart to our shadow side and meeting ourselves with truthfulness – the good, the bad, the ugly. Authenticity requires us to move into an open relationship with ourselves where we hold nothing back – no matter how unpleasant or difficult.

Satya on the yoga mat means being honest about what are and are not capable of – not striving for the impossible. It means honoring the truth of the body, the breath, and the mind – showing up on the mat with the willingness to confront our truth, embrace it, and express it. Satya is exercised in balance with the other ethical aspirations and always contextualized. It may be truthful and safe in one context but may be harmful in another – either to oneself or to another person. While your truth is not relative, it may at time not be safe to express it. Balancing truth with a practice of peacefulness will support discernment of how to apply these aspirations in balance with one another. Satya also means exploring whether something we *think* is truth, really is. When we make statements of facts, for example, are we really expressing a fact or an opinion? If we honestly look at our assertions, are they truths or are they beliefs, attitudes, biases, selective truth? Where do we get our 'facts'? Are the sources honest, truthful, and authentic. Is something we read on social media trustworthy as fact or truth? We begin to realize through satya that truthfulness is more than not lying. It is a deep investigation of how we share and assert our truths. It is a deep realization that our persona truth may not align with another's personal truth. This is not to say that there is no right and wrong. It is simply an acknowledgement that life is not simple.

Applied collectively, *satya* means that we must be truthful about all human behaviors – past, present, and future – and must make reparations for abuses of the past, sins in the present, and harmful intentions for the future. Satya at the collective level may mean owning our personal and collective contributions to societal harm such as individual, collective, institutional, and systemic racism, sexism, agism, genderism, and more. It means facing abuses as perpetrated through colonialism, war, genocide, slaughter, theft, and imperialism. Honesty in the form of satya means taking responsibility.

> **Yoga Sutra 2.36**
> **satya pratisthayam kriya phala ashrayatvam**
> **As we are firmly grounded in truthfulness, our actions will naturally accrue positive results.**
> **→ Satya cultivates a natural flow of goodness**

Non-Stealing or Asteya

Following the principle of not taking what is not freely offered, this aspirational ethical guideline invites us to embrace and create a sense of abundance, generosity, and reciprocity that eliminates the desires to take or steal from others or to have more than others. It is behaviorally expressed as appreciating abundance, cultivating contentment, and joyfully recognizing what we already have. It is behaviorally expressed as only taking what is ours to take from ourselves and from others – in all koshas – and in relationship with others. Stealing or taking what is not freely offered can take many forms, especially forms that are not material in nature. Yes, we can steal things or objects. But we can also steal time or energy from others, perhaps by always being late or by dominating relationships and taking up all the space in a room. We can steal our own or others' joy when we bring ourselves or others down with a bad mood. We can steal another's joy by not joining in their celebration when they are delighted by an accomplishment or honored with an award, kudos, or any other small or large accomplishment. We steal from self and others with jealousy. We can also steal in subtle ways – such as competing for the last parking spot and gleefully taking it before the other car can swing in. We can steal through excessive bargaining over an artist's or artisan's price; we can steal by not wanting to pay for someone's time at a reasonable and respectful rate.

Of course, *asteya* has to be balanced with the other aspirational ethics. If harm may arise from not taking something that is needed, though perhaps not freely offered, need may outweigh this aspiration. Not everyone has equal access to abundance – thus, nonstealing may not be judged from the outside but needs to be understood from within the biopsychosociocultural context in which it occurs.

Applied collectively, *asteya* means creating equal access to resources of all types. It also means making reparations and restitution for past misappropriation, theft, and imperialist occupations of lands and resources. Collectives steal in so many ways – we steal dignity, respect, honor, resources, equity, and so much more. It means becoming aware of how socioeconomic and sociopolitical systems steal from one group and favor another; how we appropriate what belongs to all to give access only to the few. We can steal in this form in subtle and explicit ways. If we block access to a natural spot by making it too expensive for many to afford, have we not stolen? If we place good and well-resourced schools only in certain neighborhoods, have we not taken away opportunity? We need to commit to creating abundance for all to truly live this limb.

> **Yoga Sutra 2.37**
> **Asteya pratisthayam sarva ratna upasthanam**
> **When we are grounded in non-stealing,**
> **treasures come our way.**
> **→ Asteya brings abundance**

Harmony or Brahmacharya

Following the principle of wise use of personal life energy, this aspirational ethical guideline invites us to be neither indulgent nor excessively restrictive when it comes to habits and desires. It is behaviorally expressed as preserving vitality or energy for what is important in life so that we can honor the true needs of ourselves – in all koshas – and the true needs of others. It is behaviorally expressed as not overdoing, overcommitting, overworking, oversleeping, overplaying, overtexting, overeating – you get the idea. This aspiration interfaces with the other aspirations. Overindulgence may also create harm; it may also be a sign of not living our truth – trying to hide some aspect of our existence behind a veil of excess. Balancing or harmonizing our desires is an aspiration that is firmly grounded in the context in which it arises. What may be considered moderate or balanced in one circumstance may be excessive in another situation or ascetic in yet another context. Staying attuned to truthfulness and nonharming may help with discerning what defines balance or harmony.

Applied collectively, *brahmacharya* relates to preservation of collective resources, to the protection of the earth for all future generations. It means stopping the exploitation of the planet and institutionalizing moderate use of precious earth resources and abandoning the plundering of the planet (which will also end the stealing of resource from future generations and other beings).

> **Yoga Sutra 2.38**
> **Brahmacharya pratisthayam virya labhah**
> **When we are grounded in harmony and energetic balance,**
> **we attain vitality, strength, courage, and vigor.**
> → **Brahmacharya balances vital energy**

Non-Possessiveness or Aparigraha

Following the principle of not being greedy about possessions, relationships, actions, and other aspects of life, this aspirational ethical guideline invites us to mindfully cultivate gratitude for what life has already provided and to thoughtfully relinquish or releasing grasping, desire, and jealousy. It is behaviorally expressed as generosity toward ourselves – in all koshas – and toward others. It is behaviorally expressed by resisting the cultivation of jealousy in relationships, by resisting the urge to hoard possessions, by resisting the need to do, have, want, need, or become more and more and more. Non-possessiveness is situated in the biopsychosociocultural context of the individual and may be hard to judge from the outside looking in. Balancing it with harmonizing our desires, truthfulness, non-stealing, and non-harming may bring some clarity to this aspiration and how to define it functionally.

Applied collectively, *aparigraha* means setting up socioeconomic and sociopolitical systems that ensure the sharing resources and power and that do not hoard or centralize access to wealth, wellbeing, health, education, employment, and other human rights among certain classes or castes of humans. It even means sharing with all beings on the planet and perhaps even more importantly preserving the planet for future generations.

> **Yoga Sutra 2.39**
> **Aparigraha sthairye janma kathanta sambodhah**
> **When we are stable in non-possessiveness and steady in non-grasping, we rest in the knowledge of a greater reality.**
> → **Aparigraha nurtures generosity**

As we set intentions, think thoughts, develop opinions, take actions, and respond in relationships based on our truth, we commit to non-harming and peacefulness. We come from a place of reciprocity, creating access to abundance and not taking away from. We commit to moderation and use energy – ours and others' – wisely. We offer our actions with gratitude for the opportunity and without grasping for a particular outcome. We come from generosity.

A lovely set of questions derived from Buddhism can help guide us in this overall process. With everything we are about to say or do, we can ask ourselves:
- *Is it true?* Does this reflect fact and authenticity?
- *Is it kind-hearted, peaceful?* Does this honor peacefulness and is it free of hostility?
- *Is it necessary?* Does this have purpose and value?
- *Is my intention pure?* Am I doing this for the right reason of creating more wholesomeness?

Limb 2: Niyamas or Life Choices for Purposeful Living

The second limb of yoga, *niyama*, involves a discipline-focused practice of yoga that encourages us to engage in insightful and clear goal-setting and purposeful action. Discipline, as embraced in the five commitments of Limb 2 described below, helps us create a cohesive change-embracing motivational set that inspires our life plans and trajectories. These principles influence the direction of our personal development in all koshas, including the capacity to access joy and bliss. They move us, ultimately, toward making lasting contributions to the world – hopefully in a manner that adds to the greater good. These principles in their fullest essence inspire us to engage in practices or lifestyles of mindful self-discipline, conscientiousness, curiosity, and intentionality that create a meaningful and purposeful life.

The mindful self-discipline and intentionality of this limb is embedded in the greater biopsychosociocultural context of our life, contributing to it as well as being influenced by it. When we create a meaningful and purposeful life, we do so not solely or simply for ourselves. Instead, we do so to create meaning and purpose for our entire community. Not surprisingly, the very essence of this limb of yoga is engaged action (which consists of the final three of the five central commitments). These commitments lead us to a conscious and discerning practice of self-care from a place of self-love and altruism to transcend self-hate and aversion. As we engage in these practices, we tend to our needs and vulnerabilities; we do not beat ourselves up for failure. Persistence in practice is key and supports healing and meaning for each of us individually, as well as for all of us collectively. Our biopsychosociocultural context helps define the content of our commitments and, in turn, is influenced by what we return to this interpersonal matrix.

An important note about the discipline cultivated by Limb 2 is that it is a balanced discipline. These principles of discipline are deeply grounded in the ideal of finding the middle way in all we do, especially if we are "householders" – humans who live in the real world, not in a cave or on a mountain top. The middle way balances effort with ease, softness with strength, firmness with freedom, commitment with contentment, intent with openness, the personal with the collective; the list could go on. For each principle, there are two extreme poles of its expression that we seek to avoid; instead, we seek to find an expression of the principle that is balanced, realistic, self-compassionate, altruistic, adapted to our biopsychosociocultural context, and appropriate for the real world and the real relationships in which we are embedded.

The Five Commitments of Limb 2

Purity or Saucha

This commitment embraces simplicity, cleanliness, positive energy, balance, order, and authenticity in intention, thought, speech, action, relationships, and environment. As a disciplined practice, it invites us to create balance, order, and pure energy in all aspects of life and in all koshas. We attend to creating pure and clean energy in our patterns of consumption, in how we structure our environments (e.g., how we attend to clutter and lack of order, toxins and dirt, distractions and overload), our relationship with our koshas (e.g., sensory inputs, food, drink, body care, thoughts, media use, work, and play). It encourages us neither to seek excessive fastidiousness (e.g., preoccupation with germs, compulsive cleaning) nor does it condone sloppiness; it suggests that we neither withdraw completely from sensory inputs, nor does it condone overloading ourselves with them.

Through *saucha*, we cultivate purity, cleanliness, and energy that is easeful, yet boundaried and committed. When we create balanced simplicity and purity in actions that feed our and others' koshas, we can access the peace and ease that comes from santosha, the second niyama.

> **Yoga Sutra 2.40**
> **Sauchat sva-anga jugupsa paraih asamsargah**
> **Purity of mind (including emotion) and body brings us closer to the deeper truth within.**
> **→ Saucha invites the natural flow of goodness**

Contentment or Santosha

This principle embraces meeting every moment from a peaceful, balanced center of gravity that allows for discernment about how to take calm and appropriate action in any context and under any circumstances. As a disciplined practice, it invites us to recognize the fullness of our life and to respond calmly to the world from this sense of having enough, rather than be reactive to circumstances. The fullness of contentment lets us take mindful note of and feel gratitude for what we have been given, for what we have received – not in a material sense only, but in a multitude of ways. We recognize the gifts we have been given and the gifts we have developed. This fullness does not imply that we give up goals or striving; quite the opposite. Contentment allows us to set clearer goals, plot paths, and revise and try again. Fullness merely means that we do not get attached to *particular* outcomes of our actions. We have a deep satisfaction simply to be on the path – to be with life as it unfolds.

Santosha encourages us to be present and calmly engaged with life presents – neither hyper-excitable, nor indifferent. This is an important understanding. Contentment (or equanimity) is a stable *being-with*, stable and clear attention to what is unfolding; it neither means not caring nor approving of horrible things in our own or others' life. Sometimes translated as acceptance, contentment means recognizing the circumstances and not becoming reactive to them. It means taking a step back; taking a moment to become calm and centered and then move forward with intention and discernment from this place of clarity. Contentment, thus defined, lets us take principled action – calmly and collectedly – when this is indicated. We are not complacent. Instead, we pause to watch and observe attentively when we are not sure how to respond quite yet. It helps us patiently weigh the options and move forward with discernment and conviction when we are ready and that we cannot be thrown off balance.

> **Yoga Sutra 2.42**
> **Santosha anuttamah sukha labhah**
> **An attitude of contentment brings us close to unmatched happiness, mental comfort, joy, and satisfaction.**
> **→ Santosha leads to true happiness**

Discipline or Tapas

This principle embraces leading an impassioned life of determined effort, accountability, and engaged practice. As a disciplined, yet nurturing, practice, it leads to the transformation of the self in all its layers, as well as of others and our environment. It does so by inviting a commitment to disciplined and conscious – not habitual or disengaged – choices in every moment. This principle encourages us neither to seek asceticism that is removed from the real world (i.e., we do not have to live in a cave or on a mountain top) nor does it condone sloth or laziness. It does not mean that we never rest. Tapas has to happen in the context of brahmacharya – of the compassionate and moderate use of energy and of replenishing our resources as needed.

Tapas means that we persevere in our practice, we apply ourselves with passion, we stick to what we do and finish what we start, and we make our best and ongoing effort to engage with ourselves and the world. We engage in this discipline with truth, nonharming, balance, non-stealing, and non-possessiveness. That is, we strive to be disciplined in a manner that reliably and consistently reflects our commitment to living our life ethically and with consideration for a greater purpose. We aspire to be disciplined in a manner that supports our wellbeing, our evolution and growth, and our compassion for ourselves and others. We are disciplined in a manner that reflects our recognition that our actions reverberate into our biopsychosociocultural context, affect others, and have the potential to change our world.

> **Yoga Sutra 2.43**
> **Kaya indriya siddhih ashuddhi kshayat tapasah**
> **Training the senses with discipline or conscientiousness burns away impurities in and enhances the functions of mind and body.**
> **→ Tapas transforms inauspicious habits and patterns**

Related News from the Research World

A sample of 2,359 participants in good health at baseline assessment were followed for five decades to look at personality predictors of longevity. Findings support the healthfulness of a yoga practice. Specifically, researchers found that individuals who were assessed to be conscientious, emotionally stable, and active lived significantly longer than their age peers.

Terracciano, A., Löckenhoff, C. E., Zonderman, A. B., Ferrucci, L., & Costa, J., Paul T. (2008). Personality predictors of longevity: Activity, emotional stability, and conscientiousness. *Psychosomatic Medicine, 70*(6), 621–627. 10.1097/psy.0b013e31817b9371

"Experiencing too much comfort will reduce your capacity for experiencing pleasure" William Irving (2019), *p. 149)* -- on toughness training as prescribed by the ancient Stoics

Self-Reflection or Svadhyaya

This principle embraces exploring personal reactions, habits, motivations, and intentions to guide us toward self-knowledge, insight, and growth. As a disciplined practice of self-inquiry, it invites us to open up to new learning from outer sources (such as books and teachers) and inner wisdom through quiet introspection. This principle does not endorse self-absorbed, narcissistic self-exploration at the expense of pondering other matters. However, it also does not condone never looking at our own motivations, intentions, needs, and inner life. When practiced in a balanced manner, this principle guides us to deeper self-understanding in the context of greater wisdom and guidance from the outside. When we arrive at this greater inner wisdom, we become clearer about our intentions and impacts on others and on the world as a whole. We begin to see our place in the world with the greater clarity of taking responsibility for a greater good, for improving the relationships and the interpersonal contexts in which we operate. We recognize the intentions for, and consequences of, our thoughts, speech, actions, and relationships.

Central to *svadhyaya* is the notion that accepts multiple sources of learning – introspection and self-reflection are one such source, but it has to rest on outer teachings. We learn from teachers and from the transmission of knowledge via reading. We consult ancient texts and modern research. We cultivate a curious mind and constantly learn, unlearn, and relearn. Our mind is open to new ways of looking at the world. We do not simply believe what we are taught either. We need to reflect on teachings and experiment in our own life to verify the truth or validity of what we have been taught. In other words, svadhyaya suggests that learning is a cycle and each step in the cycle is a way to double-check the veracity of the conclusions we and others draw. It is a process of not believing everything we hear, read, or think.

> **Yoga Sutra 2.44**
> **svadhyayat ishta devata samprayogah**
> **Self-study and self-reflection bring us into contact and alignment with a deeper reality, with spirit.**
> **→ Svadhyaya nurtures genuine spirituality**

Devotion to a Greater Good or Ishvara Pranidhana

This principle embraces creating meaning and purpose for self and others through wise discernment. As a disciplined practice, it invites us to surrender ego-driven intentions and committing to positive altruistically-oriented intentions and actions. Devotion in this sense is neither to be confused with infatuation, unquestioning loyalty, or blind obedience – nor with disconnection or lack of caring for a greater good, a larger purpose, a bigger meaning. This principle invites informed, discerning devotion that will improve all of our koshas as well as the world in which we live. We do not blindly follow a guru or preacher or other idol or icon; we explore their teachings and intentions and then make discerning choices about where to place our own devotion. This devotion is not blind – it is the epitome of clarity and commitment to a higher cause. It reflects all the other principles in this category, integrating them to create commitment that is wise, content, pure, disciplined, informed, and balanced.

> **Yoga Sutra 2.45**
> **samadhi siddhih ishvarapranidhana**
> Through contacting our collective consciousness and devotion, we move into a state of deep connection and absorption.
> → **Ishavara Pranidhana nurtures purpose and union**

Limb 3: Asana or Healing through Form and Movement

The third limb of yoga, *asana*, is comprised of physical practices of yoga that support our physical development and refinement, our nervous system responses and reactivity, and our affective presence. They also reverberate into mind and emotions, supporting awareness and wisdom based in enhanced understanding of the body and its expressions of our life experiences. The practice of asana aligns closely with the first two koshas: annamaya kosha (our physical body) and pranamaya koshas (our breath and affective or vital presence). It continues to express the commitment to the first two limbs and therefore integrates ethics and lifestyle commitments into the physical practice. Asana in this sense always reflects a deeper commitment to an integrated practice that never abandons any of the limbs.

In other words, physical practice, or *asana*, as practiced in integrated holistic yoga is always embedded in the greater context of all eight limbs and the biopsychosociocultural circumstances of students and teachers or clients and clinicians. It is important for teachers to understand that they are not simply teaching students how to attain an outer form, but instead, that they are teaching students how to become wise practitioners who can make informed, empowered, and self-efficacious, knowledgeable personal choices about the practice of yoga. It invites awareness in all layers of self (or consciousness) and great attention to how we sense ourselves from the inside out and how we sense the world from the outside in. A wholesome yoga session includes not just instruction about how to move into and out of a pose, but empowers students to listen to feedback from their body, breath, and mind and to respect this information with truthfulness and non-violence. Successful teaching is more focused on inner experience than on attaining an outer shape or form. It is focused more on inviting action and experimenting with movement than on embodying a pre-defined shape. This teaching focus invites agency and empowers students to discover their inner teacher. It invites use of variations, props, and self-determination. It always is focused on the inner experience rather than the outer expression of form and movement.

The most common asana practices are form and movement (see box on the next page). The important thing that differentiates embodied movement as a yogic practice is the application and conscious experience of the principles outlined above. We can be in a posture simply as exercise; or we can be in a posture experiencing our energetic flow, sensing our emotional reactions, and understanding our body from the inside. We can be in a posture simply to get strong muscles; or we can recognize whether we feel safe, balanced, and peaceful, or whether we are connected to a deeper experience of the shape that reaches beyond its physical manifestation.

The physical practice of yoga, called *asana* in Sanskrit, is what most people in the Western world identify as yoga. In the holistic or integrated study of yoga, posture and movement practices represent but one of eight limbs. Nevertheless, the third limb of yoga is essential due to its power to reconnect us to our bodies and to prepare our bodies for the inner practices of yoga (such as meditation, concentration, and sense withdrawal). Through mindfulness-based embodied movement, we hone insight into the physical and emotional layers of self. We create physical, emotional, and mental health and fitness, including balance, strength, stamina, flexibility, coordination, and power. Even more importantly, we come to understand physical habits, challenges, and strength; we get (back) in touch with our bodies. We learn about emotional reactions, needs, and preferences; we (re)attune to our inner world at a level that is often unconscious and thus unconsidered in day-to-day life.

Typical Asana Practices

Form – posture practices include, but are not limited to:
- Arm standing shapes (e.g., plank, downward facing dog, table top)
- Backbends (e.g., cobra, camel, bridge, wheel)
- Balances (e.g., tree, eagle, crow)
- Forward folds (e.g., downward dog, head-to-knee, chair)
- Inversions (e.g., headstand, handstand, elbow balance)
- Restorative shapes (e.g., relaxation pose, meadow brook, legs-up-the-wall)
- Seated shapes (e.g., staff, hero, lotus, easy seat)
- Standing shapes (e.g., mountain, warrior, triangle, side angle)
- Twists (e.g., lord of the fishes, supine legs around the belly)

Movement – movement practices include, but are not limited to:
- Sun and moon salutations
- Yoga kriyas
- Vinyasa

Modern science has echoed the importance of embodied movement. All of our experiences and perceptions enter through the body, including through the sense doors – our hearing, vision, taste, touch, smell, and mind. How we experience ourselves begins and ends with our physical experience of the world – be it our experience of pain, heat, fear, love, embarrassment, joy, or pleasure. Our brain is not the only part of us that responds, thinks, interprets, and understands. We produce neurotransmitters in our gut; we have neurons in our hearts. Trauma embeds itself in our tissues where it can live – ignored – for years, affecting reactions and comfort levels in our bodies, energy, emotions, and relationships. Injuries or illnesses may heal, yet their reverberations stay encoded in the body forever unless they are directly and compassionately addressed. Mindful, consciously embodied movements and actions – as well as mindful breathing, for that matter – bring us back into the body. They reconnect us, reground us, and recomplete us.

For physical practices to reach their most powerful impact, a few yogic principles apply that awaken our capacity to feel our bodies and to understand our physical sensations and emotional perceptions or reactions. Physical practice relinks us to neuroception, proprioception, interoception, and exteroception. Neuroception is our (often unconscious) interpretation of the world in which we move as safe, dangerous, or threatening. Proprioception is our ability to understand where our bodies are in space. Interoception is the capacity to feel our bodies from the inside out – being aware of the importance of inner sensation rather than focusing on outer forms. Exteroception is our sensory experience of the outside world, the environment in which we operate. Limb 3 of yoga is a powerful practice that awakens and brings to consciousness all of these ways of perceiving and experiencing ourselves.

Central Principles of Asana

- *Balance of effort and ease* – This most central traditional principle of yoga posture practice asserts the need to combine effort and ease in all physical practices. This combination of easeful steadiness allows for restful awareness combined with optimal exertion of effort, such as finding strength within flexibility and flexibility within strength; maintaining strength without gripping; finding softness without lapsing onto lethargy; finding balance in the middle between extremes, being firm and strong in the core and free and soft at the edges; or finding union in opposing forces.
- *Synergy* – This principle embraces integrated form and movement practices that link to all other limbs of yoga, clarifying that physical practices are not an end in and of themselves. This means that *asana* practices are not just about achieving physical shapes and fitness. Limb 3 is a component within a greater yogic lifestyle commitment to all eight limbs of yoga. It is always connected to all other limbs, be they ethical and disciplined lifestyle choices, or concentrated and meditative inner work.
- *Completeness* – This principle suggests that every form or movement needs grounding, expansion, and stability in all layers of self. Feeling grounded comes from establishing a firm foundation physically, energetically, and mentally. Feeling stable comes from establishing and attending to the core, or center, of each pose physically, energetically, and mentally. Feeling expansive comes from a clear line of energy that supports movement and invites radiance physically, energetically, and mentally.
- *Integration and attuned (or mindful) applications of form and movement* – This principle invites mindful attention to healthful alignment, awareness of the body in space (proprioception), awareness of how the physical body collaborates with breath and mind (interoception and neuroception), and awareness of the body's response to environmental stimuli (exteroception). It creates coordination of breath with movement into, out of, and within each posture. It creates a beautiful energetic flow through well-sequenced movement through multiple postures with careful attention to the energetic state of the body.

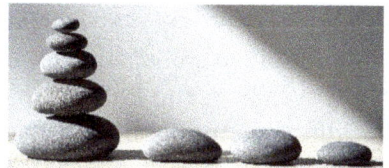

> **Yoga Sutras about Asana 2.46 to 2.48**
> (accessed 7.19.2022 at https://www.swamij.com/yoga-sutras-24648.htm)
>
> **2.46: sthira sukham asanam**
> The two essential characteristics of the sitting posture for meditation are that it must be: steady, stable, and motionless as well as comfortable and filled with ease.
>
> **2.47: prayatna shaithilya ananta samapattibhyam**
> Steady and comfortable posture comes through two means: the loosening of tension or effort to sit in the posture and allowing attention to become spacious (merging with the infinite).
>
> **2.48: tatah dvandva anabhighata**
> From the attainment of a perfected posture, there arises an unassailable, unimpeded freedom from suffering due to the pairs of opposites such as heat and cold, good and bad, or pain and pleasure.

Limb 4: Pranayama or Healing through Freeing the Breath

Pranayama is often presented as breath control. However, in integrated holistic yoga, the emphasis is more on freeing and balancing the breath. This is not contradictory with the Yoga Sutras. In fact, a tracing of the linguistic roots of *pranayama* suggests that both freeing and controlling the breath are valid interpretations of the practice of *pranayama*. Specifically, the word *pranayama* can be traced to the following roots:
- *prana*=breath or life force depending on context
- *yama*=control or restraint
- *a* in front of a Sanskrit word=the opposite of the word

This view of the linguistic roots of the word leads to a definition of *pran(a)yama* as the *freeing* of the breath (Brems, 2024b), a variation on other translations, which interpret the word to mean breath control (interpreting the *a* in the middle as being the ending of the prana as opposed to contributing its own meaning). We cannot know for certain if the ancients preferred one meaning over the other or if perhaps both meanings are implied; however, in the lineage of integrated holistic yoga, both meanings are embraced and sequenced by starting with freeing the breath in beginning practices and adding control of the breath in advanced practices.

Breathwork, almost by definition, is a practice of stress management, self-regulation, and resilience training. If we can affect the rate, rhythm, and cadence of the breath, we can affect emotions, mind, sleep, and stress perception. We can shift out of and into the various states of the autonomic nervous system by how we choose to breath. This reality makes pranayama a superb practice to support mental health and emotional resilience.

The biofeedback practice of yogic breathing, called *Pranayama* in Sanskrit, addresses a more subtle physical energy than movement as practiced in Limb 3. Breathing practices, whether breath observation, breathing awareness, or advanced breath control, invites us to become mindful and conscious of links between the breath and our emotional and physical wellbeing or experience. Yogic breathing practices help us become aware of physiological arousal and emotional reactivity; they invite us to gain an understanding of our autonomic nervous system responses. They connect us to inner sensations, recruit the parasympathetic nervous system, reduce allostatic load, and improve vagal tone. Yogic breathing practices are beautiful and inspiring ways to cultivate deeper awareness of breath that supports mindfulness, balance, and efficiency in body, breath, mind, and relationships.

Breathing practices invite awareness of how and where we breathe into the body. They help us understand that how we breathe affects and reflects our emotional and physical wellness. Breath is often an obvious indicator whether the breathing individual is at ease, in pain, tense, sad, anxious, worried, panicked, angry, and so on. Breath manifests in different ways depending on what is happening in the body. Pain may cause a shallow breath that, in turn, may worsen the pain. Anxiety may move the breath high into the chest – away from abdominal breathing – which, in turn, is likely to increase anxiety into panic. Ease moves the chest into the belly inviting a spiral of increasing calm and wellness.

Modern science has revealed that breath and physical or emotional experience are reciprocal. Just as our physical or emotional state can be read in the breath, our breath can be altered to change our sense of wellbeing. If we learn how to breathe deeply into the belly when we are anxious, we can nudge ourselves toward a greater sense of ease. If we can learn to take a long and deep inhalation and exhalation when we feel challenged, we can transform angry reactivity into thoughtful responsiveness.

Central Principles of Pranayama

The fourth limb of yoga, *pranayama*, explores the nature of breath as it manifests physiologically, anatomically, and energetically. The breath is explored from a multitude of dimensions, including the considerations related to optimal functional breathing, breath observation (including attending to timing, volume, texture, location, and resting pauses), and breath regulation (as grounded in the gunas and polyvagal theory). Through tailored pranayama that is attuned to our gunas or polyvagal states, we enhance our ability to invite either balancing, calming, or vitalizing breathing as is most auspicious in any given moment.

Central practices within Limb 4 start with *breath observation and breath awareness* (including mindful natural breathing). These are safe and readily accessible practices that, once taught, can be practiced alone in any situation or circumstance. Once observation and awareness skills are established, breathing practices can expand to include *breath regulation*. Breath regulation can proceed informed by the gunas or primary polyvagal states of students or clients and can thus be individually tailored to be optimally therapeutic.

Breath Observation and Awareness

Breath awareness and observation are inquiries into the nature of breath as it moves through us during any given moment. Awareness and observation can be free-flowing or they can be focused on a particular characteristic or several aspects of breath and breathing. A few dimensions of breath that can become the anchor for attention in breath awareness and observation are listed here.

- *Breath timing* – To create breath awareness, attention is given to the number of breaths per minute and the balance between inhalation and exhalation. Breath control includes lengthening (slowing down) or shortening (speeding up) the inhalation, exhalation, or both, which in turn may affect physical or emotional states.
- *Breath volume* – In observing the breath, awareness is expanded about how much air is moved in and out of the body with each breath. Breath control may purposefully change volume to influence physical or emotional states.
- *Breath sound* – Breath awareness is cultivated to recognize the sound or noisiness of breath, noticing if it is audible or quiet. Breath control may be used to consciously bring quietude to a noisy breath, reducing especially deliberate sounding of the breath and exploring possible pathologies or emotional aspects of breath that is not quiet.
- *Breath texture* – Breath awareness is cultivated to recognize the texture or smoothness of breath, noticing if it is choppy, interrupted, soft, smooth, or gentle. Breath control may be used to consciously smooth a choppy breath, reduce hitches and glitches in the breath, and move toward a smooth flow of air.
- *Breath space or location* – Attention is given to where breath is sensed and directed in the body, with awareness whether breath is balanced between the right and left side of the body, between front and back, and across the lower, middle, and upper thirds of the torso. Breath control may direct breath into certain body parts, sometimes via changing physical position.
- *Breath resting pauses* – Attention is given to exploring the top (between inhalation and exhalation) and bottom (between exhalation and inhalation) of the breath, creating increasing gaps or rest breaks. Rest breaks at top and bottom may be calibrated to calm the nervous system and mind.

Optimally Functional Breathing

It is a common misconception that pranayama is about cultivating a deep breath; that is, a breath that is large and full. Nothing could be further from the truth. Ancient wisdom and modern science agree that a subtle and light breath that is rhythmic and inaudible, as well as barely perceptible, is more natural and auspicious. The following characteristics mark an optimally auspicious breath and are cultivated in pranayama.

- *Nasal*: silent breathing in and out through the nose at all times (including at night and during exertion; mouth breathing in emergencies only)
- *Biasing the Diaphragm*: breathing is diaphragmatic in the sense that the primary movements notable are abdominal and low rib basket movement; upper chest, shoulder, and neck muscles stay relaxed and passive (unless purposefully or intentionally engaged)
- *Slow*: 5.5 to 10 breaths per minutes

- *Light and subtle*: inhalation is neither shallow nor forced but tailored to move just the right amount of air given respiratory rate, leading to a normal volume of 5-6 liters of breath per minute; exhalation is easeful and quiet
- *Rhythmic*: breath oscillates with a soft texture and rhythm that is neither rigid nor too relaxed; there is a balance of ease and effort; resting pauses at the top and bottom of breath may be notable but their length is adapted to the individual – there is no gasping or grasping

Optimal functional breathing optimizes all physiological systems in the body, including the respiratory, cardiovascular, immune, endocrine, and digestive systems. It invites autonomic balance with a bias toward a ventral vagal parasympathetic state and preparedness for activation of the sympathetic nervous system as needed. It maintains optimal O2 and CO2 levels in the blood and as such maintains the body's pH balance and optimal tissue oxygenation, energy production, and cellular function, including in all organs, tissues, and the brain. It supports a calm state of mind, resilient emotionality, and well-functioning cognition with good concentration and memory. It supports movement of lymph, healthy dilation of smooth muscle, maintenance of posture and spinal stability, and much more.

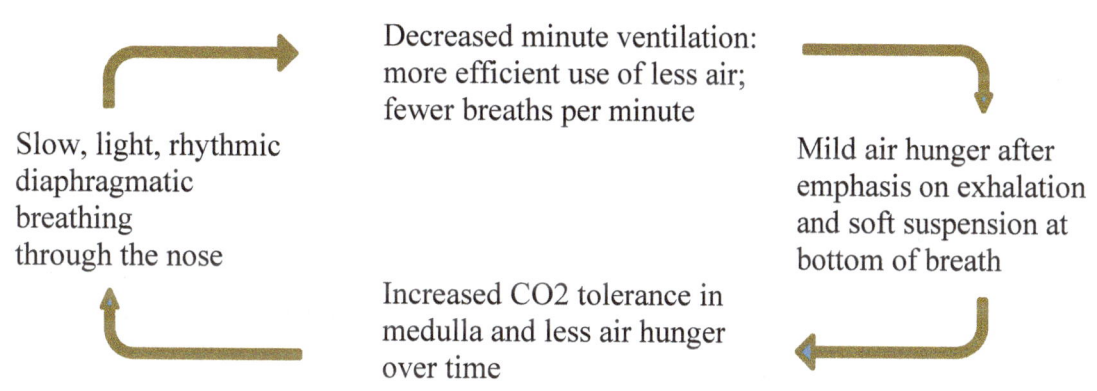

Breathing as Informed by Polyvagal Theory and the Gunas

Breath is most auspicious if tailored to the individual. One system for individualization or person-centered breathing can be framed based on the yogic gunas or modern polyvagal theory.
- *Balancing breathing* is functional breathing that supports the stabilization of the autonomic nervous system, anatomy (biomechanically), physiology (biochemically), breath (energetically), and mind (mentally and emotionally). As a bottom-up process of enhanced and accurate self-awareness and top-down emotional self-regulation, it focuses on balanced and stable inhalations and exhalations, gentle breath retention, balanced speed and vigor of breath, awareness of breath location (including interoceptive awareness of nasal versus mouth and diaphragmatic versus chest breathing), attention to breath texture, and clarity about the four parts of the breath – inhalation, pause at the top, exhalation, and pause at the bottom. It invites a parasympathetic shift in the nervous system to a ventral vagal (or sattvic) way of being present.

- *Calming breathing*, as a bottom-up process of awareness and top-down process of nervous system down-regulation to access emotional and physical balance, focuses on the exhalation, decreased speed or vigor of breath, and combining breath and resting. It recalibrates a sympathetically aroused nervous system, down-regulates mood, energy, and physical activation, provides opportunity for exploring the kleshas and vrittis, and invites gentle curiosity, calming, and relaxation. It counteracts an overly rapid breath that tends to be fast, panting, high in the chest, and through the mouth. It can also be used targetedly for a specific purpose, such as helping with inducing sleep.
- *Vitalizing breathing*, as a bottom-up process of awareness and top-down process up-regulation of the nervous system to access emotional and physical balance, focuses on the inhalation, increased speed or vigor of breath, and the combination of breath and movement. It recalibrates an immobilized or collapsed nervous system, up-regulates mood, energy, and physical vitality, provides opportunity for exploring kleshas and vrittis, and invites engagement, action, and initiative. It counteracts a tamasic breath that tends to be slowed, ineffective, high in the chest, and through the mouth.

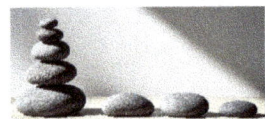

Overview of Limbs 5 to 7: Interior Practices or Healing by Drawing Inward

Patanjali's Yoga Sutras' definition of yoga is multifold. However, a central point about yoga's essence is made in the second sutra which roughly translates as *"Yoga is the stilling of the fluctuations of the mind."* Patanjali suggests that if we can still the mind, we have found refuge in our true being and our practice is complete. He then basically chuckles (if you can chuckle in writing) and lets us know that if we cannot just sit down and still the mind (and who can?), we need to follow a slightly longer path to enlightenment. Enter the eight limbs. The first four limbs are the outward practices of yoga; the final four limbs are the inward journey of yoga. The inner practices are what we have been preparing for and what we embark on – knowingly or unknowingly – as we practice yoga ethics, discipline, movement, and breath. The inner journey begins with drawing inward, then invites deep concentration and meditation, and finally leads us to a sense of connection and absorption in a greater community and purpose.

Limb 5: Pratyahara or Guarding the Senses

The first inwardly-focused practice of yoga, *pratyahara*, sharpens self-awareness of sensory inputs and consequent automatic or habitual thoughts, speech, actions, and relational patterns. It prepares the mind for concentration and meditation by halting or consciously attuning us to the constant flow of sensory stimulation that leads to stimulus overload, poor concentration, and scattered attention. It is a practice of disconnecting from the simultaneous steady flow of sensory input through eyes, ears, nose, taste buds, and other sense receptors (e.g., touch, pain, temperature, texture). It is also a practice of honing mindfulness of (or attunement to) what is happening in each of our senses, including the inner senses of interoception, proprioception, and neuroception, as well as the sensory stimuli that arise from our mental fluctuations and stories.

Pratyahara is an absolutely crucial step in the yoga journey toward stilling the fluctuations of the mind. The only way to begin to still the impact of our constantly emerging thoughts is to become aware that we have them. To do this, we have to cut through the noise of day-to-day life. How can we attend to what is on our mind, if we are distracted by the TV blaring all day? How can we attend to what is on our mind, if we keep fiddling with our phones or computers, allowing noise and distraction to enter into our life almost non-stop? How can we attend to what is on our mind, if we are walking through crowded streets, overwhelmed by sounds, sights, smells, and other sensory enticements?

The fifth limb of yoga encourages us to take a break from constant outer and inner distraction. It invites us to protect our senses – either by being fully attuned to sensory experience, without being distracted into sensory overload, or by uncoupling from certain sensory experiences, detaching ourselves from reactivity to sensory inputs. Our outer practices have prepared us for this step – we have cultivated neuroception (understanding how we achieve a sense of safety and community), proprioception (understanding our body in the physical plane of being), interoception (gaining insight into how we feel physically, energetically, and emotionally from the inside out), and exteroception (having become aware of the constant stream of outer sensory stimulation). We can now bring these practices to bear the capacity to experience sensory inputs and to attenuate our reaction to them.

Central Principles of Pratyahara

Central principles within Limb 5 of yoga explore the nature of tuning in with intention. It is a crucial step toward deeper levels of calming the nervous system, reducing emotional reactivity, and resting in a ventral vagal space of safety and peace.

- *Working with sensory inputs, stimuli, and impressions* – This process starts with becoming more familiar with the way sensory information arrives in <u>or</u> is processed outside of our consciousness. It addresses practice of attuning to and uncoupling from sensory experiences – often in combination. All humans have patterns in their sensory processing and preferences. Some sensory information is more accessible; some is partially, selectively, or even completely overlooked. Physical challenges (e.g., hearing or vision loss) and psychological processes can influence which senses are attuned to and which are attenuated, inaccessible, or ignored. Contextual factors can play a role as well, in that specific external circumstances may condition us to ignore particular inputs to support perceived needs for particular levels of performance (e.g., nurses' bladder – being so busy as to neglect to go to the bathroom, which may result in a bladder infection; turning to the need for food when stressed at work). In other words, how we manage impressions may be context-dependent and situation-specific.
- *Working with abhyasa and vairagyam* – *Pratyahara* relies on the capacity to practice with the commitment and persistent effort of abhyasa as well as the non-attachment of vairagyam. It depends on our ability to note stimuli without becoming attached, averse, or afraid of them; in other words, without activating the kleshas. This is attunement to sensory information without attachment, without reactivity, with balance and ease. We simply note stimuli for what they are, without attributions, interpretations, biases, or reactivities. As the mind begins to quiet; life force is freed up to feed and replenish the koshas.

- *Working with the kleshas* – When practitioners' attention is focused inward, the mind becomes known, affect and arousal patterns come to the forefront, and bodily sensation (including polyvagal states) are accessed. Sometimes this inward attention leads to stillness; sometimes it leads to greater awareness of inner unrest (or noise). This inner noise is often initiated by the kleshas that arise (as reactivity) in response to the sensory stimulation that enter the sense doors. As impressions arrive in our awareness, our brain begins to make predictions about how they will affect us in all our koshas. This can trigger the kleshas, our affective predilections, as well as being mediated by our gunas and polyvagal states. In turn, the gunas and kleshas flavor our subsequent mind stories (i.e., vrittis) and emotions. The impact of the kleshas is directly explored in pratyahara.
- *Enhancing awareness of habitual reactivity and its effects* – As we recognize our habits in response to sensory inputs, we also begin to appreciate the effects of these habits. We see how they affect our way of being in the world and in relationship with ourselves and others. We see the impacts on our capacity to cope, to access wellbeing, to maintain physical, emotional, and mental health. As we see the consequences of reactivity, we begin to hone our ability to transform habits and impulses into discernment and wise choice. *Pratyahara* is essential to yoga as a practice of growth and transformation, moving us beyond simply noticing into feeling empowered and inspired to create change within ourselves, our families, our communities, and our larger society. We protect our senses and transform our reactivity in service to the betterment of all.

Treat yourself gently, kindly, and honestly

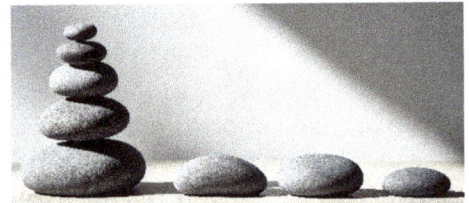

Limb 6: Dharana or Finding Single-Pointed Focus

Once we have cultivated the capacity to note and transform the influence of outer and inner distractions, we can begin to steady the mind through concentration, the sixth limb of yoga, *dharana*. This self-regulation practice of yoga integrates top-down and bottom-up processing to allow the mind to become honed and clear, like a still mountain lake.

Concentration is a practice of surrendering thought in exchange for deep inner, yet soft, attention on a single point of focus to achieve gentle mental one-pointedness. Concentration helps us transcend mental states that are disturbing, upsetting, distracting, discouraging, lethargic, heavy, agitated, or restless. Through practiced awareness of our inner states, we receive input from within – sitting with sensations from our body or emotions (i.e., bottom-up input) without the need to react. Through being able to sit with inner signals without reacting, we cultivate the capacity to formulate deliberate responses and discerning choices, instead of reactions. We hone the capacity to delay our response to a stimulus, inviting wisdom, intuition, and the ability to use reasoning (i.e., top-down processing).

Central Principles of Dharana

Central principles of the sixth limb help us move into clarity, focus, even luminosity. They invite us into a space of lucidity and concentration. They encourage attention, discernment, one-pointedness, and single-tasking.

- *Creating single-pointed focus and sustained attention* – The most central aspect of dharana is the creation of a single point of focus, the refinement of the mind to move it away from distraction, interruption, fragmentation, and dysregulation. This focus can be on an internal or external object or subject; this object or subject can be simple or complex, tangible or conceptual. It is an object or subject that holds interest to the practitioner to increase the chances that the focus can remain unwavering, steady, unfragmented, and stable. The mindfulness the practice engenders engages our attention – in its various forms – to draw us away from the default mode network.

- *Inviting concentrated and luminous mind states* – Through concentration, we begin to realize that we neither have to fight nor flee, nor obey our disorganized, distracted, confused, or lethargic mind states. Instead, we can choose simply to become aware of them, to notice what the mind is doing. In other words, we can remain attuned to our mind states through our attention practices and use them as an anchor to come back from fragmentation, distraction, or dullness. The mind states in and of themselves can become an anchor, an attentional focus that can propel us back into the present moment of soft attention and presence.

- *Disarming the default mode network and moving into wholeness* – Engaging and reengaging (however often it is necessary) focused attention is an excellent way of disarming our default mode network (DMN) and releasing us from the perpetual planning and problem-solving of the executive control network (ECN) that keeps us stuck in the past and future and that has the potential to move us into judgment, fragmentation, and negativity. The DMN and ECN continuously shift our attention and pull us out of the present moment. They are the networks that create suffering by never being fully satisfied, by being mired in habit and opinion, by being defined by wanting more and more and better and better. They are the reflection of vrittis flavored by gunas and kleshas – a mind divided, pre-occupied, and suffering. They are the networks of *doing* as opposed to *being*.

- *Working with the inner obstacles to practice* – This principle invites us to begin to deal with the inner obstacles that are under our attentional 'control' – to which we have access. They are obstacles that we can remove simply by becoming focused, attentive, and committed to the practice. The inner obstacles are, in other words, not a problem in and of themselves (unlike the outer obstacles of social injustice, oppression, racism, inequity, and so forth). The problems related to the inner obstacles come from us *being distracted or drawn into judgment and habit by them – into doing rather than being*. As we become distracted by doubt, by the stories our mind constantly spin, wanting pleasure, trying avoid things we do not like – we distract ourselves from what is meaningful and derail from the path.

- *Working with non-attachment to an outcome* – Like *pratyahara*, *dharana* relies on the capacity to practice with the commitment and persistent effort as well as the non-attachment to an outcome. Concentration practices are free from striving, expectation, desire, fear, or ego. They are accomplished – as is true for all yogic *practices* – through balanced effort, not stressful striving or overdoing. They are free of attachment to a particular outcome. Freedom from attachment to an outcome allows for a relaxed and easeful, though committed and engaged practice. Concentration is best accomplished by flowing with the inputs from mind and body; neither holding on too tight, nor holding on too loosely. It is a constant, yet softly-focused attentive practice to increase attunement to or inner mind states and our mind's tendency to shun concentration by wandering into distraction and dysregulation. It is self-compassionate and kind, not self-judgmental and harsh.

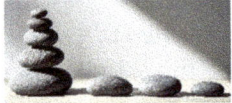

Limb 7: Dhyana or Meditative Awareness

The seventh limb of yoga, *dhyana*, refers to meditation practices in which the skills of all prior limbs come to their full flowering. The prior limbs have built the platform upon which the meditator can rest – body, breath, and mind are prepared; intuition is honed. As a spaciousness practice, meditation helps us forge new neural pathways, encouraging neuroplasticity and increasing gray matter volume in certain parts of the brain. Meditation facilitates new learning and augments the number of synaptic pathways in the brain. It is a practice of achieving an effortless state of awareness that transcends even a single point of focus. Although is not the only yogic strategy to do so, it is the most effective of the yoga strategies in facilitating new learning and synaptic pathways in the brain.

Through preparation for sitting or reclining mediation, we are able to move into spacious awareness and deep concentration that transcends even a single point of focus. The body is at ease, the breath is calm, and the mind is tuned inward; good posture supports the body; rhythmic breathing supports the calming of emotions; the mind is still and no longer serves as the constant interpreter and evaluator of experience.

Central Principles of Dhyana

From a place of preparedness, we come to understand the central principles of this limb of yoga. Through their practice, meditation invites us into deep awareness of all layers of consciousness, compassion and lovingkindness, as well as insight and wisdom.

- *Cultivation of awareness* – Meditation retrains attention via cultivating meta-awareness. It is the ability to attend to our own attention; to track where attention is landing in each moment. Meta-awareness means mindfully, nonjudgmentally, compassionately catching ourselves doing what we are doing, feeling what we are feeling, thinking what we are thinking, acting how we are acting. Meta-awareness is a background awareness that allows us to be fully present for our life at all levels (or koshas): behaviorally, energetically, mentally, cognitively, emotionally, and relationally without getting swept away (or hijacked by our amygdala).
- *Cultivation of compassion, lovingkindness, and altruistic joy* – The inner practices in general and meditation in particular, along with the values expressed in the yamas and the commitments expressed in the niyamas, call on us to acknowledge and truly sense into our generosity, kind-heartedness, social connection (and dependence), profound grounding in and responsibility for community, deep need to love and be loved, and complete dependence on other humans to live, thrive, grow, evolve, and be happy. The inner practices cultivate our interpersonal warmth, positive emotions, and recognition that all humans share the need for connection, seek happiness, and want to relinquish suffering.

- *Cultivation of insight* – The wisdom that arises from meditation is based in awareness and compassion and reflects clear knowing, a deep appreciation for our true nature, and a deep intimacy with our inner and outer world and the contributions of all of these factors to our day-to-day functioning.
- *Cultivating purpose* – The final principle of meditation is our engagement in skillful, auspicious action marked by altruism and service. Once awareness and compassionate insight have developed, the next logical step in our journey of self-realization and liberation becomes engaged action. It is this wisdom that guides us into wise and skillful action that arises out of conscious choice after discernment. It is the transformation of reactivity into responsiveness. It is engaged action, guided by all the brahma viharas and vidya, that leads to inheriting positive *karma*.

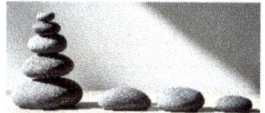

Limb 8: Samadhi or Accessing Enlightenment

Samadhi has many definitions and <u>is not a practice per se</u> despite being one of the eight limbs of yoga. *Samadhi* is a recognition of oneness, of connection. It is an experience, not a practice. Given this reality, *samadhi* is not a limb that presents us with access to techniques or strategies for healing. Instead, accessing the experience of *samadhi* is perhaps a barometer of progress in healing, of movement toward emotional resilience and mental fortitude. Some of the most common translations of samadhi are as follows:
- Enlightenment (as opposed to freedom = *moksha*)
- Freedom from desire and discontent
- Joyful and embodied presence
- Bliss and oneness
- Unraveling mental, emotional, and physical knots

With a regular and committed integrated yoga practice, spontaneous experience of the eighth limb of yoga can arise – absorption (*samadhi*). Absorption is not a practice but an experience; it is the spontaneous arising of a felt sense of integration or oneness that is beyond an ordinary state of consciousness. Purpose and interconnection arise in absorption. Practitioners gain a clear recognition of the interconnectedness of all sentient beings and a profound connection to a greater whole. A feeling of being complete, whole, or integrated arises along with the experience of interdependence or co-arising with everything. In absorption, practitioners experience mindful and joyful connection to a greater purpose and a sense of community or belonging.

Samadhi can also be interpreted as being free of desire and discontent – a definition that derives strongly from the Buddhist traditions. Joseph Goldstein shares this translation in one of his YouTube talks (Satti Patthana Sutta Session 3): "*Samadhi is the careful collecting of oneself into the present moment*". It is the receipt and experience of joy and embodied presence, an unraveling of mental, emotional, and physical knots so that we are left with bliss and an understanding of our oneness. Absorption is like coming home to ourselves and our loved ones. Absorption is unique to each one of us and defies definition.

The integration of all eight limbs of yoga allows for a greater breadth of practices. It offers us a large tool box for helping human move toward resilience, for supporting them with strategies that allow them to thrive. A wider range of practices that can support wellness means more access and more complexity. It supports the wholism of integrated holistic yoga as well as its commitment to make sure that the practice offers some for everyone, does not discriminate, and invites social engagement and self-empowerment.

Summary of the Eight Limbs of Yoga

Definition and Intention	*Central Principles and Practices*
Limb 1 – *Life Choices for Ethical Living: Yamas*	
First-person ethics that invite intentions, thoughts, actions, and relationships based on discernment and mindfulness to result in compassionate thought, speech, and action	• Nonharming (*ahimsa*) – living in a peaceful manner that seeks not to cause deliberate pain or harm • Truthfulness (*satya*) – living in an honest manner that is true to one's real and ideal self, creating authenticity and integrity • Non-stealing (*asteya*) – embracing a sense of abundance, generosity, and reciprocity that eliminates the desires to take or steal from others or to have more than others • Moderation (*brahmacharya*) – being neither indulgent nor excessively restrictive when it comes to habits and desires • Non-possessiveness (*aparigraha*) – mindful cultivating gratitude for what life has already provided and thoughtfully relinquishing grasping, desire, and jealousy
Limb 2 – *Life Choices for Purposeful Living: Niyama*	
Mindful lifestyles of discipline, motivation, and intentionality to create a meaningful and purposeful life for self and community	• Purity (*saucha*) – finding centered balance in consumption, clutter, toxins, distractions, and overload in all aspects of life, including food, drink, body care, relationships, media use, work, and play • Contentment (*santosha*) – taking calm and appropriate action, neither driven by hyper-excitability nor indifference, and of accepting life fully and calmly • Disciplined use of energy (*tapas*) – committing to making conscious – not habitual – choices in every moment that are neither hyperactive nor slothful and lead to transformation for self and others • Self-reflection (*svadhaya*) – opening up to new learning from outer sources (such as books and teachers) and through quiet introspection • Devotion to a greater good (*ishvara pranidhana*) – surrendering ego-driven intentions and committing to positive other-oriented intention and action

Definition and Intention	Central Principles and Practices
Limb 3 – Physical Movement, Activity, and Readiness: Asana	
Mindfulness-based embodied forms, movements, and actions that create physical, affective, mental, and emotional health and wellbeing, including balance, strength, stamina, flexibility, coordination, empowerment, and agency	• Attuned movement and form practices that invite neuroception, interoception, proprioception, and exteroception • Mindful movement and form practices that integrate other limbs (e.g., moving with breath; moving with non-violence and moderation) • Physical practices for strength, mobility, and/or stability • Movements that are balanced and balancing • Movements that revitalize, tonify, and energize • Movements that calm, ground, and bring peace or quietude • Practices that invite recognition and transformation of unwholesome physical habits • Physical routines – e.g., healthful nutrition, mindful eating, proper hydration, physical activity in nature (e.g., hiking, swimming, skiing), dancing, referral to medical care
Limb 4 – Breath and Breathing: Pranayama	
Breathing practices and wholesome natural breathing patterns that connect to inner sensations, recruit the parasympathetic nervous system, reduce allostatic load, and improve vagal tone	• Breath attunement practices that invite attention and awareness • Optimal functional breathing practices • Balancing or stabilizing breathing practices • Vitalizing or uplifting breathing practices • Calming or grounding breathing practices • Practices to nourish vitality (e.g., restorative practices) • Practices that invite recognition of breath, arousal or affect-related habits and patterns • Energetic routines – e.g., sleep hygiene, rest and recuperation, music, chanting or singing, referral to mental healthcare
Limb 5 – Guarding and Attuning the Senses: Pratyahara	
Becoming unperturbed by the steady flow of sensory inputs put through the eyes, ears, nose, taste buds, and other sense receptors (e.g., touch, pain, temperature, texture)	• Moving inward and tuning out extraneous stimuli to mindfully notice and understand mental habits and reactivity, to become attuned to neuroceptive and interoceptive input • Sitting still for a moment with the eyes closed to recenter and ground the mind • Reducing sensory stimulation – e.g., breaks from watching news; creating a quiet and calm environment, decluttering the home • Finding an inner point of focus on the activity of the mind's fluctuations

Definition and Intention	Central Principles and Practices
Limb 6 – Concentration and Attention: Dharana	
Inviting the mind to become honed and clear, transcending unhelpful mental states (e.g., those that are disturbing, upsetting, distracting, discouraging, lethargic, heavy, agitated, or restless) – leading to integration of top-down and bottom-up self-regulation	• Guided imagery practices that hone attention and cultivate awareness of mind states • Body scans of internal states, lovingkindness practices, and other visualizations that keep attention single-pointed, honed, and alert • Practicing an everyday, routine task with full attention and focus • An action as uncomplicated and ordinary as being fully focused on washing a dish or peeling a piece of fruit can become a concentration practice • Finding a state of flow during physical movement or action – e.g., exercise, including yoga posture practice; playing music
Limb 7 – Meditation and Awareness: Dhyana	
Achieving an effortless state of awareness, spaciousness, and peacefulness that ushers in sufficient tranquility so that sensations, emotions, and thoughts that arise no longer become a disturbance, opening a gap for making new choices and building new neural pathways	• Spacious awareness meditation • Practices that cultivate mental resilience and enhance coping through recognition of mental fluctuations • Practices for working with emotional, behavioral, and relational reactivity • Practices for shaking up mental and emotional habits or routines – e.g., puzzles for cognitive flexibility, journaling, changing up routines like taking a different route to work, time in nature, referral to insight-oriented psychotherapy • Creating a decisional gap (between stimulus and response) to invites new choices, and to exercise conscious authorship over emotions, cognitions, behaviors, and relationships
Limb 8 – Awakening to Joy and Connection: Samadhi	
Spontaneous arising of a sense of integration or oneness that is beyond an ordinary state of consciousness – not necessarily linked to practice	• Cultivation of compassion, lovingkindness, and joy – e.g., maitri meditation • Practices for the cultivation of wisdom and insight – e.g., journaling • Practices that invite taking responsibility for own and others' health, resilience, and thriving – e.g., random acts of kindness

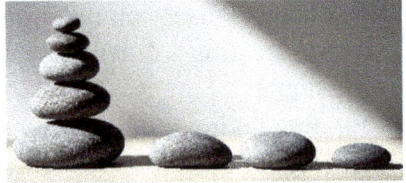

Chapter 3: Koshas or Layers of Experience

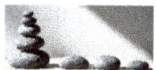

The wholism embraced by integrated holistic yoga makes a point of seeing the entirety of human beings, regardless of how or what they present when they seek out yoga, healthcare, or education. It places each individual in their context and attempts to understand their past and current circumstances, life, and embeddedness. We see ourselves, our students, our clients – everyone we encounter – in all their layers, trying to understand, honor, respect, and value their embodied self, their energetic presentation and vitality, their mind and emotional presence, their relationships and ways of expressing what is in their hearts, and their profound grounding in a particular biopsychosociocultural context and interpersonal matric. In yogic language, we recognize all koshas – or layers of consciousness – and honor these layers in our teachings and interactions with students, clients, and patients – and ourselves. A quick overview of the five layers of self or experience is shown in the box that follows; a detailed discussion follows after highlighting a few notable characteristics that apply to the koshas as a whole.

> The Sanskrit word "*kosha*" is translated as *layer* or *sheath* of the self in most Western yoga translations. However, koshas are perhaps better understood as layers of experience. The experience of an individual "self" is a construction of the mind, a way of experiencing and defining ourselves in the tangible world. Our concept of "self" is simply a construct to be able to put our many aspects of evolving and transforming experience of being into words.
>
> **Annamaya kosha** – embodied self-experiences or physical consciousness ("anna" = food)
> **Pranamaya kosha** – affective or energetic self-experiences or vital consciousness ("prana" = breath; "Prana" = life force)
> **Manomaya kosha** – verbal and social self-experiences or mind consciousness ("mano" = mind)
> **Vijnanamaya kosha** – decentered, wisely intuitive self or wisdom consciousness ("vijnana" = wisdom)
> **Anandamaya kosha** – joyful integrated self-experiences or unity/universal consciousness ("Ananda" = bliss, joy)

Koshas as Co-Arising and Interdependent Systems

The paradigm of the koshas as living, interdependent, co-arising systems is predicated on the fact that human experience and identity extends across several layers of self (more accurately, layers of experience), which develop and transform across the lifespan in community with other humans. Ancient yogis conceived of the experience of 'self' as layered – composed of several aspects or components that make up our conscious experience (to which we refer as our *self*). In Sanskrit, these layers are called *koshas*, loosely translated as "sheaths". The word *kosha* is used in this book because no English translation can quite capture the complexity of the concept. *Each kosha or layer of experience has separate and distinct functions and expressions while also being completely integrated and interdependent with the others.*

All layers of experience are with us (if only as seeds) from birth to death – yet each takes on particular significance and reaches maturation during different stages of life and development. In other words, they develop and become important neurosequentially as we begin our life in the world in relationship, learn to self- and co-regulate, and finally become beings who can reason, find purpose, and contribute to the greater good. The specific meanings and expressions of each kosha depend on the circumstances we face as we move through life and relationships.

> **Being by Swami Jnaneshvara**
>
> We are human beings.
> We are physical beings.
> We are breathing beings.
> We are sensing beings.
> We are thinking beings.
> We are feeling beings.
> We are intuitive beings.
> We are spiritual beings.
>
> *What these all have in common is that "We are Beings." Yet, paradoxically, who we truly are is none of these "beings". We want each of these, individually, to be balanced and trained so as to not disturb our peace or tranquility. Then, in silence, we want to go beyond each of these, to the center of our Being.*
>
> Retrieved from https://www.swamij.com/yoga-meditation-what-being.htm

Although they have to be discussed separately and linearly, the *koshas* are profoundly and inextricable interwoven and arise in profound interdependence with one another within the interpersonal matrix, web of life, or biopsychosociocultural context in which they develop, evolve, and ultimately transcend as we move through our lives. They are fully interrelated and never experienced in isolation of each other. They co-evolve and co-exist. The meaning of interdependence is complex and incorporates the following concepts and beyond:

- Our self and our lifecycle, as it unfolds from conception to birth, depends on the collaboration and connection among the *koshas* as well as on co-regulation and connection with others in our interpersonal matrix as defined by the biopsychosociocultural context in which we exist.
- There is no *self* that is separate from the *koshas* – there is no separate body, no separate affective experience, no separate mind, no separate relationships, no separation from the world as a whole. Although we, at times, subjectively experience aspects of self or consciousness as discrete or separate, this is an illusion. There is no body without breath; no mind without relationships; no inner world without an outer world. In fact, there is no tangible overall self at all – just consciousness of various aspects of how humans can experience themselves in relationship. Our very essence is our interconnection, our awareness, and our integrated consciousness beyond the layers of self or experience.
- Because of the ongoing and constant interdependent arising of the *koshas* within the context of our relational world, there is no permanence to our experience. We are ever-evolving, changing, emerging, and growing. We are constantly shaped and reshaped through our experiences and relationships – in all of our layers of consciousness.

- We cannot disentangle ourselves from our experiences, our context, our relationships, our world. In Buddhism, this is defined as the inherent emptiness of self. Self can only be experienced, defined, and understood in relationship, in context, in community. While this is called emptiness in Buddhism, it can also be interpreted as fullness – we are a microcosm of the macrocosm. We contain and are integrated with everything.

Experience		*Definition*	*Associated Actions or Practices*
Annamaya Kosha	d e n s e	**Physical or material experience** • Comprised of major organ systems and tissues – loosely, our anatomy and physiology	• Development of strength, flexibility, balance, and alignment; cultivation of body awareness; exercise; nutrition
Pranamaya Kosha		**Energetic or vital experience** • Comprised of processes that create energy and vitality, including affect and arousal – loosely, our physiology and nervous system	• Breathing and breathing practices; attunement to energy, rhythm, depth; synchronization of breath with movement; working with affect and arousal states
Manomaya Kosha	s u b t l e	**Mental or emotional experience** • Comprised of thoughts, attitudes, and patterns that shape us; expressions of acquired personality; emotions	• Development of awareness of mental reactions; self-reflection; guided imagery; relaxation practices; protection of the senses; concentration
Vijnanamaya Kosha	c a u s a l	**Wise or intuitive experience** • Comprised of innate intelligence, wisdom, awareness, compassion, and insight; recognition of interdependence and co-arising	• Meditation; attunement to inner promptings; reflection versus reaction; openheartedness practices; open-mindedness practices
Anandamaya Kosha		**Spirit or joyful experience** • Arises from the connection to each other, and to the greater web of life	• Compassion; lovingkindness; generosity; equanimity; joy and delight; consideration of reverberations of actions on all

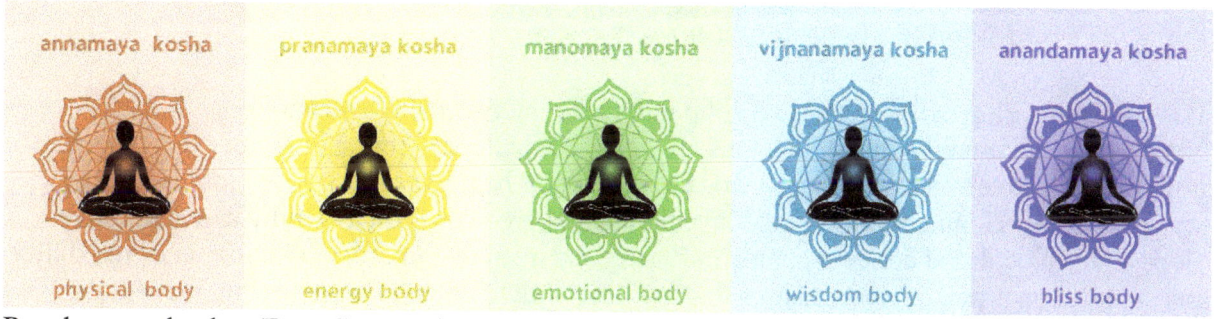

Panchamaya kosha. (Data Source: istock)

Health and Wellness and Their Relationship to the Koshas

The *koshas* combine into an integrated, interdependent, co-arising, and dynamic system that is ever-changing, emerging, and evolving, as well as all-encompassing. The *koshas* form an inner and outer human ecosystem that balances itself in response to demands or stressors that emerge in our lives and relationships. The *koshas*, collectively, represent a wholistic system that can heal itself, that has robustness, where "robustness refers not just to the strength of a system but also its ability to repair itself (p. 105)" (Stone, 2008)

Because of the interwoven nature of the *koshas*, lack of health or integration in one layer can reverberate in the others. If symptoms emerge in one layer of experience, they often bring with them challenges in another layer. However, this also means that as we repair and heal symptoms in one sheath, the others can regain balance and resilience. This interdependent arising of the layers of experience gives us access to many paths toward wellness, growth, and transformation. Balanced and integrated *koshas* facilitate optimal functioning, including accurate adaptability to situational demands, awareness and attention, flexible responsiveness (rather than emotional reactance), resilience in all realms (physical, affective or energetic, mental, emotional, and relational), and openness to change or growth.

(Re-)Balancing and (re-)integrating the *koshas* into a system of wholeness, integration, and healthy responsivity to internal and external demands and circumstances is key to wellness. Wellness can be expressed in the tangible *koshas* (body, vitality, and mind) in a variety of ways, with a few examples following.

- *Wellness in annamaya kosha*: proprioception of balance, stability, and lightness (Jones, 1976) as cited in (Payne & Crane-Godreau, 2015); neuroception of safety (Porges, 2022); strength, balance, health, and the integration of active and passive energies (Svatmarama & Akers, 2002); and interoception of physical states and changes
- *Wellness in pranamaya kosha*: affective experience of openness, confidence, and curiosity (Ekman et al., 2005); management of arousal and affect; interoception of warmth, calm, and flow (Csikszentmihalyi, 2008)
- *Wellness in manomaya kosha*: open and flexible attention (Brown & Ryan, 2003); flexible expectations, beliefs, and attitudes (Garland et al., 2015); flexible role expectations for self and others; settled mind states; lifelong commitment to learning, unlearning, and relearning; healthy expression and regulation of emotions

A Contextual Model of the Koshas

The *koshas* develop in the primordial soup that is the interpersonal matrix of our biopsychosociocultural context. Humans are born utterly dependent on resources that emerge from the collective and cannot survive or thrive without being nurtured, cared for, and deeply understood. Development through the layers of self is predicated on a healthy and supportive biopsychosociocultural collective, on a nurturing and available interpersonal matrix of reliability and support, on a web of relationships that are inherently compassionate, loving, kind, and mindfully attuned. The biopsychosociocultural paradigm invites yoga professionals to gain in-depth understanding of clients' or students' (or their own) web of life, webs of relationships, and greater connection. It reminds us that sources of challenges, difficulties, and presenting concerns, even overall life experience, are always relational and embedded in a greater context. It leads to recognition of the importance of having an understanding of biopsychosociocultural contexts that have had and continue to have a bearing on the development and experience of human beings.

Four dimensions are defined and understood with complexity from a holistic and integrated lens. They are *biological*, *psychological*, *socioeconomic/sociological*, and *cultural/familial* – or biopsychosociocultural – in nature (Brems & Rasmussen, 2019). Biopsychosociocultural contexts are in and of themselves ever-emerging, always changing, and in flux. This constancy of emergence, presence, and dissipation adds complexity, ambiguity, uncertainty, and volatility to our understanding of ourselves and our clients. In other words, our human experience is always grounded in a complex and unpredictably changeable world. A world with the features of volatility, uncertainty, complexity, and ambiguity (also called *VUCA world* – the acronym of the four defining characteristics) is inherently stressful and challenging.

Currently, we live in a VUCA world.

V = volatility
U = uncertainty
C = complexity
A = ambiguity

Such conditions are inherently more stressful and more likely to create difficulty and helplessness. However, understanding these characteristics of life and knowing how to manage them can prevent excessive suffering and distress, while enhancing resilience in body, mind, behavior, and relationships. In fact, being prepared for and open to VUCA can lead to thriving and success.

Integrated holistic yoga is one pathway for finding grounding and accessing strategic abilities in the context of human connection and co-regulation during times of VUCA. It increases our window of tolerance for VUCA and gives us the capacity to respond to it with empowerment, agency, and efficacy – recognizing our deep grounding in community and a supportive web of life. Our very interdependence (which we so often deny, especially in the Western world) is the solution to thriving in a VUCA world. It invites us into collaborative, compassionate, kind, and create relationships that support collective health and wellbeing.

Biopsychosociocultural contexts and
nurturing interpersonal relationships matter in their:
- **Influence on our developmental trajectory**
- **Influence on the layers of self or consciousness**
- **Influence on healing and recovery**

When things go wrong in the biopsychosociocultural matrix, especially in our closest and most trusting relationships, development in the koshas may be thwarted, and suffering, pain, challenge, and lack of resilience may ensue. This means that we depend on biopsychosociocultural structures of equity, belonging, and caring at the collective level and relationships of nurturance, love, and support at the familial and individual level.

> Cozolino (2015, 2024) posits that our experience of self (or consciousness) develops, is maintained, and can be healed through four crucial ingredients in our interpersonal matrix or biopsychosociocultural environment:
> - Presence or establishment of safe and trusting relationship(s)
> - Activation of experience, emotion, and cognition (bottom-up and top-down)
> - Co-construction of implicit and explicit memory, including personal narratives
> - Creation of resilience through exposure to moderate stressors and challenges
>
> These ingredients are inherent in yoga, whether yoga classes, therapeutic yoga, or yoga therapy. They are also inherent in psychotherapy and very useful in self-care and prevention activities. Most importantly, perhaps, they are the backdrop for the development of the koshas across our lifetime. At the beginning of our developmental journey, we are primarily recipients of these ingredients. As we grow and develop, relationships become increasingly reciprocal, mutual, and co-regulating. Ideally, toward the end of life, we will primarily become the givers in relationships, having achieved generativity, resilience, and wellbeing in all of our layers of consciousness.

The Developmental Perspective of the Koshas

As noted above, traditionally in modern yoga, the koshas are represented as layers or wrappings of self that define how a human being shows up in life. Using a slightly different lens, the koshas can also be viewed as a neurodevelopmental, intra-, and interpersonal journey toward self-transcendence (or a recognition of profound connection and union), a journey from non-knowing (avidya) to knowing (vidya). This allows us to understand the *koshas* from a developmental perspective. As we age, our focus shifts from physical survival and preoccupation with the physical body to our emotional connection with others, to our self-definition through how we think about and perceive the world around us, and to an ever-increasing circle of relationships with others that challenges our wisdom and intuition to make auspicious interpersonal choices.

Our development culminates in the understanding that we are part of a greater whole, that we are embedded in an interpersonal matrix of relationships that nurture us and through which we can care for others. When this realization of interrelationship becomes the primary lens through which we view the world, our understanding of life becomes panoramic and joy abounds. At the start of our lives, we are driven by our biological imperative for survival – bonding with and responding to others so we can survive and thrive. What we needed for our own physical and emotional survival when we were born, becomes what we can begin to offer to the world as we mature. Life comes full circle over and over again.

Transcendence and Integration of the Koshas

The koshas are fully integrated with one another developmentally, ever unfolding in a seemingly chronological, consecutive, and lasting way. This integration takes place in the context of the biopsychosociocultural context and therefore always happens in a web of relationships. While this journey may feel lonely at times, this is an illusion. Everything we are, we are because of relationships, interpersonal matrix, and greater context. We are co-constructed and co-regulated.

We are an integral and integrated part of a greater whole that is shaped by shared experience and integration. We develop as we do because of the context in which we evolve and because of how we receive, interpret, and integrate our relationships, experiences, and world. We evolve and grow across many lines of development, including physical, psychological (affective, emotional, cognitive, moral, and ethical), and interpersonal (social, ethical, relational, political) dimensions. Understanding the developmental natures of these various human self-expressions helps us appreciate the maturity of the individuals, their wisdom and capacity to take responsibility for contributing to the greater good through interpersonal relationships that are grounded in awareness, insight, purpose, and deep connections defined by compassion, lovingkindness, altruistic and appreciative joy, as well as equanimity.

The koshas grow and develop through a developmental model of transcendence and integration, a concept that helps us understand how humans are wired for growth, evolution, emergence, and change. In this model, nothing is ever lost – all experiences, everything we have been remains present in our consciousness. However, none of it defines us or limits us. Our life and relationships are informed by our past but not confined or constrained by it. In every moment of our lives, we can make new choices and pick new paths or directions.

To 'transcend and integrate' means that each new learning or layer of development is carried forth into the next; again, nothing is ever lost. Our personal human evolutionary process (or growth) from each level of experience (or *kosha*) begins with a glimpse of the next layer of consciousness (through relationships, new learnings, inspiring experiences) that offers a new insight, inspiration, or motivation for change. Once the skills and traits of the next layer solidify, the prior layers are integrated with the new insights and develop into a perfect union that carries with it all prior learnings, experiences, and relationships.

For example and discussed in more detail below, as we explore each of the koshas:
- Once neuroception begins in *annamaya kosha*, it remains. When proprioception is added, neuroception and proprioception become cumulative. When interoception begins to develop in *pranamaya kosha*, it is added to neuroception and proprioception.
- Our nervous system styles first express themselves in annamaya and then persist and evolve throughout the lifespan. Our affective experience of the world begins with *pranamaya kosha* and then stays with us in ever evolving ways throughout our lifespan. Language develops and helps us form the beginnings of an identity, a process that starts with *manomaya kosha* and remains with us until the moment we die. The *gunas* and *kleshas* forever influence the mental fluctuations and become manifest in our mind states.
- Moral development evidences the same journey. We move from *yamas* to *brahma viharas*, but never lose our connection to and faith in the yamas.

Understanding the *koshas* most typically starts from the outside in - from the physical body to the subtle spirit. Physical experience, *annamaya kosha*, is easiest to access and thus yoga typically starts at the level of the body. Deeper awareness and better health at the level of the body opens us up to the experience of our more subtle aspects of self - such as breath and mind. From the physical, we move to the next most accessible or concrete layer, our breath and life energy, *pranamaya kosha*, which enlivens our physical experience. Breath awareness and energetic flow are crucial precursors to working with the more subtle movements of the mind.

Our mental self, *manomaya kosha*, takes in our experiences and processes all inputs, integrating them with our greater truths and ingrained habits or understandings to help guide choices and decisions. Awareness of mental reactions and better mental health readies us to develop the capacity for discernment and wise choices.

Innate and cultivated wisdom and intuition, *vijnanamaya kosha*, build on mental awareness to help us become reflective and choose actions that are wise and compassionate. From the awakened heart and open mind of wisdom arises the experience of bliss and lovingkindness, anandamaya kosha, that is associated with being in touch with our more subtle, spiritual aspects of self. This layer of experience is connected to all that surrounds us, recognizing that we are simply a small aspect of a greater whole. *Anandamaya kosha* is the expression of our true self, the self that embodies connection to other sentient beings and our planet, the self that is loving and compassionate without condition, the self that is calm and healthy when faced with challenges or obstacles, the self that is committed not only to one being but to all that is.

Yoga guides us from the physical to the subtle; from isolation to connection; from desperation to joy. It helps us heal and be happy; it allows us to bring health and happiness to others. Yoga as a lifestyle guides us to integration and holism that brings with it a sense of joyful presence and compassionate action. This movement toward our inner truth is often graphed, as below, by showing the five *koshas* as layers that can slowly be peeled back to expose our true being. This understanding of the *koshas* indicates that our physical experience contains the seed of vitality that gives access to the breath, which in turn gives deeper expression to the physical. Breath or our energetic, vital experience contains within it emotion and the seed of thoughtful awareness that gives access to our mind, which in turn give deeper expression to breath and body. Our mental and emotional experience contains within it the seed of wisdom that gives access to our intuition and wisdom, which in turn gives deeper expression to mind, breath, and body. Our wise intuition contains the seed of bliss that give access to our joyful, spiritual self which, in turn, gives deeper expression to intuition, mind, breath, and body. Our blissful, spiritual expression of self contains the seed of oneness that integrates all aspects of being within the greater web of life.

Once we realize our interdependence and co-arising, all our actions and decisions become guided by a wise and compassionate desire for personal and collective wellbeing and thriving. We care – not just about ourselves but about everyone and everything to which we are connected. As we get to know ourselves on this deeper level, we recognize that we do not <u>seek</u> wellbeing and thriving - we <u>are</u> health and happiness. Our true definition as a human *being* is the expression of health and happiness, the experience of love, compassion, generosity, joy, and connection. We are not our layers; they are simply coverings of our true being. We are the truth hidden beneath these coverings – we experience awareness, connection, and joy; we cultivate ways of being that have at their heart the desire to create wellbeing and thriving for all who are and all that is.

Feedback and Feedforward across the Interconnected Koshas

Once understood in its developmental stage and trajectory, the current primary expression of self can reveal prominent areas of suffering (i.e., in the body, in our vitality, in how we think) and can guide us toward specific needs for change, support, and practice recommendations. Development of the practitioner (whether that refers to the student or the teacher) can make a big difference about where the most auspicious starting point for intervention and healing may be. Nevertheless, we can enter work with the *koshas* at any level because regardless of where we enter the work toward transformation, there will be reverberations and resonance throughout all the other koshas – in the same way that each jewel in Indra's net (see box below) reflects all others. When we work with the body, we automatically work with breath, even if this is not where our direct focus of attention lies. The same is true for all layers of experience. This is one of the reasons yoga can be so effective – we can create change through entering through many doors that, in the end, all lead to the same place - the whole person and beyond.

In other words, all layers of experience interpenetrate and interconnect to such a degree that what happens in one will also manifest *in some way* in the others. This interdependence and co-arising can support the process of healing in that growth in one layer of consciousness will almost automatically reverberate into the other *koshas* and will stimulate healing and transformation there as well. This interconnection works forward in development as well as backward.

For example:
- How the body develops in early childhood has an impact on the development of the mind.
- Trauma later in life will manifest in physical and breath patterns that can either profoundly ameliorate or add to suffering.
- Physical illness at any point in life can either affect development going forward or can move us into a physical crisis that leads us to a need to focus on physical wellness before returning to a forward trajectory of growth.

Likewise, all patterns of our existence are reflected in all *koshas* – even if the pattern is more clearly notable or identified in one *kosha* over another. For example:
- Inflexibility in the body may also show up as rigidity in the mind.
- Breathing patterns may reverberate in how we hold the body or how the mind responds during challenge (e.g., a shallow breath is linked to anxiety and vice versa).
- Clinging to a particular definition of the self in the mind (asmita) may show up as forced ways of moving the body or interacting with the world.

A complex example of how the layers interconnect is gained through observation of the breath. When the breath enters and leaves the body, it creates movement in the physical layer of self – the belly rises and falls as the diaphragm facilitates the flow of breath; the rib cage expands and contracts as bones externally and internally rotate in their joints to accommodate the change in lung volume on the inhalation and exhalation. How the breath flows also has direct effects on the mind; it creates movements (fluctuations, vrittis) in the mind. The mind may contract and react in fear if the breath is choppy or labored. The mind may soften and relax if the breath is long and smooth. The Hatha Yoga Pradipika states in HYP 2.2 (p. 33): "When the breath is unsteady, the mind is unsteady. When the breath is steady, the mind is steady, and the yogi becomes steady. Therefore one should [steady] the breath" (Svatmarama & Akers, 2002).

To summarize, the five *koshas* are shaped by and reflect each person's unique biopsychosociocultural experiences and contexts. They are interdependent, complex, and developmental (or emergent) in nature. They form an ecosystem that balances itself in response to demand or stress, a system that has the robustness to heal itself. Although they are discussed in sequence and have a developmental quality to them, the *koshas* coexist, co-arise, interlock, and interdepend. Everything we do and everything we experience expresses all *koshas* at once – though one may predominate. We never 'move beyond' any of the ways in which experience ourselves: we transcend and integrate our experiences (or *koshas*) to move forward developmentally, but we bring all prior layers and wisdoms of experience with us in ever-evolving, ever-changing, ever-adapting ways.

The *koshas* are not a stage model in which we outlive or outgrow a prior stage; they represent a neurodevelopmental model in which we constantly increase our complexity, add more nuance (and 'layers') to our existence, and transform and integrate all expressions of self and our experiences in our world and relationships. This unfolding and changing is completely grounded in our deep connection to the greater web of life and thus always happens in relationship, in connection with a greater whole.

Indra's Net
by Barbara O'Brian (https://www.learnreligions.com/indras-jewel-net-449827)

"Indra's Jewel Net, or the Jewel Net of Indra, is a much-loved metaphor of Mahayana Buddhism. It illustrates the interpenetration, inter-causality, and interbeing of all things. Here is the metaphor: In the realm of the god Indra is a vast net that stretches infinitely in all directions. In each "eye" of the net is a single brilliant, perfect jewel. Each jewel also reflects every other jewel, infinite in number, and each of the reflected images of the jewels bears the image of all the other jewels — infinity to infinity. Whatever affects one jewel affects all.

The metaphor illustrates the interpenetration of all phenomena. Everything contains everything else. At the same time, each individual thing is not hindered by or confused with all the other individual things."

Annamaya Kosha or Embodied Self or Somatic Consciousness

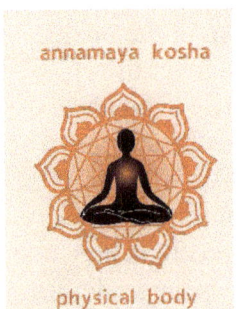

The physical layer of self consists of muscles, tissues, bones, blood, flesh, skin, organs, and more; it is the most tangible, palpable part of our existence. In yoga, this is called the gross (as in tangible) sheath of the self (the Sanskrit word is *sthula*). In science, we understand the needs and development of this layer through studying anatomy and, to some degree, physiology, with special emphasis on how the body senses, metabolizes, moves and functions. Subjectively, we experience our body through our senses – outer and inner. Many physical inputs and outputs are autonomically managed via the brain stem (of course, it is much more complex than that, but this is where we will leave it here). Others, such as deliberate movement in yoga, are under conscious control. The physical and vital layers (see more about the vital kosha below) are intimately connected and work in tandem to allow us to experience, sense, notice, and react/respond to the world around us. The physical layer embodies our most basic approach to the world, loosely defined as a tendency either to perceive and react to the world as safe, dangerous, or threatening.

The physical kosha needs to be supported by food, water, air, physical contact, and movement. It is deeply grounded in movement which, in and of itself, is strongly and genetically linked to our dopamine system (Scaer, 2012). The perception of movement as pleasurable (thanks to the link to dopamine release with movement) is crucial to human development, as movement is one of the first skills to develop (Thelen, 1995). Developmentally, movement is necessary for many subsequent developmental lines, including but likely not limited to the following:

- *Language development* – e.g., gesticulation and imitation (Esteve-Gibert & Prieto, 2014)
- *Establishment of social engagement* – e.g., through physical interaction with caregivers (Smith & Gasser, 2005; Stern, 1985), interpersonal communication (Hostetter & Alibali, 2004), and social interaction (Sebanz et al., 2006)
- *Consolidation of memory* – movement in combination with visceral and other sensory experiences leads to sensory, somatic memory consolidation at the brainstem level; this starts even prior to birth when sensory memories arise from bodily (i.e., visceral, somatic, sensory, and motor) experiences (Cozolino, 2024); this memory is non-declarative and has no source attribution; it is subject to childhood amnesia
- *Self-identity development* (Scaer, 2012; Uithol et al., 2011a, 2011b) – emerges from sensory, somatic, visceral, and motor experiences and organization; based on these experiences neural networks develop that create a sense of physical self
- *Embodied-self-development* through the experience of sensation and motor activity (mediated in the thalamus, cerebellum, and parietal cortex) – key motor milestones and experiences, such as developing eye-hand coordination, crawling, and walking, contribute to sensory and motor memory and a sense of physical self

Annamaya kosha is accessed in yoga through practices that cultivate awareness and mindfulness, as well as movement and relaxation of the physical body. Through yoga – holistically practiced – we come to understand how we process our world to feel a sense of safety (neuroception) and how we respond to the world when our physical survival and wellbeing appear threatened versus protected. Through yoga, we cultivate proprioception, so that we can understand better where our body is in space and how it moves, how we can keep it healthy, and how we maintain balance. Yoga practices also hone our interoception of bodily states, supporting our accurate understanding of our physical needs and signals (e.g., pain, hunger, thirst, discomfort, ease, tension) and how best to nourish our body in response (including with sleep, food, exercise, fresh air, self-compassion, non-violence, and much more).

Some Characteristics of Annamaya Kosha

- *Annamaya kosha* includes body awareness and physical ways of experiencing being – how we feel in the body; sample cuing elements teachers can use related to body awareness include, but certainly are not limited to the following concepts (many of which also penetrate the other layers experience, in perhaps less tangible ways):
    - *solidity* (the *earth* element in the yoga tradition): pressure, texture, hardness, softness, density, smoothness, heaviness, lightness, groundedness, stability
    - *fluidity* (the *water* element in the yoga tradition): moistness, dryness, flexibility, fluidity, cohesion, connectivity, adaptability, crying/tears
    - *temperature* (the *fire* element in the yoga tradition): heat, coolness, cold, neutral, warmth, lightness, expansion

- *vibration/space* (the *air* element in the yoga tradition): trembling, pulsation, stillness, dullness, movement/motion, pressure, mobility, integration with breath
- *senses*: scent (aromas, smells), touch (pain, ease, air on skin, earth under body, pressure), hearing (sounds, stillness), taste, vision, etc.
* *Annamaya kosha* is related to physical health and wellbeing (with significant developmental shifts in focus and needs through the lifespan):
  - development of physical health and wellbeing early in life
  - maintenance of physical health → strength, flexibility, endurance, balance, and more
  - maintenance of physical allostasis (adaptability in the face of change or challenge) and homeostasis (ability to return to a balanced physical state of being)
  - prevention of physical illness or disease
  - recovery and healing from physical illness and disease
  - overcoming preoccupation with the body and staying connected to the body
* *Annamaya kosha* develops experientially through movement and the physical experiences of being in relationship to help form an embodied understanding of self
* As noted above, *annamaya kosha* develops through movement, which is directly linked to the dopamine reward system – it is inherently pleasurable and thus self-perpetuating; this is a good thing as movement underlies many aspects of development.
* Through physical experience and embodied relationships (e.g., nursing, being held, orienting with another), the gunas – or our fundamental human ways of expressing our nature and experience (described below) – begin to emerge; see the table that follows and Chapter 4
* The yogic concept of the *gunas* is strongly related to (or overlapping with) polyvagal theory as conceptualized by Porges (2011, 2017) and Sullivan et al. (2018b)

Overview of the Gunas – Fundamental Human Ways of Being in the World			
	Rajas	*Tamas*	*Sattva*
Translation	MOTION → Passion or energy (versus drivenness or greed); passion or creation; experience of excess or overabundance	MASS → Grounding or stability (versus lethargy or dullness); darkness or destruction; experience of lack or need	LUMINOSITY → Knowledge, radiance and harmony (versus flightiness); beingness or preservation; experience of harmony
Definition	• Activity, driving force A kinetic tendency underlying change, that refers to movement versus freneticism, to creation versus greediness	• Groundedness, entropy A property of solidity, a tendency of resistance to change, that refers to stability versus inertia, to grounding versus entropy	• Knowledge, happiness Awareness-supporting quality is transparent or reflective; a way of being that is healthful, pure, open, and enlightened
Basic Manifestation	Hyperactivity, hyperarousal, hyper-engagement	Hypoactivity, hypoarousal, hypo-engagement	Balanced response, resilient arousal, healthful engagement
Positive Expressions	Enthusiasm, action, vitality, alertness, striving, movement, problem-solving, inventiveness, decisiveness, openness to change	Stability, reliability, persistence, loyalty, steadfastness, constancy, commitment, sleep, patience, restfulness, ease, stillness, groundedness	Intelligence, enthusiasm, discernment, balance, peace, clarity, openness, insightfulness, wisdom, compassion, happiness, goodness, resilience

Annamaya Kosha's Primary Neural Signatures

Annamaya kosha has specific primary neural signatures and may be somewhat akin to science's concept of *minimal consciousness*, the most basic level of awareness evidenced via reflexes and automatic bodily (somatic responses), as mediated by the brainstem and thalamus.
- It is guided by the brainstem, right hemisphere of the brain, and sensory and visceral (bottom-up) inputs from the inner and outer world (via the vagus nerve).
- It is defined by bottom-up processing that leads to visceral reactivity and instinctual and reflexive (not intuitive) reactions.
- It is mostly encoded via implicit memory, reaching all the way back to early childhood physical experiences; such implicit memories are preverbal and explain why anamaya experiences may not be easily verbalized and explained and yet are profoundly felt and experienced. It can be difficult to communicate about purely annamaya-based physical states as they are (as mentioned) based on memories that are preverbal or nonverbal and have no vocabulary associated with them that adequately express what we feel viscerally.
- It is tied to the biological imperative of physiological survival (via the polyvagal system, neuroception, and the gunas – described in detail elsewhere) and is sensory, motor, and somatically based .
- In this kosha, the subject (experienced reality) and self-identity is the body: "I am body".

Memory consolidation is implicit and has no time or date stamps. As such,
- It is subject to childhood amnesia.
- It is subject to trauma amnesia (due to high release of cortisol interfering with the laying down of explicit memory.
- Memories in annamaya kosha can be triggered by sensations that are similar to those that led to implicit physical memories, leading to reactivity that cannot be logically explained. In early childhood, this serves a useful purpose as such sensations lead to reactions that stimulate a helpful response in our caretakers (e.g., we cry because of sensations of hunger until we are fed). In adulthood, reactions triggered by such sensations can be overwhelming and startling to the experiencer and the individuals with whom they are in relationship as it may not always be clear why they are emerging given the current context (e.g., intense startle response when a car backfires; intense sense of threat when hearing a loud fan that runs continuously).

Annamaya kosha is tied to the *gunas* as the most basic and essential process that starts us developmentally. Its focus is on creating a biopsychosociocultural context of physical safety and security. There is a tie-in with proprioception and neuroception, and most profoundly with polyvagal theory (Porges, 2011; Porges & Carter, 2017) and its impacts on the development of autonomic nervous system states. *Intentionality or motivations* that arise from this aspect of experience are largely driven by fear and physical survival instincts (e.g., fearing for our life because of death, illness, injury, accidents, or aging). We integrate and transcend purely physiological survival and wellbeing as development proceeds. This integration and growth ushers in the emergence of *pranamaya kosha* and we become affective, vital beings, attuned to the subtler dimensions of the interpersonal relationships and matrix in which we exist. We begin to attune to the reverberations (even repercussions) of the biopsychosociocultural context that shapes us and that embeds us in a matrix of affective experiences and relationships.

Pranamaya Kosha or Affective or Vital Self or Affective Consciousness

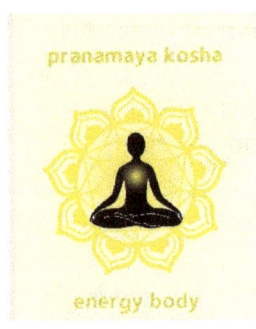

The energetic or emotional layer of experience animates and moves the body (physically, emotionally, and mentally). *Pranamaya kosha* is considered a subtle layer of self (the Sanskrit word is *sukshma*). It concerns itself with breath, energy, vitality, affect, blood flow, electrical impulses, neurochemical transmissions, and more. The energetic and physical layers inseparably and jointly process incoming signals from inside and outside of the body. There is no separation in experience of *pranamaya* and *annamaya koshas*. The physical is vital; the energetic and affective is also physical. Together, they form the emotional motor system, which is marked by an intricate interaction and mutuality between movement and posture with breath, energy, affect, and arousal. Shifts in movement or body position can lead to changes in affect and arousal; shifts in affect and vitality leave imprints on our physical form and movement. Our affective issues have imprints in our physical tissues; imprints in our physical tissues perpetuate (and even create) affect and arousal.

The vital aspect of the self is tied strongly to our limbic system and interoceptive network (including the salience and default mode networks). Layering on top of the *gunas* that began to be active in *annamaya kosha*, sensations now translate not only into state of nervous system arousal and (re)action, but also carry with them a particular affect. Experiences not only have an impact on nervous system arousal (ventral vagal/sattvic; sympathetic/rajasic; dorsal vagal/tamasic) but are also perceived as having a feeling tone (or *vedana* in Sanskrit) that is positive, negative, or neutral. Thus, *pranamaya kosha* holds, shapes, and expresses our vitality, our sense of arousal or engagement (i.e., integrates the gunas or polyvagal states), our affective tones (pleasant, unpleasant, neutral), and prepares us for the emergence of affective predilections (i.e., *kleshas*), and attachment styles. Like all layers of self, our vital being is highly interpersonal and develops (grows and matures) through socially and affectively engaged relationships, especially early in life.

At the most basic level of definition, this vital layer consists of the physiological systems in the body that create affective and energetic awareness (i.e., respiratory, cardiovascular, nervous, endocrine, circulatory, immune, and lymphatic systems). In ancient yoga tradition, this is also the layer that houses the five vayus (or vital airs) of prana, apana, samana, udana, and vyana (more about this below). Sensory experiences and somatosensory organization are now developmentally supplemented by affective experience (i.e., feeling tones of neutral, pleasant, or unpleasant) and energetic experiences (i.e., arousal, hyperarousal, hypoarousal).

Organization of somatic and affective experiences lead to affective memory (in addition to sensory and motor memories). Sensations and motor activity are paired with pleasant, unpleasant, or neutral affects in the context of childhood experiences, trauma, and stress. They are greatly affected by the presence of adverse childhood experiences (ACES; Brems & Rasmussen, 2019). The affective self that begins to emerge at this developmental stage is tied strongly to sensory, motor, and somatic experiences, rhythms in the brain stem (Badenoch, 2018), and midbrain-mediated primary process emotions (Panksepp & Biven, 2012).

In yoga, we work with the vital layer through increasing interoceptive awareness of affective tone, arousal, and reactivity, and its expressions as sensation and wellbeing in the body and as their consequences for the states and contents of the mind. Neuroception of *affective* safety, danger, or threat to existence is added to neuroception of *physical* safety, danger, or life threat. Practices such as conscious breathing, movement for perceiving inner responses to inner and outer signals and sensations, and creating awareness of our inner valuation (or valence) of experiences promote accurate self-perception, other-perception, and predictions of physical and vital (energetic and affective) needs. Yoga practices that support this layer also help us develop exteroception, which promotes accurate reading of relationship cues and other signals that meet us from the world around us. Exploring whether we respond with grasping and desire versus anger and hatred versus fear or lack of accurate understanding is an important part of the yogic work of this layer.

Some Characteristics of Pranamaya Kosha

- *Pranamaya kosha* represents our vitality, our energetic as well as affective awareness and ways of being – how we feel energetically and affectively; sample cuing of related concepts may revolve around affective and energetic awareness and can include some of the following and more (Brems, 2024b):
  - exhaling to release, to find quiet, to access ease
  - inhaling to nourish or nurture, create vitality and aliveness, rejuvenate and sustain
  - linking to body: feeling breath as movement in the body, vibration, pulsation, reverberation of energy, pain versus pleasure versus neutral sensation, ease of energy in the body, life force, vitality
  - linking to mind or mental states: letting go, releasing stress, moving beyond the primary affects of pleasant/unpleasant/neutral to the secondary (more nuanced and granular) emotions
  - linking to emotionality expressed in the mind states and understanding the valence contributed to mental fluctuations by arousal and affect
  - linking to kleshas (i.e., our emotional predilections or the roots of suffering):
    - pleasant affect linked to attachment (e.g., joy, ease, happiness versus grasping, clinging, jealousy)
    - unpleasant affect linked to aversion (e.g., clarity, steadfastness, engagement versus judgment, rigidity, anger)
    - confusion and lack of clarity about whatever is experienced
  - linking to wisdom and community: feeling energies of connection, codependent arising, interdependence, shared vibration, communal affect and arousal, tranquility, peace
- *Pranamaya kosha* contains the *pancha vayus* – or the five vital winds of the lifeforce:
  - *prana vayu* = most central of the five winds of *Prana* as it sets everything in motion and moves us forward; it is central to the creation of vitality and moves energy inward and upward, even forward
  - *apana vayu* = the vital energy deep in abdomen that supports elimination (ridding us of what no longer serves) and reproduction; it moves energy downward and outward
  - *samana vayu* = the central stabilizing energy that imbues heat and warmth, especially at the center of our being; it moves energy from the edges to the core

- - *vyana vayu* = most central energy to circulation at all levels, in all koshas; it is central to absorbing the benefits of what we take in and moves nourishing energy outward from the center to the periphery
  - *udana vayu* = primary positive energy that invites life to unfold – inviting growth and spiritual transformation; it moves energy upward, to the head, senses, and mind
- *Pranamaya kosha* is related to affective, vital, and energetic health and wellbeing (with significant developmental shifts in focus and needs through the lifespan):
  - development of affective health and wellbeing early in life
  - recognition of affect (positive/pleasant, neutral, negative/unpleasant), which ultimately moves us toward emotional and affective granularity and complexity
  - recognition of energy/arousal (hyperarousal, hypoarousal, nervous system regulation), which is supported by keen neuroception and interoception
  - expression of the gunas and recognition (and once integrated with higher koshas, transcendence) of the kleshas
  - recognition of emotional nuance and increasingly mature processing of emotion as relevant developmentally (once integrated with higher koshas)
- *Pranamaya kosha* develops relationally or interactively (and movement remains a key aspect of experience and encoding) – the infant begins to experience sensations tied to wellness (feeling good, bad, neutral – very rudimentary) and arousal level (hypo, hyper, regulated) in relationships with caretakers
- Developmentally, *pranamaya kosha* relates to affective ways of being/experiencing the self from a perspective of an early developmental stage where the individual needs affective nurturance and caring to integrate
- Our interpersonal matrix, especially its affective (*vedana*) and arousal (*gunas*, polyvagal theory) characteristics, has a profound impact on the development, transformation, and maintenance of *pranamaya kosha* throughout our lifespan
  - all the biopsychosociocultural factors and influences that arise in our interpersonal relationships have profound effects on how we learn to show up affectively – in relationship, alone, at school, at work, everywhere, and with everyone

Pranamaya Kosha's Primary Neural Signatures

Pranamaya kosha has specific primary neural signatures and may be somewhat akin to science's concept of primary (or core) consciousness, a transient, present-moment awareness of self and environment based on sensory stimuli that bring along particular emotional or bodily states. This level of consciousness is mediated by the brainstem and thalamus, as well as regions of the cortex such as the posterior cingulate and insular cortex. For example,

- It is guided by the emotional network in the brain (including, yet not limited to, the limbic system, right hemisphere, and amygdala). It remains tied to the biological imperative, now in the form of affective survival (via the polyvagal system, neuroception, and interoception).
- At the emergence of *pranamaya kosha*, experience is mostly encoded via implicit memory stemming from early child physical and affective experiences – just as memories in *annamaya kosha* are encoded in pre-verbal forms, so are memories in *pranamaya kosha*.
- *Pranamaya kosha* is strongly sensory, motor, and somatically based – bottom-up signals trigger survival-based affects and states of arousal.

Later in development, top-down processes are added to include contextual appraisal of sensory, motor, somatic, and affective experiences to inhibit reactivity and move us into responsiveness and discernment instead. Thus, in this *kosha*:
- The subject (i.e., experienced reality and self-identity) is our experience of our energy, affect, and arousal: "I am my affect/my sense of energy or vitality/my attachments/my aversions".
- Intentionality or motivations in this layer are largely driven by desire (and/or aversion) in the service of affective survival instincts (grasping for affective wellbeing via material things, success, wealth, pleasure, renown and more).
- The *gunas*, or autonomic nervous system states, are expressed in pranamaya kosha from a perspective of affective (in addition to purely physical) arousal and survival.
- The *kleshas* (see the table that follows and in Chapter 4) are the essential processes that, based on affective and vital experiences of the self, lead to preferences and aversions and begin to identify with affect as a representation of reality, of how things really are (when, of course, they actually comprise so much more that we cannot yet see because of the developmental stage we are in at this point in our life).

Overview of the Kleshas – Emotional Predilections or Roots of Suffering					
	Raga	*Dvesa*	*Asmita*	*Abhinivesha*	*Avidya*
Translation	Attachment, greed, desire	Aversion, enmity, hatred	Egoism, ego-attachment	Fear of death or change	Confusion, delusion
Definition	Wanting pleasure, desiring positive outcomes; attached to having what we want	Intolerant of pain or discomfort; wanting things differently than they are; anger as default response	Ego-absorbed individualism and self-absorption; worried about losing one's identity or roles	Holding on to how things are; not accepting impermanence of things and experiences, denying our mortality	Lack of wisdom, incomplete understanding, misinterpretation, limiting views, literally 'not seeing correctly'

As development moves toward increased language skills, different consolidation of memory, and the capacity to take perspective, our cognition and emotional experiences become more complex and nuanced. We begin to glimpse that there is more to our experience than the physical and affective and can move forward developmentally to integrate new parts of our consciousness and self-identity. We integrate our physical and affective world and transcend them, moving forward into *manomaya kosha*.

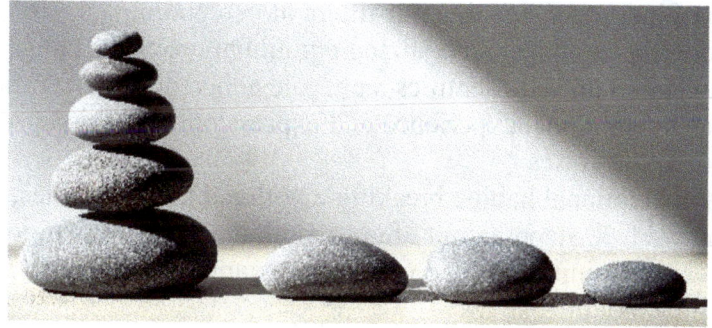

Manomaya Kosha → Verbal and Social Self or Mental and Emotional Consciousness

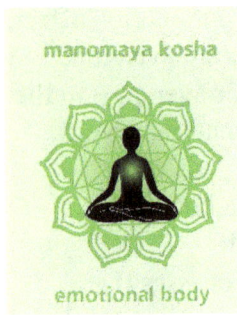

Manomaya kosha, the mind layer, comprises perceptions, thoughts, labels, emotions arising from mental interpretations, and expressions of acquired personality. Like *pranamaya kosha*, *manomaya kosha* is considered subtle (or *sukshma*), yet still affected by and expressive of all five senses. This *kosha* is linked to language, memory, and prefrontal cortex development. It encompasses our (emerging and always evolving) perceptual and cognitive understanding of the world, including our and others' perceived roles within our communities and in our relationships. Through the mind and its perceptions, we begin to gain clarity about our habitual (stimulus-response) reactions and can transform habit into conscious choice. As we progress along this layer of self, we improve our capacity to analyze cause-and-effect and to make subsequent behavioral and relational choices and changes.

Yoga strategies that work with thoughts and emotions focus on calming the mind through self- and interpersonal awareness, mind-based mindfulness interventions, and concentration and meditation practices for recognizing inauspicious habits and transcending them into conscious choices. Yoga for this layer of awareness deals with introspection to understand what drives our perceptions, mental biases, and cognitive habits, such as getting caught up in the past (in memories), anticipating the future (via constant planning), labeling experiences, misperceiving or misinterpreting events and relationships, or ways of distracting ourselves from the present moment (e.g., day-dreaming, zoning out, over-working, and more).

Some Characteristics of Manomaya Kosha

- *Manomaya kosha* reflects our cognitive and emotional awareness and ways of being – how we perceive the world and our experiences cognitively/mentally and emotionally; sample language around cognitive and emotional awareness:
    - *cognitive*: noticing thoughts, recognizing mental reactivity, monkey mind, cow mind, preoccupations with thoughts, planning, memory, being caught in the past or worrying about the future, finding grounding in the present moment
        - to transcend cognitive habits: breaking mental habits or rules, not believing everything we think, stepping out of our story, letting go of hardened views, re-examining beliefs, paying attention to intention, reexamining automatic thoughts, letting go of judgment, opening our filters of perception
    - *emotional*: noticing emotions, recognizing emotional reactivity, attachments, aversions, fears, clinging to certain self-identities, ego, role adherence, differentiating emotions, finding nuance in emotional experience and expression, recognizing various gradients within emotional categories
        - to transcend emotional habits: breaking emotional habits or rules, not believing everything we feel, stepping out of our emotional story, letting go of hardened emotions, re-examining reactive feelings, reexamining relational patterns, reexamining emotional styles

- *Manomaya kosha* is related to cognitive and emotional health and wellbeing (with significant developmental shifts in focus and needs through the lifespan):
  - development of language and labels, along with development of expectations, biases, attitudes, and beliefs
  - development of self-agency and self-determination
  - development of role definitions and ego or self-identity
  - emotional development leads to the rudiments of social engagement and social self-development
  - instrumental morality that then evolves to decenter and become more altruistic
  - emerging wisdom and self-determination
  - evolution of experiencing, perceiving, understanding, interpreting, and engaging with the world and relationships around us
  - integration of affect and increasing granularity (nuance) of emotion
- *Manomaya kosha* develops out of the capacity for representational learning, especially as mediated by language development; thus, it is strongly language- and communication-based – within our interpersonal matrix and within our biopsychosociocultural context
- Biopsychosociocultural factors strongly shape how we think, what we believe, how we identify others, how we label and perceive ourselves, how we show up in relationships
- Depending on our biopsychosociocultural context and interpersonal influences, *manomaya kosha*, or mental and emotional experience, can lead to prejudice, bias, and misunderstanding if it is based on perception without mindfulness and deeper understanding of the interdependence with context; without the recognition of how environment, context, and circumstances affect how we perceive, label, and experience our world and relationships, we see only the surface of things (we can only see an apple as red or green, missing the white color on the inside)
- Perception as labels, memories, and habits that, via expectations, flavor how we view and understand the world but miss the deeper context, the complexity of the object, relationship, or concepts being perceived – this can lead to bias, prejudice, and misunderstanding; when we add the wisdom and insight of context, we move toward *vijnanamaya kosha*
- Later in life, an increasing recognition of the greater context and a less self-centered focus on others is developed with increasing empathy and altruism, readying us for the next developmental step (*vijnanamaya kosha*)

Developmental Layers within Manomaya Kosha

Manomaya kosha contains within it several developmental stages of the mind (verified by modern developmental psychology) as it moves from narrow to broader, alongside neurological/brain development and readiness for increasing altruism and decentering:
- *Manas* (thoughts, labels, reactions) – basic differentiation of objects and experiences (e.g., the ability to use names and basic labels for things and for relationships or roles); limited recognition of context or bias in our use of labels and reactions
- *Ahamkara* (self-identity, roles and ego, personality, identification of self as separate from other) – identity is derived for self and others by societally-normed roles; there is little questioning of the roles with which we identify or that we ascribe to others; there is little recognition of how identity definitions are shaped by context and environment (the biopsychosociocultural matrix)

- *Emerging buddhi* (more objective and reflective, moving toward awareness and wisdom, naturally pauses to reflect and make more discerning choice – ushers in vijnanamaya) – we increasingly take into consideration the experience and contexts that helped shape us and everyone else; we let go of calcified opinions, ideas, biases, and prejudices and exchange them for a desire to understanding the interdependent arising of everything within its context, environment, and relationships; we see clearly societal and personal biases, prejudices, and harm perpetuated by decontextualized understanding and ignorance of impermanence, emptiness, and interdependent arising

Manomaya Kosha's Primary Neural Signatures

Manomaya kosha has specific primary neural signatures and may be somewhat akin to science's concept of *higher-order (or extended) consciousness*, a much more complex level of awareness that includes self-reflection, explicit memory, and the ability to plan for the future, as mediated by the prefrontal cortex and default mode network. For example,
- *Manomaya kosha* is possible due to increasing cortex maturation; the parietal, occipital, and temporal lobes collect data and integrate new neural pathways. We begin thinking about our life history, work on solving problems, and become able to imagine hypothetical scenarios.
- Top-down processing begins to emerge as the frontal lobe begins to engage in analysis of sensations and translates them according to the context in which they arose. That is, behavior becomes more planful and actions more discerning and tailored (less reactively driven).

Beginnings of hemispheric integration lead to increasing cognitive complexity and nuance. Communication between hemispheres leads to integration of emotional context and cognitive understanding; learning becomes contextual and context broadens over time. We increasingly decenter across the developmental span, taking larger and larger perspectives and increasing cognitive capacity to considering and integrated increasing complexities.

Thanks to ever-growing language skills, *manomaya kosha* is mostly encoded via explicit memory consolidation of various forms, hippocampus- (not amygdala-) driven, and time and date stamped; this encoding and the various types of memory lead to self-identity consolidation:
- Language memory – learning labels
- Episodic memory – encoding processes
- Narrative memory – encoding self-identity through time- and place stamped memories
- Autobiographical memory – encoding a story of self that becomes increasingly expansive and decentered, increasingly prosocial and altruistic

Increased memory encoding via the hippocampus leads the way to the development of explicit declarative memories that help us to remember the past and predict the future – a key human survival skill. In fact, with *manomaya kosha*, the brain becomes the prediction 'machine' that it is – many of our thought processes are about predicting what will happen and taking action in response to these predictions. In *manomaya kosha*, the subject (our experienced reality and self-identity) is our experience of mind:
- "I am my thoughts, labels, emotions" – identification with *manas*
- "I am my roles" – identification with *ahamakara*
- "I am my responsibilities to my greater community" – identification with *buddhi*

Manomaya kosha remains tied to the biological imperative; physical and affective survival are joined by self-identity preservation (e.g., clinging to role-definitions, being viewed as a moral being [good girl/good boy]). This early in our cognitive and perceptual development, we often miss the bigger picture and are driven by selfish, habitual, and reactive perceptions and needs:
- We see solidity instead of recognizing complexity
- We see the forest and miss the trees; then we see the trees and miss the leaves; then we see the trees and miss the veins and chlorophyll, and so on
- We mistake the surface, the concept, the label as the reality
- We create concepts like "self" and "other" and start to mistake them as reality instead of seeing the ever-evolving, ever-changing, interdependent nature of everything

Gunas and *kleshas* carry into this *kosha* in a profound manner, expressing themselves in new ways – linked to verbal development, cognitive development, and changing self-identity. Intentionality or motivations that arise from this aspect of experience are largely driven by duty (wanting to do the right thing, to be responsible) and ego (wanting to fulfill one's role in society; wanting to feel to be accepted, to be part of a group) in the service of social and emotional survival and being accepted and cared for. As *gunas*, *kleshas*, and brain mature, increasing executive control is gained in relationship to these physical and affective experiences.

Manomaya kosha then leads to the conscious processing and expression of mental fluctuations (*vrittis*) and pattern locks or habits (*samskaras*), as well as recognition of the mind states, as the essential processes that mediate the verbal and social self. The *vrittis*, namely, the five expressions of fluctuation of mind and mental consciousness (or the ways in which we perceive, process, label, and organize our experiences of the world and our relationships) are profoundly affected by the *gunas*, *vedanas*, and *kleshas* and shaped by our biopsychosociocultural context and interpersonal matrix. The *vrittis* are summarized in the table that follows and explored in detail in Chapter 5.

As we begin to realize others' perspective and begin to decenter from a personally-focused perspective on the world, we integrate physical, energetic, affective, cognitive, and emotional aspects of self to expand our understanding of who we are yet again. We transcend our exclusive focus on the prior layers conscious and development moves toward empathic connection and deeper understanding of our deep dependence and inter-being with others. We expand into the expansive and intuitively compassionate world of vijnanamaya kosha.

> **Our memory is made up of our individual memories and our collective memories. The two are intimately linked.**
> **Haruki Murakami**

\	Overview of the Vrittis – Fluctuations of the Mind
Vritti and Translation	*Positive and Negative Manifestations*
Pramana = right perception, verifiable knowledge	*Positive Expression of Pramana* o Clear perception is the capacity to see reality as it is o We construct our reality without flavoring via direct experience, via inference, via testimony o We discern or spot our misidentifications as they arise and do not get sucked into them o We penetrate our mental constructions to recognize when they have become neither truth nor reality o We practice the Buddhist joke/principle of "don't believe everything you think"
Viparyaya = misperception, faulty or illogical thinking; cognitive distortion	*Viparyaya is essentially the negative expression of pramana* o Getting trapped in opinions, values, ideas o Getting lost in rigid perceptions of roles and relationships o Imposing our view and skewing reality into the direction of our preferences o Psychological protective mechanisms kick in (e.g., projecting of emotions and thoughts) o We forget that our thoughts are just constructions, not reality o We get lost in thinking that beliefs and identifications are truths
Vikalpa = fantasy, imagination, creative thinking, future thinking, daydreaming	*Negative Expression of Vikalpa* o Getting trapped in the future o Getting lost in daydreams and then not acting o Clinging to wishes and desires for particular outcomes of developments o We forget that the future is not yet real – that our future as we construct it in the mind, is simply a thought in the present *Positive Expression of Vikalpa* o Power of imagination gives us wings of creativity o Dreams for the future, impetus for trying new things, creation of change, emergence of new ideas, development of new solutions o Mental capacity to imagine the future and learn from the past. o Mental skills that supports our ability to be altruistic, take mental and emotional perspective of another being, sense into experiences of another being (i.e., vicarious introspection). o Decentering from our own experience to take a vaster perspective
Smriti = memory, recollection, remembrance	*Negative Expression of Smriti* o Getting trapped in the past, getting lost or stuck in old stories and narratives o Getting attached to old identities, memory as a habit or rut – as a narrowing of possibilities o We forget that the past is no longer real – that our past as we recollect it, is simply a thought in the present moment

\	Overview of the Vrittis – Fluctuations of the Mind
Vritti and Translation	**Positive and Negative Manifestations**
	Positive Expression of Smriti ○ Remembrance and mindfulness to allow us to reflect on the past and be in the present ○ Time-stamped and place-stamped memory that is explicit (as opposed to implicit) ○ Ability to reflect on past experiences to create change and growth ○ Memory as a helpful guide in the present and as we plan the future
Nidra = deep dreamless sleep, absence of thought, emptiness, absence of the other *vrittis*	*Negative Expression of Nidra* ○ Getting trapped in escapism or avoidance ○ Getting lost in spaciness ○ Sleeping (or sleepwalking) through our lives *Positive Expression of Nidra* ○ Consolidation of memory during deep sleep (triaging short-term memories accumulated in the hippocampus during the day, connecting some to lasting neural pathways and rejecting or letting go of unnecessary ones) ○ Creativity may emerge during deep sleep leading us to waking up with a new idea ○ Sleep is a crucial aspect of life, allowing rest and rejuvenation in body and improving brain function ○ Nature of our sleep may also give us hints about the nature of mind, or our mind states

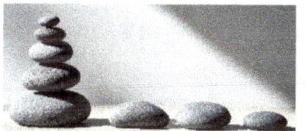

Vijnanamaya Kosha → Wise, Reflective, Decentered Self or Wisdom Consciousness

The wisdom layer comprises our deep understanding of and sense of responsibility for community. It is the place where innate intelligence, talents, traits, and natural inclinations (or innate temperament) meet emerging and growing wisdom and deeper understanding. *Vijnanamaya kosha* is considered a subtle (or *sukshma*) layer of conscious; however, it is even subtler than *pranamaya* and *manomaya koshas* as it is no longer affected by outer sense experiences. To reach conscious awareness of this *kosha* (which many of us do not until late adulthood), we need to have achieved cortical and hemispheric integration. In other words, our brains need to have matured and become capable of synchronous processing of experience. When we have achieved this level of integration, we become an observer of our own (inner) reactions and responses to the world and in relationship. We begin to perceive our roles and responsibilities with more clarity, recognizing our place in the world as one that can invite joy, lovingkindness, compassion, and equanimity. We apply ethics and morality with discernment and a large lens that allows complexities and contexts that might easily be missed. We live out our highest intentions with generosity and gratitude, and we fully embrace our deep interconnection to all that is. We have integrated and understand ourselves in relationship to our own and others':

- Affects and emotions
- Attention and awareness
- Behavior and actions
- Relationships and connection

It should be noted, however, that even this description of *vijnanamaya kosha* is deceptive because in writing we still have to use a *subject* to describe the experience. However, at this level of consciousness, there is no more subject (no more self-referencing) – only shared and mature experience of a connected and interdependent web of life. Consciousness and experience at this level is a flow: an arising, knowing, and dissolution of experience in an instant, over and over, clear and lucid, vividly reflective of what is, without object or subject. That is the nature of knowing or experiencing in *vijnanamaya kosha*. Grammar choices can reflect this somewhat when we use witness or observer language (passive voice) rather than active voice.

"*A thought is present*" – rather than "*I am* thinking"
"*A sound is heard*" – rather than "*I am* hearing"
"*A pain is felt*" – rather "*I am* feeling"
"*Thoughts are coming and* going" – rather than "*I am thinking*"

There is no I, there is no subject.
There is simply knowing, feeling, doing, caring, loving

Yoga at the level of *vijnanamaya kosha* invites individual and collective transformation through conscious lifestyle choices, mature emotions, commitment to a greater purpose in the service of others, and clarity about human interdependence. Meditation, concentration, and mindfulness are typical practices and begin to permeate our work on and off the mat.

Some Characteristics of Vijnanamaya Kosha

- *Vijnanamaya kosha* leads us toward spacious awareness and open-heartedness– a greater wisdom emerges that can see the larger web of life (beyond the biopsychosociocultural factors that influenced us earlier in life) and our interconnection with everything. From here, wise choices and enlightened decision-making can emerge as we transcend the chains arising from cravings and aversions (kleshas) and transcend emotional and mental fluctuations and habits (vrittis).
- *Vijnanamaya* is the *kosha* of interconnection – of the conscious recognition that there is no solo self, no self at all – but only a relative self that helps us navigate life. This relative self, however, is entirely dependent on context, emerges from relationship and collective experience, and is spaciously aware, mindfully attuned, and intentionally compassionate, loving, and concerned about collective wellbeing.

- *Vijnanamaya kosha* transcends narrow definitions of what constitutes our interpersonal matrix, our biopsychosociocultural context, our view of the world and what is possible expands – as do our perceived responsibilities to others and their wellbeing.
- *Vijnanamaya kosha* is related to societal, social, environment, and ecological health and wellbeing – concern is no longer for the self, but for all.
- In *vijnanamaya kosha*, discernment becomes intuitive and facilitates healthful and reciprocal relationship, as well as strong community-mindedness and increasing altruism. Activism in this kosha comes from a neural platform of social engagement and wisdom (*sattva*, ventral vagal complex), from resilience and altruistic motivation, mindfulness, awareness, and compassion.
- An individual in *vijnanamaya kosha* moves from needing nurturance and support to providing it to others; tied in with the development of mature emotions (brahma viharas) of equanimity, compassion, lovingkindness, and altruistic as well appreciative joy.

Vijnanamaya Kosha's Primary Neural Signatures

Vijnanamaya kosha has specific primary neural signatures and may be somewhat akin to science's concept of *meta-cognition or self-consciousness*, the ability to think about one's own thoughts and awareness, fostering introspection and self-monitoring. It is mediated by the anterior prefrontal cortex and midline structures like the anterior cingulate cortex. For example,

- *Vijnanamaya kosha* is facilitated by the increasing cortical integration, memory encoding via hippocampus, hemispheric integration, and integration of bottom/up and top/down processes
- As evidenced in meditators, the following neural signatures show up (Gerritsen & Band, 2018; Goleman & Davidson, 2017):
  - enlarged insula (i.e., enhanced attunement to internal states and emotional self-awareness; increased capacity to attend to and note internal signals)
  - enlarged somatosensory cortical areas (i.e., enhanced capacity to note sensations of touch and pain)
  - enlarged areas in the prefrontal cortex (i.e., greater capacity to pay attention and to rest in spacious (or meta-) awareness
  - enlarged anterior cingulate (i.e., enhanced self-regulation)
  - decreased activity in the posterior cingulate (i.e., downregulation of default mode network and reduction in self-referencing/self-preoccupation; less self-concern and more compassion)
  - more activity in the orbitofrontal region of the prefrontal cortex (i.e., additional capacity for self-regulation and top-down control; less mind-wandering and better attention)
  - less brain shrinkage in prefrontal cortex and hippocampus as age advances (i.e., younger brains compared to same-age cohorts)
  - increased connectivity in brain circuits for empathy and compassion (i.e., greater compassion and greater likelihood to lend assistance)
  - shrinkage in the nucleus accumbens (i.e., lessening attachment, clinging, wanting,, and self-focus)
  - decreased stress reactivity (lower cortisol levels; greater connectivity between amygdala and regulatory prefrontal cortex circuits)
  - among super-meditators, there is increased gamma wave activity (even at rest) and greater synchronization of brain waves across all brain regions; neuroplasticity

Vijnanamaya kosha develops out of the capacity to begin to think perspectively, facilitating theory of mind and transcending (and also integrating) the biological imperative. The existential imperative becomes primary, allowing us to consider the greater good and higher meaning. In vijnanamaya kosha, the subject (our experienced reality) and self-identity becomes more collective and includes our ever-widening circles of important people: *"I am my family/my community/country/world/planet".*

Intentionality or motivations that arise from this aspect of consciousness are inspired by love, by wanting to care for others, by the urge to be of service, and to express an existential imperative of creating a better world for everyone. Intentions of this kind are expressed with gratitude and generosity. *Vijnanamaya kosha* brings with it the full capacity to express the mature emotions of equanimity (the fruit of wisdom and the seed of the other brahma viharas), lovingkindness, empathic or altruistic joy, and compassion. We awaken to the desire to serve, to engage in seva (selfless service). We begin to give of ourselves, our time, our energy, and our goodness simply to give and to serve without expectation for reciprocity and transactionalism. We take the opportunity to improve the human condition, at times even at our own expense or suffering (consider the monks who have set themselves on fire in protest of human rights violations).

> "We are all connected; to each other, biologically.
> To the Earth, chemically.
> And to the rest of the universe, atomically."
> Neil DeGrasse Tyson (astrophysicist)

Anandamaya Kosha → Joyful and Connected Self; Union or Unity

The joyful and connected self is also called the bliss layer and refers to the realization of deep inner, unconditional joy and awakened living. It is the causal layer of self – being even subtler than subtle in that is has no matter associated with it. Like vijnanamaya kosha, it is not affected or ruffled by the senses. This kosha is not one we consciously work on through yoga "strategies". It *emerges* as a state of flow, connection, clarity, ease, and peacefulness. It is our deepest and most spontaneous way of expressing who we are (in a collective sense, not as a solo *self*), of how we are embedded in a greater web of life, and of living our most compassionate, kindhearted, and loving truth. When we rest in anandamaya kosha, we are no longer separate; we have achieved union and understand deeply that there is a greater connection, interrelationship, interdependence, and coexistence that transcends each of us individually. We even transform our fear of death. We experience a deep quietude; suffering is transcended and we rest in a serene sense of joy and happiness. It may also be noteworthy to point out that this layer of consciousness also brings with it the capacity for playfulness, joyfulness, and spirited presence.

In anandamaya kosha, we access the profound recognition and experience of interdependence, connection, and oneness. This realization at all levels of our experience and ways of being in the world leads to social activism and a vast understanding of the need to preserve and promote all life. Essentially, union and bliss emerge as duality is transcended – the subject (i.e., what we may perceive as our *Self)* now includes everything there is and is thus completely decentered. We recognize our deep and profound connection and its meaning: namely, that there is no *self* that is independent of anything. This recognition of co-arising and interdependence as the true definition of who we are is the basis for the Buddhist concept of *non-self* (clearly not at all a concept of nihilism, a common misunderstanding).

Habitual Identification with a Particular Kosha

Most of us are firmly anchored for the bulk of our lives in one of the first three or four koshas. One way to think about it is that we are likely at the developmental level of the kosha in which we spend at least 50% of our time each. Deep identification with a particular kosha can intensely flavor how we are in the world, how we relate to ourselves, how we think, how we feel, and how we relate to others. This identification, in a way, is a habit – a *samskaras* or our habitual ways of responding, often based in distorted cognitions and harmful habits. Samskaras and habits are based in the scientific principle of what fires together, wires together and is related to the default mode network.

A cursory overview of how we might realize where our primary preoccupations lie is as follows:
- Identification with *annamaya kosha* – we may find ourselves preoccupied with material elements, with things, with form and safety. Primary preoccupations may include:
  - our body (preoccupied with, worried about, or extremely interested in health, wellbeing, illness, disease, pain, pleasure, weight, and other aspects of our embodied being)
  - our and others' physical activity and actions (e.g., preoccupied with, worried about, or extremely interested in exercise, eating, or sleeping)
  - the physical or material world (e.g., architecture in the sense of soundness of construction, sturdiness of material things, accumulation of stuff, distress over the vulnerability of material things [e.g., getting upset if an item breaks or is lost])
- Identification with *pranamaya kosha* – we may find ourselves preoccupied with affect, with energy or vitality. Primary examples include:
  - getting caught up in pleasure or displeasure
  - sensing the energy of things
- Identification with (developmentally early) *manomaya kosha* – we may find ourselves preoccupied with the perception of things and relationships. Common examples include:
  - getting caught up in aversions to the way things manifest
  - getting attached to particular ways of being
  - having a strong sense of aesthetics and wanting for things to be a certain way
  - being preoccupied with beauty or lack of beauty of people and things
  - getting caught up in labels and adjectives (the outer appearance) rather than the inner nature of things
- Identification with (developmentally middle) *manomaya kosha* – we may find ourselves preoccupied with interpretations, obsessive thoughts, and worries about relationship, actions, events, and role conformity (or lack thereof). Examples of these preoccupations include:
  - getting distracted by your own thoughts
  - getting caught up in emotions
  - approaching everything with a strong sense of volition – wanting to just get things done
  - having rigid expectations about how others *should* behave, react, and relate

- having rigid expectations for our own capacity to meet our identified roles and identities
- feeling threatened when others critique or criticize our expression of our perceived roles and identities

• Identification with (developmentally late) *manomaya or vijnanamaya kosha* – we may find ourselves preoccupied with conscious living and compassionate relationships. Examples include:
  - thinking things through with care and with consideration of possible outcomes, advantages, and disadvantages
  - setting not only intentions but also planning with consequences and impacts in mind
  - considering the needs of others in decision-making
  - making sure that we are in the world with kindness and compassion
  - placing a high value on meeting challenge with equanimity

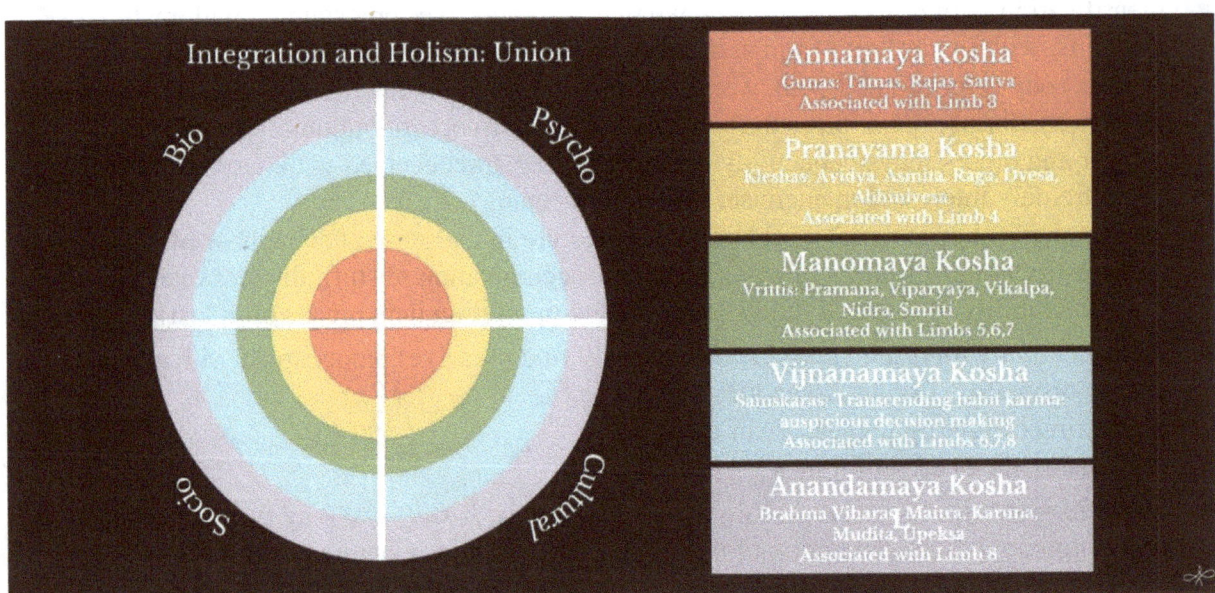

Chapter 4: Connecting to the Deeper Dimensions of Being

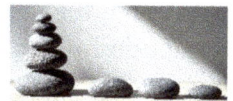

The deeper dimensions of yoga psychology are designed to take students on a path of transformation, self-inquiry, and conscious decision-making toward a life and teaching infused with intention and purpose. They are applied personally – on the mat and in day-to-day life – as well as in the design and implementation of yoga sessions. The path into yoga starts with the intellectual understanding of yoga psychology, continues with the practice of all limbs, and results in awareness, compassion, and wisdom – all to be applied to reality off the mat. Integrated holistic yoga is a path that leads to awareness (or mindfulness as it is more typically called in the Western world), insight, connection, and purpose. It is a journey into wisdom, accompanied by keen insight into our interconnection, our suffering, our interdependent nature, and the ways we can move into peacefulness, quietude, and equanimity. It is a journey of cultivating compassion and transforming not-knowing (or avidya) into a deeper understanding and wisdom (or vidya). It is a constant process of learning, unlearning, and relearning. A process of rethinking and discernment; a whole integrated path not a single skill.

As noted previously, the basis of any dedicated yoga practice grounded in the eight limbs and five koshas is sankalpa, the setting of intentions for the practice and our lives. The Sanskrit word is sankalpa, where *kalpa* means vow and the Sanskrit root word *san* refers to the highest truth. Setting a sankalpa means that we vow to orient our practice to the search for truth; we resolve to search for the deeper meaning of our individual and collective lives; we commit ourselves to a deep search for purpose. Intentions signal commitment and dedication; they anchor us to a deeper meaning so that we can stay with our practice when it becomes challenging – which it will. Intentions infuse our actions with volition and motivation. They set in motion thought, speech, and action that will infuse the outcomes and impacts of our actions (though intention and impact must not be confused – we can have a positive conscious intention [that may be flavored inauspiciously by other unconscious processes] and yet set off a negative impact).

Intention setting is woven into yoga practice, psychology, and philosophy from beginning to end. We can set an intention for an individual practice; we can set an intention for our practice across a lifetime; we can set an intention for a particular timeframe; we can set intentions in many different ways. Intentions are – in a way – a drishti for life – a focal point for our attention and concentration that orients our thoughts, speech, behaviors, and relationships. They provide structure, clarity, and scaffolding to our efforts.

Intentions are an important step or stage in committing to a spiritual practice and in aspiring to a more enlightened and compassionate way of being in the world. Intentions in this sense are aspirations – a very different type of commitment than concrete goal-setting. They are central to the first and second limb of yoga, the personal life commitments toward living an ethical and inspired life (more about this in the Limbs of Yoga section). They contain within them a commitment to do no harm, to be gentle and kind, and to be of service; they encourage us to live with an open heart. Once we have intention, we can integrate additional aspects of yoga psychology to create an increasingly meaningful practice. Such a practice will serve the greater good by enhancing our purpose and meaning in life. This chapter begins this exploration with yoga psychology concepts that take us deeply into the most hidden and perhaps most influential aspects of being human, our fundamental qualities of nature and our emotional reactivities that are often considered the very roots of our suffering.

Gunas or Fundamental Qualities of Nature

Ancient yoga psychology recognizes three fundamental expressions of nature, or *gunas*, that are inherent in everything, including human bodies, energies, and mind or emotions. The *gunas* are articulated most commonly in some combination with one another: *sattva* (or lucidity and clarity), *rajas* (or motion, enthusiasm, action, and activation), and *tamas* (or groundedness, quietude, and inertia) (Iyengar, 2006). These three *gunas* are the fundamental qualities or expressions of nature that manifest in all aspects of nature and sentient beings. They are the natural expressions and manifestations of spirit in nature (as compared to *purusha* and *Ishvara*; (Boccio, 1993). They reflect humans' fundamental ways of being in the world as well as the fundamental nature of all things, including weather, climate, activities, food, animals, plants, music, movies, water … everything. All *gunas* are manifest from the moment of birth and express themselves first in *annamaya kosha*, as we are born as embodied selves. They then quickly also express themselves in *pranamaya kosha* as our energy and vitality is almost immediately linked to our greater web of life that sustains and cares for us.

Sattva refers to wholeness, wholism, or wholesomeness, as well as luminosity or clarity (the literal translation is "goodness"). It is a way of being in the world that allows us to connect to others, to feel safe, to be in a state of trust, and to cope with resilience and stamina. It involves a state of harmony, balanced responsiveness, resilient arousal, and healthful engagement with the world. The sattvic individual is neither too fast nor too slow to respond to a situation, is discerning without being discriminating or judgmental, seeks careful awareness when making decisions, and exudes a sense of equanimity and peacefulness. In many ways the sattvic temperament combines or balances the best of rajas and tamas.

Tamas, on the other hand, refers to a state of lethargy, inertia, or exhaustion, that may bring with it bluntedness in emotional responsiveness, withdrawal, and a stance of distrustfulness toward the world and others. However, tamas can also be a grounding force that allows us to settle into the moment with solidity, when it invites us to rest and restore with clarity and intention. People who are tamasic tend to be solid and deliberate, with little perceived need for change or action. They are reliable and can be counted on for their presence and stability. They tend to be committed to their way of life with little motivation to rock their boat.

Rajas refers to a state of energy and activation; it can bring with it enthusiasm or hyperactivity. Generally speaking, it is associated with readiness for action, especially in the service of self-protection and self-defense. Rajas is useful when it ignites passion and enthusiasm, encouraging us to engage vigorously with the world. It may show up at work, in play, and in sports. Individuals who have a default operating system that is rajasic are passionate, goal-oriented, and always ready to take charge of a situation. They can be enthusiastic and fast to come up with new ideas. Their minds are sharp and always active.

For many of us in the Western world, we pivot between the extremes of *rajas* and *tamas*, rather than finding our sweet settled and balanced state in *sattva* or even engaging with *rajas* and *tamas* in auspicious ways. We over-engage and over-activate at work, in sports, in our hobbies and our relationships – or we collapse into exhaustion, lethargy, and dullness when we feel tired and worn out. Ideally, we find our balance in *sattva* – in a state of clarity and openness that allows us to be in the world in an engaged and balanced way, finding a bit of rajasic energy to get up and get going when we need to and releasing into a bit of tamasic rest, stability, and solidity when we need to recover and ground.

Overview of the Gunas – Fundamental Human Ways of Being in the World			
	Sattva	**Rajas**	**Tamas**
Translation	LUMINOSITY → Knowledge, radiance and harmony (versus flightiness); beingness or preservation; experience of harmony	MOTION → Passion or energy (versus drivenness or greed); passion or creation; experience of excess or overabundance	MASS → Grounding or stability (versus lethargy or dullness); darkness or destruction; experience of lack or need
Definition	→ Knowledge, happiness → An awareness-supporting quality is transparent or reflective; a way of being that is healthful, pure, open, and enlightened	→ Activity, driving force → A kinetic tendency, underlying change, that refers to movement versus freneticism, to creation versus greediness	→ Groundedness, entropy → A property of solidity, a tendency of resistance to change, that refers to stability versus inertia, to grounding versus entropy
Basic Manifestation	Balanced response, resilient arousal, healthful engagement	Hyperactivity, hyperarousal, hyper-engagement	Hypoactivity, hypoarousal, hypo-engagement
Positive Expressions	Purity, intelligence, enthusiasm, discernment, peace, insightfulness, openness, clarity, happiness, compassion, wisdom, goodness, balance, resilience	Enthusiasm, action, vitality, alertness, movement, striving, problem-solving, inventiveness, decisiveness, openness to change	Stability, reliability, persistence, loyalty, steadfastness, constancy, commitment, sleep, ease, patience, restfulness, stillness
Moderate Expressions	Order, cleanliness, health, self-restraint, contentment, humility, fearlessness, happiness, intellect	Activism, passion, ambition, arrogance, competitiveness, agitation, obsession, struggle	Indecisiveness, confusion, apathy, procrastination, fear, irrationality, grief, deceit, depression
Negative Expressions	Self-satisfaction, conceit, complacency - these are limited in negativity, as all actions are motivated by spiritual awareness and basic goodness; flightiness, spiritual bypassing	Craving, hoarding, anger, desire, contempt, proneness to variable emotions/moods, greed, mania, phobia, worry, anxiety, non-reflection, impulsivity, aggression, ruthlessness	Inertia, obliviousness, lethargy, dullness, idleness, disease or unease, sluggishness, quiet anger, harshness, violence, depression, resistance, torpor, lack of initiative

Overview of the Gunas – Fundamental Human Ways of Being in the World			
	Sattva	**Rajas**	**Tamas**
Stress Response	SOCIAL ENGAGEMENT→ Associated stress response with this nature is social connection, non-alarm state, and maintaining a sense of security and calmness	MOBILIZATION→ Stress response associated with this nervous system style or nature is fight or flight, taking defensive action	IMMOBILIZATION→ Stress response associated with this nervous system defense or nature is shut-down or collapse (freeze and submit) in self-protection
Relationship to Polyvagal Theory	Associated with the ventral branch of the parasympathetic nervous system; a stance of perceived safety leading to social engagement, resilience, ability to downregulate, and action commensurate with need and context; puts the brakes on sympathetic arousal	Associated with sympathetic nervous system arousal; a self-protective style in which the individual tends to expect danger, living in a near-constant state of sympathetic arousal, isolation, and physiological overload or break-down	Associated with the dorsal vagal branch of the parasympathetic nervous system; self-protective style in which individuals expect life threat and develop a habitual pattern of shrinking back from life – associated with trauma events or complex trauma experiences if predominant
Nervous System Regulation	Ventral innervation pathways include the face, throat, and upper chest (to activate muscles of social connection and engagement); associated with adaptive regulation of the nervous system and allostasis and homeostasis; capacity to be socially engaged, to grow and restore, and adapt, grow and evolve – the embodiment of resilience	Sympathetic innervation pathways are distributed along the spinal cord (to activate all muscles necessary for fight or flight); associated with hyperarousal of the nervous system and with mobilization or activation (readiness for action); useful manifestations are the capacity to act in response to threat; the capacity to respond to life challenges	Dorsal innervation pathways include the heart, diaphragm, and viscera (to bring neuroceptive and activate only body areas necessary for immediate survival); associated with nervous system hypoarousal and immobilization; useful manifestations are the capacity to pause to restore, the ability to feel grounded and steady, a willingness to persist

Rajas in Yoga Psychology

A possible translation is motion; *passion or energy* versus *drivenness or greed.*
- Kinetic quality, facilitating change, evolution, and enthusiasm; unhealthy expression may be craving or hyperactivity
- Self-protective style in which the individual tends to expect danger, living in a near-constant state of sympathetic arousal, isolation, and physiological overload or break-down; linked to the sympathetic branch of the autonomic nervous system (sympathetic nervous system)

- Sympathetic innervation pathways are distributed along the spinal cord (to activate all muscles necessary for fight or flight)
- Associated with hyperarousal of the nervous system and with mobilization or activation (readiness for action)
- Stress response associated with this nervous system style or nature is fight or flight
- Useful manifestations are the capacity to act in response to threat, the capacity to respond to life challenges
- Possible challenging manifestations may include phobia, worry, anxiety, mania, addiction

Tamas in Yoga Psychology

A possible translation is mass; *grounding or stability* versus *lethargy or withdrawal.*
- Property of persistence, facilitating steadiness and stillness; unhealthy expression may be couch-potato syndrome or indecisiveness
- Self-protective style in which the individual expects life threats and develops a habitual pattern of shrinking back from life, withdrawing – even dissociating – from human experiences
- Linked to the dorsal vagal aspect of the parasympathetic branch of the autonomic nervous system (dorsal vagal, parasympathetic nervous system) – can be associated with trauma events or complex trauma experiences if this is the predominant response style of the individual
- Dorsal innervation pathways include the heart, diaphragm, and viscera (to bring us input from the inside about our state of alertness and to activate only those body areas that are necessary for immediate survival)
- Associated with hypoarousal of the nervous system and with physical immobilization
- Stress response associated with this nervous system defense or nature is shut-down or collapse (freeze and submit)
- Useful manifestations are the capacity to pause to restore, the ability to feel grounded and steady, a willingness to persist
- Possible challenging manifestations may include emotional numbness, mental spaciness, depression, dissociation, derealization

Sattva in Yoga Psychology

A possible translation is wholism or wholesomeness; *radiance or harmony* versus *flightiness.*
- Integrated quality that facilitates self-knowledge, purity, peace, and balance; unhealthy expression may be fantasy or spaciness
- Sattva integrates the best of both tamas and rajas to result in wise action
- Interactive self-protective style in which the individual tends to perceive safety, living more commonly in a relaxed, socially engaged, and restorative ventral vagal space; linked to the ventral vagal aspect of the parasympathetic branch of the autonomic nervous system
- Ventral innervation pathways include the face, throat, and upper chest (to activate muscles of social connection and engagement)
- Associated with adaptive regulation of the nervous system and allostasis and homeostasis

- Stress response associated with this nervous system style or nature is social connection, non-alarm state, and maintaining a sense of security and calmness
- Useful manifestations are the capacity to be socially engaged, to grow and restore, and adapt, grow and evolve
- Possible challenging manifestations may include flightiness or spiritual bypassing (pretending to be fine when one is not)
- Yoga helps us recognize when we have moved out of sattva, out of our ventral vagal space, and into *rajas* or *tamas*; then we learn how to re-regulate from hypo- or hyperarousal to a steady state of non-alarm and regulation; we find the balance between heroic effort and defeated surrender

Most of us are neither pure *rajas*, *tamas*, or *sattva*. Instead, most of us have mixed traits, with one temperament being predominant and somewhat tempered by the other two *gunas*. Pure *sattva* is a desirable operating system, but is very rare indeed. Only advanced yogis or enlightened beings can maintain the wise and mindful presences of harmony, reflection, compassion, and love at all times. Most of us have brief moments of *sattva*, and many moments of rajas or tamas. *Rajas* and *tamas* in and of themselves are not negative traits or temperaments. They become challenging only if they do not balance each other to some degree or if they occur without the illuminating influence of sattva. Pure rajasic temperament can lead to burnout, being driven, being overly competitive and ambitious and can create a way of being in the world that reflects greed and craving rather than compassion and generosity. Pure tamasic energy, on the other hand, is sluggish, with little drive to create something new and leads to diseases of excess (such obesity, cancer, or metabolic syndrome). It is also associated with a sense of deprivation and lack that leads to depression as well as being a dark energy for those who interact with the tamasic individual.

Gunas Interacting with Koshas

For integration across the five *koshas* to become a healthful and happy reality, the *koshas* each need to be balanced within themselves. The *gunas* are a helpful framework for exploring such balance. As noted above, the *gunas* reflect our primary way of being - a general energetic style, temperament, or default operating system that expresses itself automatically when we are called upon for a reaction or response.

The *gunas* express themselves in every aspect of self, that is, in all koshas. Our physical experience (*annamaya kosha*) can express the *gunas* through the type of physical actions we favor, ranging from rajasic hyperactivity and high-impact exercise to tamasic inactivity and physical laziness. *Gunas* can even express themselves physically at a physiological level, with rajasic individuals having a very fast metabolism that allows them to eat a lot of food without gaining weight versus tamasic individual having a very low metabolism that leads to overweight and associated illnesses. Rajasic individuals are more likely to burn themselves out; tamasic individuals are more likely to suffer from diseases of inactivity, such as heart disease or metabolic syndrome.

Our vital experience (*pranamaya kosha*) can express the *gunas* through the energy and emotions we exude. Rajasic individuals often have a driven and agitated energy that may feel irritating or overwhelming to others. Tamasic individuals, on the other hand, may have a dark energy that can be depressing and off-putting, resulting in lonely lives. The mental self (manomaya kosha) reflects the gunas in terms of openness to new learning, creative thought, and openness to change. Rajasic individuals have quick minds, love to learn, and create new ideas with conviction and ardor. Tamasic individuals are content with few learning opportunities, do not avail themselves of chances for learning, and tend to have some resistance to new ideas.

The intuitive and wise expression of self (*vijnanamaya kosha*) reflects *gunas* in the way individuals interact with the world at a very spontaneous and basic level. Rajasic individuals are naturally passionate and engaged; tamasic individuals are naturally slow to engaged and tend to expect the worst. All *koshas* of sattvic individuals express balance, flexibility, strength, wisdom, basic goodness, and positive, compassionate intention.

	Gunas Expressed in the Koshas		
	Rajas	*Tamas*	*Sattva*
Annamaya Kosha	Restlessness, hyperactivity, speed, high energy, fast metabolism, fast reactions, burnout, drivenness	Lethargy, sluggishness, weakness, inflexibility, lack of endurance, slow metabolism, slow reaction	Ease, flexibility, strength, balance, endurance, health, balanced metabolism, balanced movement, balanced reactions
Pranamaya Kosha	Energy that seeks to accomplish, achieve, and create; energy that exudes passion or agitation	Energy that expresses inertia, slowness, and decay; energy that is dull, dark, and depressive	Energy that reflects and creates balance and purity; energy that is meditative, peaceful, and serene
Manomaya Kosha	Good general knowledge, skepticism; a restless but creative mind; a mind that is preoccupied with desire and wanting	Ignorance, illusion; a dull, lazy, uninformed, and fickle mind; a mind that is preoccupied with rejection and resistance	Discerning knowledge, illumination; a peaceful, serene, stable mind; an open mind that is accepting and understanding
Vijnanamaya Kosha	Naturally passionate, pleasure-seeking, and engaged; guided by a basic fondness for goal-oriented and productive activity	Naturally inclined toward restful pursuits and settledness; guided by a basic fondness for recuperation and rest; able to slow down	Naturally devoted, compassionate, loving, calm, and spiritual; guided by fondness for wisdom, compassion, and learning
Anandamaya Kosha	Creativity and vitality as expressions of joy and compassion	Loyalty and patience as expressions of love and connection	Connection, love, joy, bliss, compassion, equanimity, spirituality

Gunas in Nature and the Environment

Gunas do not just express themselves through human beings. *Gunas* are inherent in nature; everything in nature is endowed with energy and this energy affects us directly. External stimuli, such as food or weather, have a temperament or primary style in and of themselves (i.e., are sattvic, rajasic or tamasic). Everything we perceive, stimulates our senses and creates energy within us. For example, wind has a rajasic energy that is active, wild, and restless. A dry, hot day at noon can feel oppressive and has a tamasic energy that leads to idleness and stillness. A fiery sunset can be rajasic, while a warm sunrise can be tamasic or sattvic. A dark, moonless night has a tamasic, dark effect; a bright, cool sunny day with a mild breeze can be sattvic. A dark snowy day in winter with low light is tamasic, whereas a spring day with a blue sky and fresh snow is sattvic.

Even the atmosphere we create in our homes will express the *gunas* to varying degrees. A home in which there is constant noise and activity from TVs, radios, video games, a steady coming-and-going without time for shared meals is clearly rajasic and less than peaceful. A home where windows are always closed, rooms are small and dark, furnishings are large and heavy, or décor is large and cluttered will have a tamasic and downward energy. On the other hand, a home that is light and bright, has fresh flowers and live plants, open windows, wide views or beautiful artwork, little clutter, and warm colors will exude sattva and will uplift its inhabitants.

Even food and how we eat can be classified according to the *gunas*. Rajasic foods are spicy and exciting to the palate. They stimulate the appetite and the senses and may overwhelm. Tamasic foods, on the other hand, reflect a heaviness that derives either from the consistency, age, or source of the food. Foods that resulted from aggression or violence toward a sentient being (e.g., slaughterhouse meat) is considered tamasic. Heavy foods, such as whole-fat milk, ice cream, French fries, or cakes are equally dulling and tamasic. Any food that is old, stale, and over-ripe has tamasic properties. Sattvic foods are those that are derived healthfully from nature, such as fresh fruits, luscious salads, sprouts, or nuts. No matter what the food, if we eat it too fast, we create rajas. If we eat too much, we create tamas. More examples of how the *gunas* are expressed in nature and our surroundings are shown in the table that follows.

	Gunas Expressed in Nature and the Environment		
	Rajas	*Tamas*	*Sattva*
Foods	Stimulating, energizing, excitatory foods, including such foods as onions, garlic, and hot peppers; pungent spices; spicy, bitter, sour, acidic, hot, dry, or fried food; caffeinated food or drink; fast food; prescription drugs; sugary food or drink	Heavy and enervating foods such as meats, dairy, and junk foods; alcohol; stale, over-ripe, decaying, or spoiled food; overcooked food; processed, packaged, canned, or reheated food; food laden with pesticides or preservatives	Well-balanced diet with wholesome foods; mainly fruits and vegetables, water, herbal teas, sprouted or whole grains and legumes, nuts; fresh, juicy, simple, light, easy-to-digest, close-to-nature, nourishing food; organically grown food

Gunas Expressed in Nature and the Environment			
	Rajas	*Tamas*	*Sattva*
Eating Style	Eating too fast; eating without attention; eating at one's desk, while working; eating in a rush without really tasting	Overeating; eating to self-soothe or self-medicate; unconsciously overeating or constant snacking	Eating mindfully; eating with gratitude; eating with gratitude and appreciation; fully attuned to food's flavor
Home Environments	Noisy, lots of artificial light, constant activity and a sense of hectic, 'loud' colors, constant running of TVs or radios; no time for shared meals or joint activities; disorganization	Dark colors, clutter or hoarding, lack of natural light; stale air, high humidity, or hot dry air; ; lifeless; no common space for family togetherness; closed windows	Natural light, quietude or soothing sounds (e.g., fountain, classical music), living house plants, calming colors, mindful floor plan that encourages connection, uncluttered
Colors and Light	Red; bright or loud colors; neon colors; bright artificial lights; perpetual or very bright sunlight	Black; dark or dull colors; dreary colors or lights; arctic "day"light in winter; lack of sunlight	Bright yellow or white; soft or natural colors; adequate natural daylight; well-lit balanced light at home
Hobbies or Activities	High-speed or high-violence sports; heavy exercise or hot exercise; frantic or noisy video games; shopping without real purpose; loud music; noisy restaurants or bars that interfere with conversation	Sitting in front of the television without purpose or attention; drinking or taking drugs; frequent napping or sleeping late; watching violent movies or soaps; activities that tune out or turn off	Hiking in beauty, beach walking, going to a park, cooking healthful food, reading peaceful books, volunteering, yoga, visiting a farmer's market, spending meaningful time with friends
Relationships	Distrustful, confrontational, conflictual, argumentative, belligerent, superficial, transactional, demanding	Symbiotic, co-dependent, controlling, manipulative, oppressive, judgmental, habitual or unchanging, non-nurturing	Equal partners, respectful, honest, clear, open, kind, compassionate, sharing, ever-evolving, nurturing mutuality
Neighborhoods	Inner cities with lots of noise and activity where there are always lights and sounds that distract or arouse or even frighten	Neighborhoods that are dark, dirty, and dank with high rates of crime where people are disconnected and fearful; threat of crime	Clean neighborhoods with peaceful gardens, open spaces, tranquility, and human connection; access to natural and beautiful spaces, art
Work Environment	Hectic, full of deadlines, driven, competitive, angry, hostile, harmful, dangerous, cut-throat, controlled or controlling with lots of stress and overpowering responsibility	Boring, dull, senseless, violent, dealing with death, isolating, passively harmful to self or others, lots of stress without agency or control over the situation, paralyzing	Collaborative, team spirited, for a higher/good purpose, meaningful, caring, positive, with stress and commensurate means for resilience and problem-solving

Gunas Expressed in Nature and the Environment			
	Rajas	*Tamas*	*Sattva*
Animals and Pets	Monkeys, cats, dogs, lions, eagles	Spiders, bats, snakes, snails, lizards, sloths	Cows, elephants, deer, swans, tortoises, whales
Weather or Climate	High and turbulent wind; hurricanes or tornadoes; thunderstorms; rainstorms with flooding; hail storms; arctic summers with endless daylight; cool, windy island climates with constant ocean breezes; river ice breaking up at spring time	Rainy, damp, humid weather; very still (maybe even stale) air; snow and ice; arctic winter climates with perpetual ice and snow; very hot summer days; climates with oppressive heat and humidity; little movement of air without a sense of freshness	Warm sunlight with adequate humidity; bright, warm days with mild airflow; temperate or balanced climates with natural cool-warm cycles; warm spring days with returning sun and moist air; perfect fall days with sunshine and morning dew
Nature	All expressions of fire; volcanoes, raging rivers, chaotic or fast waterfalls, hot springs, craggy rocks, towering mountains, choppy ocean waves or high surf, spiny cacti	All expressions of darkness; deep forests, dark canyons, stagnant ponds, damp caves, decaying leaves, dying vegetation, barren fields, dry meadows or creek beds	All expressions of light; open meadows, clear rivers, blue lakes with clear water, new spring growth, blossoming trees, gentle mountains, beautiful sunsets, tranquil oceans

When we encounter and perceive (take in) external expressions of the *gunas* through food, weather, nature, work requirements, music, plants, animals, or other people, we react to these energies. Our reaction reflects not only the guna of the external stimulus, but its interaction with our own primary energetic style. If a rajasic individual is placed into a home environment that is chaotic, noisy, and overstimulating, the person will become overburdened and even more driven or hectic. The same person placed into a calm house with live plants and soothing music will have a chance to counter the innate rajasic nature and will become more balanced and sattvic. Balancing the gunas, then, is an important endeavor and can take advantage of the expression of the various gunas in nature in general.

Finding balance is not the same as finding perfection, flawlessness, or completeness at all times. Finding balance does not even mean being pain-free. Balance is a flexible concept that is more about the intention that underlies it than the moment-to-moment expression. As humans, we will not be perfect at all times; we can simply hold the intention in our heart to be compassionate, luminous, kind, loving, generous, and committed to our own and everyone's health and happiness. Then we accept that we will fail in this endeavor over and over again, only to resume with commitment our striving toward balance. Balance thus also includes acceptance of and compassion for our failings and transgressions, with a clear commitment not to give up when we fail, but to dedicate ourselves with even greater ardor to trying again and again. There are many ways to balance the gunas and achieving balance is a life-long endeavor. Below are a few examples of interactions and attempts at achieving or failing to achieve balance.

	Examples of Attempts (Successful or Unsuccessful) to Balance the Gunas
Method	*Example*
Balancing rajas with tamas	A busy executive (rajasic temperament) has been trying to keep up with work and home demands by drinking coffee and eating sugary snacks (rajasic food). After a while her adrenals burned out (rajasic disease). Now she balances her hectic work schedule (rajas) with restorative yoga practice in the evening (tamasic exercise), an extra hour of sleep (tamasic self-care), and a cup of warm chamomile tea before bed (tamasic food).
Balancing tamas with rajas	A middle-aged college professor with a laid-back, at times unmotivated, (tamasic) temperament and sluggish metabolism (tamasic physical self) has been skipping breakfast all his life and recently started gaining weight and was diagnosed with metabolic syndrome (tamasic disease). He has begun to get up a little earlier every day to take a brisk walk before work (mildly rajasic exercise) and then has a breakfast that includes a cup of coffee (rajasic food). He now also listens to energizing music (rajasic hobby) on his way to work and has started to exercise in the afternoon with a colleague who is an avid racquetball player (rajasic exercise).
Balancing rajas with sattva	A 10-year-old boy with an active (rajasic) temperament was called hyperactive and attention-disordered by a teacher (rajasic disorders). He got up early each day, watching TV before school and playing video games (rajasic activities) while eating a breakfast of sugary cereal and chocolate milk (rajasic food). After school, he played soccer (rajasic sport) and more video games. He went to bed late (rajasic sleep cycle), after watching TV. Instead of placing the child on Ritalin as recommended by his physician, his parents changed his lifestyle and diet. They developed a new bedtime structure that allowed for at least eight hours of sleep (sattvic sleep cycle). They limited TV and video time in favor of time outdoors, joining his dad with bird-watching once a week, and volunteering with his mom at a homeless shelter every weekend (sattvic activities). They changed his diet to include more fresh fruits and vegetables, along with unsweetened goat dairy and sprouted grain breads (sattvic foods). They limited soccer to twice weekly and added yoga (sattvic sport) and gardening chores (sattvic hobby).
Balancing tamas with sattva	A 6-year-old girl was referred for assessment for depression (tamasic disorder). She spent her non-school time drawing and cuddling (tamasic activities) with her depressed single mother. She often overslept (tamasic sleep cycle) and came to school late or missed it altogether. She ate poorly, often no breakfast at all, and only prepared and packaged foods like TV dinners, soup or tuna from a can, and ice cream (tamasic foods). She was overweight (tamasic physical state) and unmotivated, spent no time outdoors and had few friends. With the help of a parent educator and a school counselor, the family made many changes, including putting in a garden (sattvic activity), getting help with creating dietary changes to include fresh fruits and vegetable and freshly prepared meals (sattvic foods). They enrolled the girl in swimming classes and bought her a bicycle, teaching her how to ride (sattvic sports). They hired a babysitter who took her for beach walks, going tide pooling and playing in the sand (sattvic play).
Burning out rajas with more rajas	A stressed-out graduate student holds down a part-time job, while engaging in a demanding course of study in chemistry. They keep up with all their work requirements, make sure to hand in all assignments by their deadline, never miss a beat on work or academia. To balance their stressful work and academic life, they have decided to run three miles every morning as a way of clearing their mind by moving their body. In the evenings, they attempt to remain active in their social circle, attending and hosting functions and get-togethers as often as their work and graduate school schedule allows. One Sunday morning, they woke to a racing heart, sweaty palms, extreme anxiety, and hyperventilation. (rajas, rajas, rajas, leading to illness of imbalance)

Examples of Attempts (Successful or Unsuccessful) to Balance the Gunas	
Method	*Example*
Collapsing tamas with more tamas	A 21-year-old college student with a profound history of adverse childhood experiences is having a hard time keeping up with their college studies and has become socially withdrawn and isolated. They have begun to attempt to stay out of severe state of depression for several weeks by using rest, staying home and saying no to all social invitations. They have also found that they feel more settled if the nurture themselves with comfort foods, heavy on take-out and ready-made meals, left-overs, and sweets, especially ice-cream.
Encouraging the expression of sattva	A family of four, with a 15-year-old boy and 10-year-old twin girls, was having a hard time developing a healthful family rhythm. The mother was working full-time as floor manager of a manufacturing plants in charge of over 50 employees (rajasic employment), and when home tended to all chores and responsibilities in the household and yard (rajasic home life). The father was unemployed, depressed, and withdrawn. The son was in a heavy metal band (rajasic music), played football (rajasic sport), ran with a rough crowd (rajasic peers), and was starting to experiment with drugs (rajasic influence). The twins were very focused on each other, playing for hours quietly in their room (tamasic play), avoiding others, and rarely interacting with their brother (tamasic relationships). They were withdrawn and quiet (tamasic temperament), with few interests in anything involving the outdoors. Their favorite pastime was reading (sattvic leisure activity). The family rarely had meals together, with mom and son eating on the run and the girls fending for themselves for breakfast and eating whatever fast food (rajasic food) mom brought home after work, often in front of the TV. The son rarely ate at home, generally eating on the run between activities (rajasic eating). Realizing the risk for their son to develop an addiction (rajasic drug use and lifestyle) and their daughters to develop social isolation or even depression, the family decided to make major lifestyle changes. The dad agreed to begin to prepare a healthful breakfast for the family, which they ate together. The girls were enrolled in a skating class and an after-school program that was focused on helping children volunteer in their communities.

Given the concept of balancing the *gunas* and expressing who we really are, balance in the five *koshas* is neither tied to achieving *perfection* nor to achieving health and happiness in the conventional sense. For example, balance in our physical self expresses itself in optimum strength, flexibility, balance and stamina given the physical realities within which we exist. In other words, the balance we achieve in the physical realm is predicated and measured on the physical realities we face. A measure of strength is not equal for all - we have different body shapes, sizes and capacities. We develop balanced strength not in comparison to someone else's body, we develop the optimum strength that is appropriate for the body with which we were born. Developing our strength beyond that limit will likely make our body inflexible. The same holds true for flexibility, stamina, or any other physical self-expression. We appreciate and develop our physical being within the parameters of the physical reality we are given, not pushing painfully past our boundaries (*rajas*) but also not stopping short of them (*tamas*).

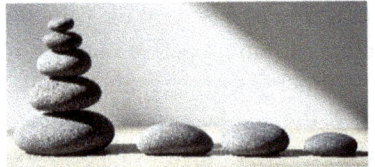

We will return to the concept of individualized sattvic expression in detail below. For now, it is simply important to understand that balance builds from the outside in and that creating balance in one aspect of self helps build balance in the others. Yoga psychology suggests that:
- Once the body is balanced (optimally strong, flexible, and so forth given our personal reality - but not necessarily always pain-free or without limitations), breath can be accessed
- Once the breath is balanced (optimally regulated, calm, rhythmic and so forth given our personal reality - but not necessarily always perfect or without restrictions), mind can be accessed
- Once the mind is balanced (optimally relaxed, discerning, accepting, and so forth given our personal reality - but not necessarily always completely still or without judgment), wisdom can be accessed
- Once wisdom is balanced (optimally peaceful, nonattached, knowing, and so forth given our personal reality - but not necessarily always in the present moment or without habitual reactions), spirit can be accessed
- Once bliss is balanced (optimally joyful, compassionate, loving, and so forth given our personal reality), truth (i.e., health and happiness) can be accessed

Gunas in the Context of Polyvagal Theory

Neuroscience research has revealed how ancient yoga texts are closely aligned to our modern understanding of the mammalian nervous system. This research provides us a modern understanding or interpretation of yogic principles. One recent neuroscience theory that is extremely helpful in understanding the *gunas* is polyvagal theory developed by Steven Porges (Porges, 2009, 2011, 2017). Following is a brief overview of polyvagal theory, followed by its application to, and integration with, the yogic principles of *gunas*.

Polyvagal theory (PVT) came to life in the 1990s based on Porges' groundbreaking research that updated scientific thought about how humans react and adapt to environmental inputs and stressors. Prior to PVT, it was thought that humans had **two** hardwired autonomic nervous system (ANS) branches and types of responses to ensure personal and species survival:
- Parasympathetic *rest-and-digest* (also called breed-and-feed) response
- Sympathetic *fight-or-flight* reaction

These two branches of the ANS were shown to work together to help humans achieve allostasis and homeostasis – the capacity to adapt to changing environmental demands in a sufficiently adaptive manner (allostasis) and to return to a state of balance (homeostasis). The sympathetic nervous system typically takes over when fast reactions are needed for the safety (i.e., physical survival) of the organism, mobilizing the organism into action and initiating the infamous "*fight-or-flight*" reaction in response to stress. The sympathetic nervous system activates skeletal muscles in preparation for mobilization. The parasympathetic nervous system comes into play when fight-or-flight mobilization is not needed. It allows the organism to lower its defenses, regain a state of calm, and return to the business of being a thriving organism, prepared to "*rest and digest*", "*feed and breed*", heal and rejuvenate, and connect and stay safe.

The vagus nerve is responsible for mediating nervous systems responses, being the nerve that is responsible for activating the parasympathetic nervous system response by inhibiting (via the vagal brake) the sympathetic nervous system response. With Porges' research on the vagus nerve, the understanding of the autonomic nervous system, especially its parasympathetic branch, expanded, became more complex, and became *less reciprocal* (or mutually exclusive) and *more interactive and integrated*. The primary nerve that transmits and organizes signals within the autonomic nervous system is the vagus nerve (i.e., the 10th cranial nerve). It innervates all major organs, the only cranial nerve that reaches (or wanders) this far into the body (the others being mostly focused on the neck and head, especially the face). The vagus nerve is an integral aspect of the ANS – the part of the human nervous system that functions outside our conscious control to surveil and regulate bodily functions such as breathing, heart rate, and arousal. The vagus nerve has afferent and efferent fibers, with fibers dominating that bring sensory signals to the brain. In fact, 80% of the information conveyed by the vagus nerve is sensory information coming from the body and being carried to the brain.

The vagus nerve thus is our body's surveillance (or appraisal) system, an unconscious, subcortical process relying on implicit memory and procedural memory to assess or appraise any and all situations we find ourselves in at all times and readying us for an action-based response. The vagus nerve collects and sends (from the bottom up) sensory signals from within the body, endocrine release, and other internal and external signals of environmental threat or danger (e.g., sensory information coming from the outwardly-oriented senses that provide input about others' facial expressions, gestures, voice quality, and actions). This information (collected and conveyed to the brainstem by the vagus nerve) is the foundation of what Porges calls *neuroception* – the ability to read our internal physiological reactions, along with exteroceptive inputs, translate them into an assessment of our sense of safety, and react to them quickly and efficiently to mitigate possible dangers or threats to life or safety. All of this happens outside of our conscious awareness or control, being based in our pre- or subconscious and not mediated by conscious cognition.

Porges' work revealed that the vagus nerve has two distinct branches that surveil and regulate the parasympathetic nervous system, resulting in two profoundly different ways to cool down (or put the brakes on) the sympathetic nervous system response of mobilization (i.e., fight-or-flight) or to help us exist and stay safe in the world. These two separate and distinct, yet interactive and integrated, branches are the dorsal vagal (DVC) and ventral vagal (VVC) complexes. Both originate in the parasympathetic branch of the nervous system; yet, they mediate intensely different responses to inner visceral and outer environmental sensations, inputs, or stimuli.

The *dorsal branch of the vagus* nerve responds to perceptions of extreme danger and life threat, and results in immobilization (e.g., playing dead, fainting, dissociating, or shutting down behaviorally and/or emotionally). This branch of the vagus nerve is very ancient and can be seen very readily in the behaviors of reptiles who are under life threat. It is linked to sensory nerves below the diaphragm and hence relates to visceral responses.

The *ventral branch of the vagus* nerve responds to perceptions of safety and results in prosocial behavior. Through increased neural complexity first noted phylogenetically in mammals, the ventral branch of the vagus nerve evolved a *social engagement system* (Porges, 2009). It is linked to the sensory nerves above the diaphragm and, as such, is associated with the heart and hypothalamus-pituitary-adrenal (HPA) axis. The social engagement system facilitates prosocial behavior, verbal and nonverbal communication, and adaptive emotional responses to occurrences around us and inside of us. In humans, this profound social connection and embeddedness, coupled with complex reasoning ability and multifaceted brain power, likely paved the way to the development of human culture, language, technology, politics – and sadly to the human assertion of power over other creatures and the planet.

Neuroception of sensory inputs from the environment and visceral inputs about our internal state can result in three basic perceptions of what is happening: *safety*, *danger*, or *life threat* (terror). Based on the types of stimuli received via neuroception and their lightning-fast, unconscious interpretation as indicating either safety, danger, or threat, the autonomic nervous system activates either the sympathetic branch (danger) or the ventral vagal (safety) or dorsal vagal branch (life threat) of the parasympathetic nervous system. This ANS activation, regardless of branch, affects, alters, and adapts all organ systems to be prepared for the most appropriate response given the incoming stimuli. These effects are particularly notable in the respiratory, cardiovascular/circulatory, endocrine, musculoskeletal, and gastrointestinal systems, as well as in voice, hearing, and metabolism.

Neuroception of Safety

Neuroception of *safety* activates the *ventral vagal complex of social engagement*. The social engagement system ties us to one another. When we are in a ventral vagal state of safety and connection, the vagus nerve literally connects us to the physiology above the diaphragm, especially the region of our faces. We become attuned to one another's facial cues, nonverbal communication, tone of voice, expressiveness of the eyes, and meaning of gestures. We are attuned to human voices and tune out auditory ranges of lower sounds. When we are in a ventral vagal state, we are in a state of co-regulation – or natural habitat. We are evolved to be embedded in an interpersonal matrix, a connected web of life. Infants need parenting, community, embeddedness. Only when they internalize a sense of trust and safety, can human children move out and explore their world increasingly freely – with periods of rapprochement to reconnect and refill their tank of human connection.

Neuroception of safety results in physiological recovery, emotional processing and interoception, mental regulation, and prosocial behavior (including socially engaging voice and facial expressions, and relaxed posture). The breath is soft and gentle, heart rate and blood pressure are calm and within typical limits for the individual, digestion is chugging along, endocrine hormones for social engagement are released (e.g., oxytocin), facial muscles relax, the voice is melodic and has the prosody of relaxation, and hearing is optimally attuned to human voices. We relax into contact with other human beings, ready for conversation, connection, interaction, collaboration, even playfulness and shared joy.
- The ventral vagal state is our wholesome, restorative, and resilient way of being in the world. It is our coping state that allows us to create relationships and to stay connected.
- When we are in a ventral vagal space, we are open-hearted, ready to communicate, non-defensive, and emotionally balanced. We are ready to be in relationship and to give and receive love, kindness, and compassion. We can engage in easy conversation, relax in the presence of others, and enjoy our connection to our community. We are ready to play and have fun. We sense into our connectedness, our interdependence.

- When we are in our ventral vagal space, the vagus nerve puts the brakes on the sympathetic nervous system, communicating safety and no need to rev up our heart rate, increase respiration, or prepare skeletal muscles for fight or flight. The vagal brake on the SNS leads to optimal opportunities for developing and maintaining health, cultivating resilience, facilitating growth, supporting restoration and regeneration, and sustaining healing.
- However, because life has challenges and ups and down, none of us ever stays in a ventral vagal state forever. We move to other states as needed when the environment or relationships throw us a curve. However, if all goes well, we return to the ventral vagal space when the crisis has resolved.

Neuroception of Danger

Neuroception of *danger* releases the vagal brake (moving us out of the ventral vagal state of social engagement) and activates the sympathetic nervous system, mobilizing a fight-or-flight response to increase likelihood of survival. In other words, if arousal increases due to increased perception of danger of challenge, our VVC response may transform – our vagal brake loosens its grip on the SNS. Playfulness may turn more aggressive, dance may turn into preparation for a show of strength and fierceness, and collaboration may turn into competition. We shift our focus of attunement; our attention turns to different aspects of our experience – away from faces and eyes; away from hearing human voices. We move into auditory hypersensitivity for sound ranges of potential danger (e.g., a tiger's low growl) and away from being able to hear human voices.

Release of the vagal brake on the SNS results in increased muscle tone, redirection of blood flow from the periphery to the core, inhibition of the gastrointestinal system, dilation of the bronchi, and increased heart rate and respiration (among other physiological responses) to ready the organism for a vigorous, proactive survival response. Breath and heart rate increase, skeletal muscles tense in readiness for action, digestion is turned down or off, stress hormones are released (e.g., cortisol), the voice becomes hard and threatening or insistent and alarming (to relay perception of stress to others), and hearing shifts to optimize the reception of extremely high and low sounds of threat (shifting away from optimal perception of human voices).

- When we are in an acute sympathetic state, we see the world as dangerous and are more likely to interpret the actions of others as aggressive or threatening. Given this perspective, we are preparing to fight and defend ourselves, our loved ones, and our tribe. If we cannot defend successfully, we are ready to flee to escape our dangerous circumstances. We lose our social connection beyond our tribe and lose our willingness to negotiate or talk with those to whom we do not feel we belong. We are less interested in communicating to resolve conflict; we are ready to pounce and defend instead. We are in survival mode and care more about our own and our tribe's survival than the wellbeing of others who are seen as a potential threat or danger. This reactivity sets up a vicious cycle of potential interpersonal disconnection, even violence. We threaten, express rage and anger, we defend and fight; we scream, and stop listening; we become physically threatening or aggressive – all actions that only serve to bring others into their own sympathetic nervous system response.
- When we are in a chronic state of hyperarousal (as many of us are due to ongoing chronic stress or perception of stress), over time, our physical and emotional health becomes compromised. Because we cannot seem to get back to the ventral vagal space, our blood pressure may stay chronically high; our digestion may start to fail and our gut flora might

suffer; we may always be on alert or prone to anxiety and excessive worry; we might resort to drugs or alcohol to try to calm our nerves; we are always on alert and ready for action and self-defense. In time, our adrenals may wear out and we lose energy and start to feel worn out and unable to cope. We want to muster our resources to stay in the fight, but we cannot do it anymore. We burn out; we lose our resilience – our ability to bounce back.
- Only if the threat or danger is neutralized (by whatever means, including having received help from someone) can we return to a ventral vagal state, put the (vagal) brakes on the SNS reactivity, and return to a neutral and socially connected state.

Neuroception of Life Threat

Neuroception of *life threat* activates the dorsal vagal complex of immobilization. The sense of terror it instills results in shutting down, freezing, or "playing dead"; decreased muscle tone and decreased cardiac output; reflexive defecation and urination; and other physiological responses that reduce life functions to the least amount needed for survival. This nervous system state is a profound departure from our natural evolution as co-regulators. In an extreme dorsal vagal state, we disconnect from co-regulation, from one of the most basic traits of what it means to be human (or a mammal). It is much harder to reemerge from dorsal vagal collapse or immobilization than from sympathetic arousal. It is important to remember that we do not consciously choose the nervous system state that is activated in response to neuroception.

Neuroception is unconscious and non-cognitive, rooted in implicit memory – the same is true for our response (reaction, rooted in procedural memory). Moving into a dorsal vagal state is as much (or even more so) a survival or self-protective mechanism as is the movement into a sympathetic state. Evolution has clearly demonstrated the effectiveness of the dorsal vagal collapse and immobilization to self-preservation.
- If a perceived danger cannot be resolved (via fight or flight or social engagement) and turns into a perceived threat to our lives or psychological integrity, *and* we see no solution for escape or potential for supportive and helpful others, we become overwhelmed, feel alone, and shut down – physically, energetically, mentally, emotionally, and relationally.
- When we are in an acute dorsal vagal space, we perceive the world as distant and others as removed, emotionally unavailable, unhelpful, and not supportive our very (physical, affective, mental, or emotional) existence. Given this (unconscious, subcortical, non-cognitive) perspective, we shut down – we are no longer able to or interested in communicating; we have given up on defending ourselves. We have become physically or emotionally immobilized or numb; we cannot muster any resources other than withdrawing, even playing dead (literally or figuratively) to try to save ourselves.
- When we have experienced significant or complex trauma, we may move into faulty neuroception of life threat when there is none. From this neural platform, we begin to live in a chronic dorsal vagal state. Because we cannot return to the ventral vagal space of human connection and trust, we develop emotional difficulties and a myriad of physical challenges, even illness.
- Physical challenges arise related to the shut-down of physiological processes and negatively affect our immune system, digestion, cardiovascular health, even sleep hygiene.
- Emotional distress takes us out of supportive relationships. We expect to be re-traumatized and hurt. We may develop pains and aches that keep us inactive and disengaged from life; we

may lose our drive to create a better life; we might give up on feeling connected again. We may move through life in a depressed and defeated way. We may even become suicidal.
- Only if the threat to our life or psychological integrity is neutralized (by whatever means, including having received help from someone or having been able to mount an escape after all) can we return to a ventral vagal state, reconnect to others, and return to a state of wellness and ability to heal and recover. More often than not, escape from dorsal vagal collapse occurs through sympathetic arousal (as opposed to movement into social connection). We regain the capacity to fight; from there, if successful, we might move into social connection.

Mixed Polyvagal States and Gunas

Ventral vagal, sympathetic, and dorsal vagal responses can show up in their pure form; however, perhaps more commonly, they interact. The three branches of the ANS are not mutually exclusive; rather, they are balanced with one another, allowing for smooth transitions from one to the other, as well as allowing for a mixture of polyvagal states. To understand this, it is important to remember that the autonomic nervous system overall is not a system of defense – it is a **system of allostasis and homeostasis**. It is a system that evolved to maintain our health, restore our functioning after disruption, facilitate growth and regeneration, and support wellbeing. Mounting a sympathetic nervous system response in a defensive state is therefore different from mounting a sympathetic nervous system response in a socially engaged state. Identically, collapsing into a withdrawn and distant dorsal vagal state in a moment of self-protection against life threat is not the same as moving toward dorsal vagal quietude and inhibition of movement while also remaining socially engaged.

There are pure states of SNS – these serve defensive or self-protective functions – and mixed states of SNS arousal that happen within a context of social engagement. Mixed SNS/VVC states are what we enter into during competitive sports, vigorous (especially movement-based) play, and moments of interpersonal assertiveness. There are pure states of DVC – serving a last-ditch self-protective function – and mixed states of dorsal withdrawal and quietude in a context of social engagement. Mixed DVC/VVC states are what we enter during moments of physical stillness of intimacy (e.g., nursing a baby, cuddling with a loved one) or in moments of deep relaxation, such as in meditation or contemplative yoga practices. There are even mixed states of SNS/DVC. This mixture of nervous system states can serve as a final attempt at creating safety or as a way of releasing from dorsal vagal collapse and returning outward. A summary of the three pure states (VVC, SNS, DVC) and several mixed states is shown in the table that follows.

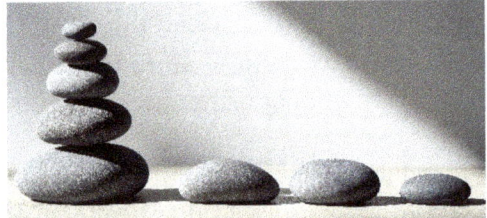

The Many Polyvagal States – Our Physiology of Safety
(with gratitude to Stephen Porges as experienced in workshop environments)

- **Pure VVC → Perception of safety**: live in a socially engaged parasympathetic nervous system; relaxed, engaging, and restorative (myelinated) ventral vagal space – SOCIAL ENGAGEMENT

- **VVC + SNS → Perception of the need for safe and interpersonally engaged action with mobilization** in the service of personal or collective growth, health, competition, and play (especially play involving physical movement); sympathetic arousal that is slightly downregulated and accompanied by the desire or need for social engagement; assertiveness (as opposed to aggressiveness) that leaves open a door for collaboration – PREPAREDNESS, PLAY

- **SNS + VVC → Perception of the need for safe and interpersonally engaged action with mobilization** in the service of assertive (as opposed to aggressive) self-defense, self-protection, or defense and protection of loved ones or one's community; this assertiveness leaves open a door for collaboration and negotiation; emotions stay regulated and manageable; opportunity remain for finding peaceful solutions and social reconnection outside of tribe – ASSERTIVENESS

- **Pure SNS → Perception of danger**: prepared for danger, live in a near-constant state of sympathetic arousal, isolation, and physiological overload or breakdown; mobilized sympathetic NS state of fight or flight – MOBILIZATION

- **SNS + DVC → Perception of the need to survive by ceasing mobilization** in service of survival in the face of being overcome; a collapse into a dorsal state with echoes or traces of the urge to flight or flee; an inadvertent effort to ensure physical and psychological survival – FREEZE, SUBMIT

- **DVC + SNS → Perception of the need to survive by increasing mobilization** in service of bringing physical, energetic, mental, emotional, and social engagement functions back on line; active effort to rally resources of the SNS to reemerge from dorsal collapse – RALLYING, HOPE

- **Pure DVC → Perception of life threat**: develop a habitual pattern of shrinking back from life, withdrawing, disengaging – even dissociating – from human experiences and relationships; parasympathetic NS is at an extreme state of withdrawal, of surrender and hopelessness – IMMOBILIZATION

- **DVC + VVC → Perception of the need for safe immobilization without significant active interpersonal engagement** in the service of rejuvenation (e.g., healing from an injury, supporting growth or immunity, regeneration of physical or energetic resources); a dorsal state of calm and of letting go, a state of deep relaxation or surrender as might be experienced in yoga or meditation, a state of concentrated mind with physical immobilization; this nervous system state may be accessed in a solitary or communal setting – RELAXATION, TRANCE

- **VVC + DVC → Perception of the need for safe, trusting and interpersonally engaged immobilization** in the service of prosocial activities (e.g., child birth, nursing, sadness, collapse in laughter); a dorsal state of surrender or relinquishment of control and effort, accompanied by strong human connection and engagement – INTIMACY, SHARED STILLNESS

Neuroception and Autonomic Reactivity as Related to Rajas, Tamas, and Sattva

The gunas are mediated by the branches of the autonomic nervous system or polyvagal system for meeting the world and, as such, are tied into our threat, self-protection, and defense circuits through amygdala activation and reactivity. They may represent our habitual or preferred/conditioned self-protective strategies. These strategies or styles manifest as tendencies from birth and reflect the past and the future in the present moment. They can be aligned with the autonomic nervous system states of sympathetic arousal or parasympathetic arousal – either in the healthful expression of a ventral vagal state or the more challenging expression of a dorsal vagal state.

As such, the gunas can be understood – like our autonomic nervous system (or polyvagal) states – as the basis of vigilance to be prepared for and responsive to life's challenges:
- Scanning the environment for threat, danger, and safety
- Tuning into the need for mobilizing self-protective strategies
- Withdrawing into self-protective strategies of emotional blunting and relational withdrawal, even dissociation
- Moving into profound interpersonal connection with a sense of safety, openness, and joyful engagement with the world

The gunas and polyvagal states may begin to develop and express themselves in utero, but certainly begin to be noticeable by three months of age (when response styles of the infant begin to mirror those of the primary caretakers). They refine and continue to evolve through interactions, experiences, and learning histories over the entire developmental span. Top-down and bottom-up mechanisms are set in place that perpetuate these defensive and self-protective styles and thus can also become the mechanism for change. The gunas manifest in each of the tangible koshas; they begin to fade in vijnanamaya and are transcended in anandamaya.

The gunas and PVT, in combination, support a better understanding of our own and our students' nervous systems, allowing us to adapt yoga practices, especially movement and breathing practices to our nervous system needs (Brems, 2024b; Schwartz, 2024). We can learn to become aware of our reaction and to read our own signals of when we have slipped into SNS, VVC, or DVC. With awareness, we become more knowledgeable about our physiology and what it signals about our nervous system adjustment. We can begin to read ourselves as well as others. Once we recognize our physical, affective, arousal, cognitive, emotional, behavioral, and relational patterns, we can also begin to retrain our nervous system (Sullivan et al., 2018a).

The process of retraining our nervous system and physiology starts most auspiciously with sensing into our body, our energy (i.e., breath), and our affect, along with accessing strategies that engage our ventral vagal complex. Physical embodiment and movement as well as breath work are extremely supportive to resetting the nervous system, to exercising the social engagement system, and to returning into a ventral vagal space. Everyone can access movement or breathing to reset, most easily through shaking and wiggling or through lengthening the exhalations. Even just letting people talk something out can be helpful – especially if they can talk without being interrupted, until their arousal rebalances and their affect neutralizes.

	Overview of the Gunas – Relationship to Polyvagal Theory		
	Rajas – SNS	*Tamas – Dorsal Vagal*	*Sattva – Ventral Vagal*
Stress Response	MOBILIZATION → The stress response associated with this nervous system style or nature is fight or flight, taking defensive or evasive action	IMMOBILIZATION → The stress response associated with this nervous system defense or nature is shut-down or collapse (freeze and submit) in self-protection	SOCIAL ENGAGEMENT → The associated stress response is social connection, non-alarm state, and a sense of security and calmness
Relationship to the Autonomic Nervous System	Associated with sympathetic nervous system arousal; a self-protective style in which the individual tends to expect danger, living in a near-constant state of sympathetic arousal, isolation, and physiological overload or breakdown	Associated with the dorsal vagal branch of the parasympathetic nervous system; self-protective style expecting life threat and develop a habitual pattern of shrinking back from life; associated with trauma events or complex trauma experiences if predominant	Associated with the ventral branch of the parasympathetic nervous system; perceived safety leading to social engagement, resilience, ability to downregulate, and action commensurate with need and context; puts the brakes on sympathetic arousal
Nervous System Regulation	Sympathetic innervation pathways are distributed along the spinal cord (to activate all muscles necessary for fight or flight); associated with hyperarousal of the nervous system and with mobilization or activation (readiness for action); useful manifestations are the capacity to act in response to threat, the capacity to respond to life challenges	Dorsal innervation pathways include the heart, diaphragm, and viscera (to activate only body areas necessary for immediate survival); associated with hypoarousal of the nervous system and immobilization; useful manifestations are the capacity to pause to restore, the ability to feel grounded and steady, a willingness to persist	Ventral innervation pathways include the face, throat, and upper chest (to activate muscles of social connection and engagement); associated with adaptive regulation of the nervous system and allostasis and homeostasis; capacity to be socially engaged, to grow and restore, and adapt, grow and evolve – the embodiment of resilience

Gunas, Polyvagal Theory, and Attachment Styles

- Safety (*sattvic* orientation): most likely to develop when there is access to caring adults who themselves have healthy, secure attachment styles; sattvic individuals have greater likelihood to perceive safety, live in the socially engaged parasympathetic nervous system and are more commonly in their relaxed, engaging and restorative (myelinated) ventral vagal space– *social engagement* – they can develop **healthy, secure attachment styles:**
  - e.g., baby spontaneously reacts positively to caretaker; shows appropriate fear of strangers
  - e.g., toddler plays nice with other children if they feel safe; or leaves the play situation if it feels unsafe

- Danger/risk (*rajasic* orientation): most likely to develop when surrounded by primary caretakers who themselves have insecure-resistant or anxious-ambivalent attachment styles; rajasic individuals are always prepared for danger, live in a near-constant state of sympathetic arousal, isolation, and physiological overload or break-down – mobilization of the of the sympathetic nervous system – fight or flight/*mobilization* – they might develop **insecure-resistant, or anxious-ambivalent attachment styles**

- Life threat (*tamasic* orientation): most likely to develop when surrounded by primary caretakers who themselves have disorganized or anxious-avoidant attachment styles; tamasic individuals develop a habitual pattern of shrinking back from life, withdraw – even dissociate – from human experiences; they are in their parasympathetic nervous system in an extreme state of withdrawal – freeze or submit/immobilization – they might develop **anxious-avoidant (fearful) or disorganized attachment styles**

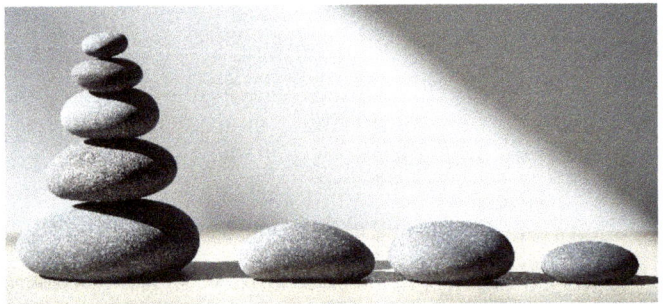

Evening Gatha (a Zen Buddhist verse)
Let me respectfully remind you,
Life and death are of supreme importance.
Time swiftly passes by and opportunity is lost.
Each of us should strive to awaken...
Awaken... take heed! Do not squander your life!

Kleshas or the Roots of Suffering

The next developmental stage after the establishment and expression of the gunas is the experience of vedana or affective tone, which is linked to the arousal stemming from the particular guna (or polyvagal state) that is emerging as primary. The experience of vedana is the simple differentiation between sensations or arousal that are pleasant, unpleasant, or neutral. These affective tones lead to emotional preferences as expressed in the yogic concept of the *kleshas*. The word *klesha* has many translations and meanings, all juxtaposing these potential challenges to the concept of vidya, or clear understanding.

Here are some translations (implying slightly differing interpretations) of the word *kleshas*:
- Hindrances, causes, or roots of suffering; root instincts
- Affective or energetic sources of confusion from which suffering, pressure, friction, problems, and stress (i.e., dukkha) arise
- Emotional conditioning or predilections that flavor (or tint) experience and understanding of life in combination with the gunas (and ultimately in combination with our *vrittis*)
- Fetters or impediments that get attached to experience – rather than experiencing what is, we develop preferences for what we would like to experience instead, for something different than what we have – we live an ideal world rather that the real world; in clouded mind, rather than clear mind
- Distractions that prevent us from being with life as it is – from being present for what is

In the yogic tradition, five *kleshas* are enumerated (defined in detail below), namely, attachment (*raga*), aversion (*dvesa*), ego (*asmita*), fear of death and change (*abhinivesha*), and confusion and misunderstanding (*avidya*). In various Buddhist traditions, some list three primary root kleshas and some list as many as seven *kleshas*. Given the yogic context, the five kleshas model is presented here. Regardless of ancient tradition, the *kleshas* stand in opposition to vidya, the capacity to accurately see, understand, and be present the reality of each moment. When we transcend the *kleshas* and move into *vidya* we are liberated from clinging, grasping, wanting, not wanting, worrying, and more.

The kleshas may find their origin very early in life with the simple sensation of affect and arousal. They emerge as we move from simply perceiving our physiological (arousal) and affective (valence) state to developing preferences for particular affects or types of arousal. Simply being with or noting things as pleasant, unpleasant, or neutral is hardwired into our being; the interpretation of these affects (*vedana* in Sanskrit), on the other hand, is a developmental process that starts in relationship with caring others.

The development of the *kleshas* begins in pranamaya kosha with the experience of something (an object, a relationship, an interaction, a circumstance) as pleasant, unpleasant, or neutral (valence) along with a sense of arousal (hyperarousal, hypoarousal, natural arousal). If there is no value judgment about it, the experience in and of itself is neither problematic nor reactive - it is simply the affective tone (or flavoring) of our experience (*vedana*) – a reality that is always with us. When we notice *vedana* (i.e., affect and arousal) and understand that this is all it is, often the experience will arise and fall away; it will come and go without reactivity or consequence. We can simply enjoy what is enjoyable and move on when it is over. We can simply be with what is unpleasant, trusting that this too shall pass. We can endure the neutral without getting bored or confused. However, if we experience displeasure and want to move away from it and perceive it as problematic or if we experience pleasure and we want more of it and perceive as meaningful, important, or even essential, the *kleshas* have been born.

When we recognize our affective state or level of arousal and develop a preference about how we would like to feel, we begin to cling to or grasp for affective experiences of pleasure and to push away the experience of displeasure or neutrality. The development of preferences for particular affective experiences can arise in all sense portals. That is, we might develop preferences for what arises visually, auditorily, gustatorily, olfactorily, tactile, perceptually, and so on, including preferences for mind states and relationships (though the latter two come later developmentally). Following are some examples of the *kleshas* in the various sensory portals – obviously these lists could be endless:

- *Visual*: hating or being proud of how we look, liking some types of art but not appreciating others, judging some people as ugly or unattractive and others as gorgeous, judging a scenery as magnificent or unimpressive, looking for beauty or seeing ugliness
- *Auditory*: hating certain sounds, loving particular types of music but not others, judging people by the sound of their voice, being bothered by certain noises and unencumbered by others
- *Olfactory*: loving particular perfumes or scents, being grossed out by particular smells, judging people for body odor, having bad or good memories in response to certain aromas
- *Gustatory*: loving certain foods – perhaps to the point of addiction, hating the taste of particular drinks, judging a food by its taste or lack of taste
- *Tactile*: seeking certain sensations of pleasure, rejecting certain types of touch, judging items by how they feel

The *kleshas* are sometimes referred to as the *second arrow*. The first arrow is the reality of human suffering and challenge. Life always present obstacles, pain, stress, difficulty, or concern. The *kleshas* overlay with the pain of life – the second arrow, which adds suffering to pain. If we fail to notice the sensation for what it is (impermanent and empty), it will lead us to the second arrow, or dart, the *kleshas*. We either fight the sensation (with aversion or fear) or get attached to it (with clinging, craving, pride, ego) and/or we blame the object, circumstance, or relationship that gave rise to the sensation. We want the noise, the smell, the rudeness to stop; we get mad at the people making the noise, the smell, the rude comments; we want to leave the situation. Or we get attached to pleasure, do not want it to stop and begin to seek it out over and over. We begin to want, cling, grasp, desire. We may also begin to fear the loss of pleasure, loss of relationships, loss of our identity, and begin to feel existential fears and anxiety, even death anxiety.

In other words, the experience of pleasant, unpleasant, and neutral sensations (affects and arousal, or *vedana*), is natural and in Buddhism is called the first arrow. It does not have to harm us as long as we are aware of the sensation, as well as it arising and dropping away. If the experience is transformed via conditioning into craving (in the form of attachment, wanting more) or aversion (wanting something different), the second arrow has been launched and it is this dart that makes the kleshas and binds us into a cycle of suffering. It is only if we recognize that it is simply a sensation arising in us (impermanent and empty), that we can let go of that second dart, of the *kleshas*.

The *kleshas* may be linked to our dopamine-driven reward, pleasure, and emotion circuits of the ventral striatum which activate when we seek pleasure or want to avoid pain – they can be like a gas pedal for the activation of motivation. Thus, not surprisingly, once cravings or desires flavor our perceptions, we begin to impose our perspective on reality instead of seeing life as it really is – we begin to misunderstand ourselves and our world. In other words, once the kleshas awaken, they are the energy and affect that we carry into everything. They become the energy and affect that tint out motivations, intentions, thoughts, speech, actions, and relationships. This happens unconsciously, at a habit-driven level, until we notice this predilection and how it unfolds in a way that happens mindfully and discerningly (this topic will be revisited later, when we dive into the transcendence of habit). The pull of wanting and craving can ruin our lives – in yoga and Buddhist traditions the overcoming of craving, the liberation from clinging (and its flip side of aversion) is enough to bring us enlightenment.

Developmentally, the first *kleshas* we are likely to experience are the developmentally more 'primitive' forms of *raga* and *dvesha*. The sutras list them more in the order in which they still manifest for most adults – but for tiny humans, as soon as they get a taste of something good, they want more of it (food, relationship, calm environment, etc.) because these good things fuel our survival. We are, in a way, hard-wired for the kleshas. Clinging ensures embeddedness in relationships; aversion might keep us safe. That is how the field of cravings, of clinging gets started. The *kleshas* may be necessary in early life to support social affinity – connection to others through affection, attachment, and wanting.

In later development, we become able to realize there are affects and energies that are pleasant, unpleasant, and neutral that are <u>not</u> rooted in or lead to the kleshas. Instead, these affects or experiences of pleasantness or unpleasantness are based in renunciation of sense pleasures. For example, generosity is a pleasant affect arising from renunciation of greed. Quietude arises from embracing simplicity, renouncing excess. All *yamas*, *niyamas*, *brahma viharas*, and generosity (if felt purely and without clinging) can fall into the categories of pleasant or unpleasant sensations that are not confounded by the *kleshas*, by clinging, aversion, ego, or confusion.

In a way, the kleshas can be understood (approximately) as affective extensions of the *gunas* (physical survival now linked to affective survival) and *vedana*:
- *Tamas* is most likely to translate into intense survival fear (the more developmentally basic form of *abhinivesha*)
- *Rajas* is most likely to translate into aversion; also likely related to avoidance-related fear; less likely to relate to clinging to sense pleasures; but possibly related to clinging to certain ego identifications
- *Sattva* is most likely linked to clinging, especially to relationships, protection, and connection; can also be related to clinging to certain ego identification
- All contribute to *asmita* as all are going to lead to the self-protection of a particular aspect of self/ego (*tamas* – physical and affective self; *rajas* – physical, affective, and verbal self; sattva – verbal, social, relational self-identity)
- All contribute to *avidya*, non-seeing, misunderstanding, confusion, and not knowing

The five *kleshas* of the yogic tradition are the direct consequence of our experiences in our biopsychosociocultural context, along with the resultant gunas or polyvagal adjustment, and our affective and vital experiences in relationships that result in affective tones or flavorings of all of our experiences (*vedana*). The first four *kleshas* (*raga, dvesha, asmita,* and *abhinivesha*), to be explained next, are the expression of the fifth, which is avidya or lack of clear understanding. When we move into clear seeing and begin to understanding the world as it truly is, the other kleshas are very naturally transcended.

Raga or Craving, Clinging, Grasping, Wanting

Raga is about seeking sense pleasures. It can be defined as a form of attachment to a thing or an experience because of misidentification of that thing as the source, requirement, or catalyst for happiness. The root of this *klesha* is greed, wanting, or passion.
- The first wanting will likely be for sense pleasures – craving for or clinging to food, being held, being comforted, being in relationship
- Craving taps into our dopamine reward system and becomes self-sustaining
- Then there comes the desire or craving for certain occurrences or outcomes (I cry because I am in pain and I want someone to do something so there is less pain; I cry because I am hungry and I want food to arrive, etc.)
- As we age, wanting gets more complex – sense pleasures include all kinds of desires – even addictions, expectations to have things and relationships a certain way, greed for getting what we want when we want it; what we crave or cling to may be flavored by the primary *koshas* we inhabit or the *kosha* to which we aspire
- *Raga* can even show up in the form of hope – we mistake hope for a particular outcome or cling to a way things were. True hope, however, is like faith: it is a remembering of our strength and resilience; it is a trusting in the process and patiently learning from it; it is a recognizing of opportunity for growth – it is not driven by wanting, but a reflection of a deep faith in the impermanence of experiences
- There is a subtle nuance worth mentioning that differentiates craving from clinging:
   - craving is thirsting or reaching for something you want and do not (yet) have
   - clinging is hanging on to something you already have and feel attached to
   - we even cling to craving itself when we look for things to want… (in his dharma talks, Joseph Goldstein calls this *catalog consciousness*)
- Not all craving and clinging is bad. Concentration and other yoga practices are a skillful form of clinging – we hang on to them to move toward deeper wisdom. We do not give them up until we have arrived at enlightenment
- There are many parables for this: we cling to the boat (of the dharma or the sutras) until we have reached the other shore of the river; Thanissaro Bikkhu gives the example that we keep the banana in the peel (hang on to the peel) until we are ready to eat the banana

Dvesha or Aversion, Anger, Hatred

Dvesha is the flip side of the same coin as *raga* that breeds wanting or craving for sense pleasure; wanting for something *not* to be or not to happen; aversion to a thing because of misidentification of that thing as the source or catalyst of suffering; the root here is hatred; and can manifest as jealousy.

- Anything that takes us out of our comfort zone becomes a target for *dvesa*
- This is a state of resistance, rejection, even destruction – at its core is hatred (dislike, if you prefer) of something, someone, an experience, a state of mind, a physical sensation, an energy or aura
- We can flip-flop from craving/wanting to aversion, if we are disappointed; we have all had people we liked, and then hated; we have all eaten a food until we could not stand it anymore
- The pull of aversion to pain, hatred, enmity, and so on can be incredibly strong and can easily sweep us away
- What we resist or resent may be defined in part by the primary *kosha* we inhabit
- Of course, at times, aversion can be helpful, such as pulling our hand away from a flame
- We crave for an "out" – we want to get away from a particular way of:
  - experiencing the body (pain, thirst, hunger, effort, the way I feel in handstand or plank)
  - feeling (e.g., bored, uncomfortable, challenged, even excited)
  - being (e.g., alone, around too many people, overstimulated, under-stimulated)
  - being in a relationship (e.g., having to confront someone and want to avoid the confrontation, wanting to break up with someone but not want to face their pain)

Asmita or Clinging to Ego, Rigid Role Identities for Self and Others

Asmita is about wanting an identifiable, separate self; a misidentification with our roles, our mind, our body. It is a desire for becoming 'someone' – to have a role and importance. It is a failure to see our basic essence and our connection as codependently arising from collectives or communities. In a way, we resist the reality of who we are as human beings. *Asmita* can carry with it a certain amount of conceit and is mired in the need to have an ego identity that is to be admired, that has status, reflects competence, and invites the admiration, approval, or appreciation of others. *Asmita* means that there is attachment (with conceit) to *I was..., I am..., I will be ...., I could be ....*

- This is a klesha of *raga* and *dvesa*, tied to ego (*ahamkara*) – we identify and want to be loved for certain roles we play, for certain self-identities we have, for self-definitions to which we are wedded
- We feel very threatened when we do not feel validated in those roles or identities (by others or by ourselves) – it feels like a little death each time we are threatened in our self-identity
- The more threatened we feel, the more separate we feel – there is a strong tie-in with *gunas* and attachment styles here
- If our basic worth and essence is not interpersonally validated, our attachment style can become insecure or disorganized and we cannot see ourselves (or others for that matter) as worthy or part of a collective
- If we feel a threat to our self-identity, emotional or mental existence; we may flee into defense (*rajas*, sympathetic nervous system arousal) or give up (*tamas*, dorsal vagal state)
- *Asmita* is the home of egoism, ego-absorbed individualism, identification with a rigid way of being in the world – with a particular role or roles
- *Asmita*, when combined with *dvesa* (or fear), may kindle our many -isms (racism, sexism, agism, oppression, White supremacy); may lead to hatred of the "other" by clinging to "self"

Abhinivesha or Fear of Change, Fear of Loss of Life, Fear of Loss of Self

Abhinivesha is about fear of change and uncertainty, especially fear of death; misidentification of impermanence as the source of suffering; not coming to terms with impermanence, clinging to the past or waiting for the future, craving for permanence; wanting a future/permanence

- Thinking that having something (like a fun event, a piece of cake, a romantic fling) brings happiness leads us to have FOMO (fear of missing out) and to cling to things, not realizing that they are impermanent and hence a source of unhappiness if we attach to them
- Not coming to terms with impermanence leads to holding on to life, to roles, to relationships – to many things that are in actuality ephemeral and unreliable
- Loss of what we perceive as crucial to our survival leads to fear of change because of fear/anxiety about the new or unknown
- Having certain desires for the future creates or allows for (false) sense of permanence – leads to craving (raga in a way) for certain goals or outcomes
- This fear can be viewed as a craving for becoming – for wanting a tomorrow, for wanting the next thing as a way of denying impermanence and death
- Fear in this way has a grip on us (and thus essentially overlaps with the kleshas of raga or dvesa) – whatever we fear, we in essence perpetuate:
  - if we fear death, we die 1000 deaths
  - if we fear poverty, money will forever have a grip on us
  - if we fear the loss of others, we will forever worry about being left out or behind
- When fear grips us, one way to release it is to practice lovingkindness

Avidya or Non-Seeing

Avidya means not seeing reality as it is. It is a lack of clarity, dullness, or failure to investigate thoroughly. At times, it is translated as ignorance, though this is a harsh translation. However, it is a state of not seeing clearly, as evidenced by the three roots of the Sanskrit word *avidya*:

- <u>vid</u> which means seeing clearly,
- <u>a</u> which negates whatever word it begins (in this case it negates *vid* or clear seeing into unclear seeing), and
- <u>ya</u>, which is an activating suffix for any word (akin to the English gerund of -ing, that indicates that something is happening in this very moment).

When we consider *avidya* in this way, the word suggests that in this moment, we are actively not seeing our reality or our truth clearly. We are caught in illusion or misunderstanding. We are looking to the wrong things to lead us out of suffering. We mistake the important for the unimportant, the essential for the non-essential; because of this we are constantly distracted by temptations for our attention that are, in the end, less than meaningful or useful. We waste our time on things and pursuits that are not important; we get confused about what really matters. *Avidya* leads us into less than wholesome action and can manifest in many ways. It might result in misidentification of what is real and what is true; in seeking pleasure and release from suffering from the wrong sources; misunderstanding, bias, or prejudice; or simply not being present with what is happening in the moment.

Avidya may be due to lack of clarity, misperception, ego, attachment, aversion, fear, or simply forgetting. However, sometimes it is grounded in a lack of desire to really know, to really understand, to truly pursue insight and wisdom. At times, we really do not want to be informed, we lack curiosity, we lack the stamina to seek out facts and double-check our opinions and ideas. We prefer to chitchat or watch TV; we go shopping, surf online, pull the covers over our head, and pretend not to know that is happening around us. We seek *avidya* to avoid responsibility for our own lives and the lives of others. The collective plays into this avoidance of clear seeing by offering us constant distraction – tempting us with false promises of fame, pleasure, wealth, entertainment, bliss, and so much more.

- *Avidya* is at the root of all the other *kleshas*; it means that we are mistaking various aspects of the self (various layers) as reality (identification with that layer as the subject, instead of the object). In early development this makes sense, of course – we simply begin to gain awareness of our self and its unfolding layers; as we mature and age, however, clearer understanding has to emerge because from here the *kleshas* work hand-in-hand with our way of perceiving and processing the world via our mental fluctuations, the vrittis (*avidya* rears up in all the mental *vrittis* as will be explored in Chapter 5)
- *Avidya* is tough to see in ourselves, but we can so easily see it in others
- *Avidya* is a lack of wisdom – we cling to our thoughts (or our way of thinking -- e.g., western versus native ways of knowing) and ideas as if they were truth, not realizing their subjectivity, their impermanence, and their context
- *Avidya* manifests as limited understanding – we misinterpret our opinions as truths; often the more unexamined an opinion is, the more we cling to it
- *Avidya* shows up as misinterpretation – do not believe everything you feel; do not believe everything you think; do not believe everything you think you need in relationship
- *Avidya* means we are likely losing out on the mystery of life by not having a sense of the present moment – not being in the present; we miss out on a sense of awe for each moment

In Sutra 2.5, Patanjali highlights four particular forms of avidya (which are also central to Buddhist psychology where they are sometimes called the four great hallucinations). Understanding these four forms of *avidya* helps carefully differentiate between relative (or provisional) truth and ultimate (or unconditioned) truth.

Confusing the Impermanent with the Permanent

We think things, relationships, emotions, thoughts, and other experiences will last forever and define reality. The denial of temporariness leads us to denying our own mortality and a longing for the future as if there were always another tomorrow to be had. Not living consciously with the ephemeral nature of everything takes us out of the present moment, forgetting that it may be the only moment left to us (this truth is also recapped in abhinivesha – wanting, taking for granted, a future). We forget that everything arises and everything dissolves. Through this forgetting, we get caught up in wanting (*raga*) and aversion (*dvesha*), escaping the present moment instead of either savoring it (if it happens to be pleasant) or being in it (if it is neutral) or accepting or being inspired by it (if it is unpleasant).

Confusing the Story with the Truth

In this form of *avidya*, we would rather believe an illusion than search for reality. We believe in illusion of everlasting pleasantness and positivity that lead us into clinging and craving; we get lost in illusions that move us toward aversion, hatred, anger, and loathing. This form of *avidya* can take the shape of stories immobilizing ourselves. We rationalize staying in bad situations by telling ourselves that this is just how it is. We stick with ideas, beliefs, and opinion, telling ourselves we *know* what is right. Our conviction in our own story takes us away from seeing things as they are or even might be. We confuse relative reality with ultimate reality. We certainly need to live in our relative reality – it is our human nature to respond to our circumstances and to have stories and beliefs about them. However, we greatly increase our suffering by believing that *our* story is the only true one or even that our *current* story is the best one (losing track that our stories and our perceptions of what is good and what is true has actually evolved and changed across time).

This form of *avidya* can also manifest as mistaking our story as the only possible story, either disregarding the stories of others or twisting reality on its head. We misinterpret (without noticing) what is not beautiful or not attractive to be beautiful or attractive or vice versa – we get tied up in exterior definitions and fail to see the deeper truth or reality. Often, but not always, these mistaken stories are fed to us by our environment, by media, and other influences. This can lead to shared delusions at a societal level, in which we can construct stories (i.e., history) based on the perceptions or experiences of the few, rather than the whole.

Confusing Pleasure with Pain

In this form of *avidya*, we mistake what is suffering, unsatisfying, unhappiness for nonsuffering, satisfying, happiness (and vice versa), or we mistake something as happiness that is actually causing harm. For example, we might believe that material things can make us happy; we might believe that everything that feels good in the short-term must also be good in the long; we might believe that what feels good to us is also good for others. We overlook the challenge in positive experiences for the *temporary* pleasure they bring (at the personal level, this might be overlooking the long-term effect from eating too many processed, sugary foods; at the communal level, this might be ignoring the consequences for the planet of overconsumption and pollution).

We might overlook the benefit of tough situations for the *temporary* challenges it presents (at the personal level, we might overlook the positive effects of a higher education because of the shorter-term stress it may create; at the collective level, we might ignore the long-term payoff for the planet and all beings from enduring the short-term challenge that arise as we switch to a sustainable energy economy). This form of *avidya* puts blinders on us and wraps us up in decision-making at a level that fails to consider all perspectives. It takes us away from discerning consciously what is or is not of benefit to each of us and the ecosystem as a whole.

Confusing Roles and Superficial Identities with Who We Really Are

In this form of *avidya*, we mistake what is not self to be self – signaled by our belief we are our body, our affect, thoughts, our feelings. For example, when we feel fear, we turn this into "I am a fearful person" (fear=self) or when we forget something we turn this into "I am an idiot" (forgetting=self). We mistake mind states for reality, for self, and build a story of self around them. In fact, we cling so much to how we define ourselves in any given moment that we lose track of the fact that there is a deeper reality underneath that is begging for attention. We get lost in our bodies, our emotions, our roles, our relationships and mistake them for truths. We create an idea of ourselves or of the identities of others and then cling to them even if they do not really fit what we are experiencing or observing. This form of misunderstanding takes us away from our deeper inner truth, from our truth as connected and co-arising beings (this truth is also recapped in asmita – clinging to an identifiable, separate self). Constructs of "I" and "you" become fixed and lose flexibility and pliability.

By identifying with false identities, we create suffering when we or others do not conform to these ideas. In reality, we are constantly changing and transforming:
- We are not our bodies (because our bodies constantly change anyway). If we were our bodies, what would we be? Our leg? Our head or chest? Our neurotransmitters or blood cells? A cancer cell or a macrophage? We do not own any part of our body; it responds to each moment. We get hungry, then we feel full. We are warm, then hot, then cold. We are heathy; then we are ill. We have an injury, then we heal. We grow old, then we die.
- We are not our minds (because our minds constantly change anyway). If we were our minds, what would we be? Our remembrances of yesterday? Our planning for tomorrow? Our worries or fears? Our perceptions of having been hurt or loved? Our ideas about politics or history? We do not control our mind. We have one thought only to note it being replaced by another. We hold a belief as sacred only to have implode. We develop a certain understanding of something only to see it fall apart. We are angry, then scared, then relieved. We feel sad, distraught, and then joyful. From moment to moment, thoughts and emotions come and go; beliefs and opinions evolve and change.

We are temporary constellations of experiences. We can be patient or healer; student or teacher; daughter or mother; father or son; lover or hater. When we realize this changeability in ourselves and others, we can let go of the suffering that comes from holding on to preconceived notions of who and how we and others should be. No, it does not hold us harmless of our actions and their consequences; that is a story for another moment.

Three personality types (habitual ways of being in the world and in relationship) emerge from the *kleshas* (Kornfield, 2009) and are revisited in the section on behavioral, affective, emotional, and mental habits or pattern locks (*samskaras*), which is essentially what these personality styles are.
- *Greedy, desirous*: we go through life, the world, our relationships mostly paying attention to and seeing what we like and what we want; we are mired in wanting, grasping, and clinging; this can be transformed into *faith and devotion*
- *Averse, angry*: we go through life, the world, our relationships mostly paying attention to and seeing all the things we do not like or do not want; we are mired in aversion, hatred, anger; this can be transformed into *discerning intelligence*
- *Confused, deluded* - we go through life, the world, our relationships mostly confused and not clearly seeing what is happening; we are mired in misunderstanding and tend to be oblivious; this can be transformed into *profound equanimity*

Summary of the Kleshas – Emotional Predilections or Roots of Suffering				
Raga	*Dvesa*	*Asmita*	*Abhinivesha*	*Avidya*
Translation				
Attachment, greed, desire	Aversion, enmity, hatred	Egoism, ego-attachment	Fear of death or change	Confusion, delusion, ignorance
Definition				
Wanting pleasure, desiring positive outcomes; attached to having what we want	Intolerant of discomfort or pain; wanting things to be different than they are; anger as the default	Ego-absorbed individualism and self-absorption; worried about losing one's identity	Holding on to how things are; not accepting impermanence of things and experiences, fearing change	Lack of wisdom, incomplete understanding, misinterpretation, limiting views, confusing story for reality
Basic Manifestation				
Expectations to have things and relationships a certain way	Rejecting attitude, lack of satisfaction, trapped in anger and aversion in daily life	Identification with roles for self and others; upset if role expectations are not met	Anxiety about the unknown or new, worrying about change, ambiguity, uncertainty	Inability to see impermanence, to recognize suffering and interdependence; misunderstanding
Attitude				
We go through life, the world, our relationship mostly paying attention to and seeing what we like and what we want	We go through life, the world, relationships mostly paying attention to all the things we do not like or do not want	We go through relationships & life mostly based on our concepts of who we and others should be and the roles that define us	We go through relationships & life adhering to the old and familiar, ever afraid of what might be, of anything new	We go through life, the world, our relationship mostly confused and not clearly seeing or understanding what is happening
Transcendence				
Faith and devotion	Discerning intelligence	Fluidity in and non-attachment to identity	Openness to change and ambiguity	Equanimity and understanding

Collective Expressions of the Kleshas

Just as the *yamas* have collective expressions in addition to personal or individual manifestations, so do the kleshas. Societies can be mired in attachment, ego, aversion, fear, and delusion. *Modern economies are based largely on greed, clinging, and grasping.* Because of the acceptance of money as a shared delusion, humans develop greedy attitudes, cavalier approaches to finite resources, and unrealistic notions of economic growth. Societal kleshas contribute to hate crime, war, othering, all -isms, climate crisis, economic policy that is selfish and exploitative, social policy that is exclusionary, educational systems that are elitist, and the list goes on almost endlessly. Confusing possession with happiness is a great delusion of societies.

What is needed instead is a collective that is based in the recognition and honoring of our utter interdependence with one another, all other beings, and the entire planet – a deep ecological understanding of the reality that we do not exist inherently without a context, without others, without the collective; a collective that thinks, speaks, and acts from a basis of compassion, lovingkindness, joy, and equanimity; a collective that that courageously embraces compassion; that calls out attachment/greed, aversion/hatred, and delusion. We need a shared, co-constructed "story" (i.e., a reality) that includes many perspectives, that honors our shared experience, that hears all voices, that is infused with a commitment to an ethical and values-based foundation that invites compassion, kindness, joy, and equanimity in the services of all and everything. We need to transcend stories (delusions) that are based on a small segment of the population, that represent only certain perspectives, that have closed minds and cold heart toward any experience that seems different.

The *kleshas*, given full rein at the societal level, are likely to lead to the demise of our (and many other) species. Each one of us is responsible to call out societal expressions of the *kleshas* – in all four quadrants of our interpersonal matrix and in each individual relationship – to dismantle the negative impacts of the collective expressions of the *kleshas*. We each have to do this with kindness and compassion, yet we do have to call it out to create an engaged practice of yoga that leads to action for the betterment of our social and environmental context.

A Modern Psychology Perspective on Avidya

Avidya can also be captured, at least in part, via the psychological construct called defense mechanisms, or as I prefer to call them, self-protective mechanisms. These self-protections initially grow out of an attempt to keep ourselves safe, supported, and accepted in our biopsychosociocultural context to assure that we are accepted by our community, our tribe, our family. They often serve a valuable purpose – until they no longer do. They lose their value when they become overgeneralized and transferred into contexts to which they are actually irrelevant. What may have served our wellbeing at one point in time (say, when we were 3 or 10 or even 15 years of age), no longer serves us (say when we are adults). The table on the next page provides a listing, by no means comprehensive, of psychological mechanisms that we develop to protect ourselves and to create safety.

These self-protections in particular, and *avidya* in general, are ways to prevent us from having to face truth, reality, the situation and relationship at hand. We, in some ways, have learned to fool ourselves, to lie to ourselves, to blind ourselves to what is. Interestingly, these psychological protections can also manifest in the collective. Denial, repression, displacement, avoidance – all can be engaged in by whole groups of people, by whole societies, when we choose to live in illusion rather than reality – often to keep us from having to deeply acknowledge our failings, from having to wake up from our illusions of comfort. Through *avidya*, we perpetuate suffering in ourselves, in others, in our families, communities, tribes, and societies.

Psychological Self-Protective Mechanisms	
Definition	*Example*
Repression	
Unconsciously pushing distressing thoughts, memories, or desires out of awareness	A person who experienced childhood trauma has no conscious recollection of the events
Denial	
Refusing to accept reality because it is too distressing	A smoker insists that smoking does not harm their health despite medical evidence
Displacement	
Redirecting emotions from the original source to a safer target	A man who is angry at his boss comes home and yells at his children
Sublimation	
Channeling unacceptable impulses into socially acceptable activities	A woman with aggressive tendencies becomes a professional boxer
Rationalization	
Justifying behaviors or thoughts with logical but false explanations	A student who fails a test blames the professor for making it too difficult, rather than admitting they did not study
Regression	
Reverting to a behavior from an earlier developmental stage when faced with stress	An adult throws a temper tantrum when they do not get their way
Intellectualization	
Focusing on facts and logic to avoid dealing with emotions	A person diagnosed with a terminal illness researches medical treatments in great detail instead of processing their emotions
Reaction Formation	
Acting in the opposite way of one's unacceptable thoughts or feelings	A person with same-sex attraction outwardly expresses strong anti-LGBTQ+ views
Identification	
Adopting characteristics of another person (e.g., someone admired or superior), often to cope with feelings of inferiority or fear	A child bullied at school starts dressing and behaving like their bully.
Projection	
Attributing one's own unacceptable thoughts or feelings to someone else	A person who feels hostile toward a coworker believes that the coworker is actually hostile toward them
Projective Identification	
Projecting unwanted feelings onto another, and then subtly influencing that person to adopt these projected feelings or behaviors as their own; unlike in simple projection, the recipient begins to feel or act in ways consistent with the projection	A person who feels deep insecurity may act in a way that makes others feel inadequate, causing them to doubt themselves—thus expressing the original person's unconscious belief or fear (essentially on their behalf)

Chapter 5: Moving Toward Transformation

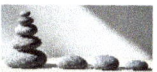

The next developmental step beyond the *gunas* and *kleshas*, which were linked developmentally to *annamaya* (our somatic or physical consciousness) and *pranamaya* (our vital, affective, and energetic consciousness) *koshas*, respectively, is the emergence of language, increasingly conscious processing and recognition of external stimuli, and the beginning of explicit memory consolidation. These cognitive developments are linked to the emergence of manomaya kosha and the increasingly direct expression of our mind contents (which can now be shared via language and shared experience). We become aware of our mind (or self) – we shift our identity from body and energy-based identification to mind (or self)-based identities.

Before going much farther, let us explore what is meant by 'mind' or 'self' in modern terms. Mind can be considered the sum total of all information that is available in our nervous system and that is used to construct our day-to-day reality arising from our interpersonal experiences and contexts (Damasio, 2012). Mind reflects the interpretation of all incoming stimuli in the context of stored memory (implicit and explicit) and of our greater biopsychosociocultural context (with all its values and expectations). It is deeply collective, interdependent, and co-arising from our interactions with the people and world around us. Our history and context, our experiences and relationships over the course of our lifetime help shape our store of information and how the mind accesses and uses it to make predictions and guide actions. Our memory, history, reasoning, and experiences allow the mind to create an enduring and subjective sense of self, a narrative or autobiographical representation of who we are and how we function and fit into the world at large (Cozolino, 2024; Damasio, 2012). Some of the stored information is directly known and knowable (conscious); some is unknown and yet recoverable or accessible (preconscious); some is unknown and perhaps unknowable (unconscious).

Many physical processes will never be conscious – and for good reason. We would not want conscious control over most of our autonomic nervous system; we would not want to have to consciously beat our own heart, metabolize our food, or rally our immune systems in the face of an invader. Many early childhood experiences are stored in implicit memory stores to which we do not have clear access (Badenoch, 2018; Brems & Rasmussen, 2019). We have reactivities (*gunas*, polyvagal states) and felt senses (*vedanas*), but without clear parameters or memories about them. These types of memories affect our intentions, thoughts, actions, and relationships in indirect ways and often cannot be easily talked about because they are created and laid down during a time in our life that was pre- or non-verbal insert (Badenoch, 2011a; Cozolino, 2024). They may bubble up unexpectedly in *asana* or *pranayama* practices as surprising, overwhelming, curious, or uncomfortable physical sensations or releases, or as emotions and affects that we cannot quite process easily. They can emerge during inner practices as we observe ourselves with compassion and kindness, without judgment.

Yoga practice over time can help us become more familiar with more hidden aspects and patterns of ourselves and can help begin to reshape these memories within a new context of safety, support, and acceptance. Our mind begins to recognize these states as a meaningful and important part of us, integrating previously unknown information about ourselves into our current identity. We internalize new realities about who we are, how we think, what we believe, why we develop certain types of relationships, and where we can go from here. We begin to change our mind; we change our perceptions, our attitudes, our actions, our relationships with ourselves and others, even our identities. We recognize that nothing is permanent; everything is constructed and co-constructed with others through shared experiences moment-by-moment.

Vrittis or the Yogic Expressions of Mind

In yoga psychology, mind contents are organized into five vrittis, or mental impressions or fluctuations (*vrittis* = revolution, revolving). It is one of the crucial tasks of yoga to still the fluctuations of the mind to move forward on the path to awareness, wisdom, and insight. This notion is expressed in the second Yoga Sutra of Patanjali, *yogas citta vritti nirodha,* translated as "yoga is the calming or stilling of the fluctuations of the mind". In brief, the five fluctuations of mind are correct knowledge or perception (*pramana*), incorrect knowledge or perception (*viparyaya*), memory (*smritti*), imagination or creativity (*vikalpa*), and deep sleep (*nidra*), all explained in much more detail below.

Development of the Vrittis

The mind layer of human experience encompasses perception, recognition, and memory storage (which are the first developmental steps) and, ultimately, volition, motivation, emotions, and all things related to information processing. As language develops in leaps and bounds, it becomes central to communication with others and creates shared experiences across time and space. It builds a bridge to increasingly refined and complex mental skills that allow us to construct a representational verbal and social self. From the mental constructs made possible by language and informed by our biopsychosociocultural context, we slowly begin to build and then constantly evolve and transform identities for ourselves and others. These identities and understandings are centered around (i.e., heavily influenced by) our familially and culturally transmitted and shared connections and the beliefs, attitudes, values, and ideas contained within those collectives.

As the rudiments of language begin to develop and as we learn to label emotions, sensations, perceptions, and thoughts, a representational self (i.e., mind) emerges. Labels and concepts become important to how we perceive and interpret the world and we begin to add valuation (even judgment) to our experiences – again, all heavily marked by the interpersonal context in which we grow up. As memory consolidation becomes increasingly language-bound, time-linked (or time-stamped), and place-stamped, explicit memory emerges and is added to the implicit memory of the *gunas* and *kleshas*, further creating stories of self, increasingly calcified narratives of who we are, how we are, and what we are.

Our mental perceptions and impressions lead to self-identification with mind (moving beyond physical and affective self-identification and survival instincts) at various levels of cognitive development. Our self-identity starts narrow and slowly; over many decades, it begins to broaden in perspective, taking into account more and more viewpoints, more and more possibilities, and more and more considerations of others. We decenter and open up to the possibility of a more perspectival mind. As our mind expands, our intentions shift. This is a very important recognition as our intentions shape our speech and actions; our speech and actions profoundly affect our relationships and our impact on our communities.

The developmental nature of the vrittis may be captured from the following features:
- When language first begins to emerge, we identify with our thoughts and labels – *we are what we think*, label, imagine, and feel. We consolidate language and episodic (procedural) memory, learning new behaviors and routines.
- As memory becomes more time- and date-stamped, we identify with our habit powers and ego, mistaking them for a self, a personality. Especially in combination with the kleshas' flavoring, we can become powerfully attached to this self-identification and can get stuck here for much of our life. We consolidate a narrative self; *we begin to tell stories of "I"*.
- As our perspective broadens to include the unique and personal viewpoints of others, we begin to transcend our identification with individual labels, thoughts, emotions, beliefs, and ideas, even with our individual personalities or egos. *We begin to glimpse a greater wisdom* (still tied to mind but beginning to be more expansive). We stop resisting what is by letting go of ego and embracing the reality of human life – with all its challenges and limitations. We begin to consolidate an autobiographical self that slowly can expand in terms of what it considers part of the autobiography, part of the self. The more decentered the definition, the more movement there is toward *vijnanamaya kosha* and the *brahma viharas*. The decentered viewpoint of *vijnanamaya kosha* is clear of the *gunas* and *kleshas*; it considers all other beings, even the entirety of the planet. Our view of the world becomes wise and inclusive.

Stickiness of Identifying with Our Mind Contents

As stories of self and our life are created and flourish, things get tricky. We might come to believe all of our narratives as the truth rather than seeing the possible misperceptions and biases that are contained in them. Anytime we believe there is only one single narrative (or way of understanding our perceptions and experiences), we need to get suspicious of our own mind and need to remember that typically there are multiple viewpoints. As stories of self and other develop, so do interpretations of thoughts and physiological responses as emotions and truths, influenced by the *gunas*, *kleshas*, and biopsychosociocultural contexts. Our default mode network kicks in – we get lost in our habitual thoughts when attention or concentration is not honed; when left to our own devices, we get trapped in our selfish perspective on the world (mediated by the posterior cingulate cortex).

As we begin to attach emotions and identities to simple labels, we ascribe inherent nature to things, experiences, people, and occurrences based on how we have labeled them. The label becomes the identity of the experience, object, or subject; we lose the connection to the reality of our experiences and relationships. For example:
- We define ourselves with a particular role and lose all other aspects of ourselves, e.g., we are a "parent" at the exclusion of every other role we have (confusing role with identity)
- If we label someone as belonging to the category of "other", we become frightened or biased or ascribe traits (e.g., "all Germans are antisemitic")
- We think of a visit to the dentist as terrifying and painful, and we begin to avoid going to our annual check-ups

- We come to think of ourselves as *"lazy"* and, as a result, we might not even try to be proactive and engaged anymore
- We label someone as a *"perfectionist"* and now that becomes all we perceive when we interact with them

As our mind emerges, thoughts, desires, clinging, and cravings become increasingly verbal and culturally shared. They are influenced (tinted or flavored) by our grasping and clinging, our aversions and fears, our egos or perceived identities, and our lack of clear seeing and our misunderstandings and confusions. We develop not only our own vrittis flavored by the kleshas, but we also absorb the flavored and tinted thoughts and beliefs of the collectives in which we are raised. For example:
- Memory may be tinged or flavored by past pleasures (*raga*), leading to longing or nostalgia; memory may be controlled by self-identifications (*asmita*), leading to narrow definitions of how we are or even who we can be
- Fantasy may be flavored by the future and becoming (*abhinivesha*), or wanting pleasure (*raga*), or avoiding pain (*dvesa*)
- Misperception may be colored by opinions, values, and ideas (*avidya*) or self-identifications (*asmita*)
- Sleep may reflect our *gunas* or linked to escape or avoidance of what causes displeasure

Our labels become sticky and they begin to entangle us in rigid beliefs and unexplored opinions and attitudes. Some of this stickiness is also driven by our implicit (unconscious or preconscious) memory linked to the *gunas* and *kleshas* we have developed through our life experience and embeddedness in a larger context and Zeitgeist. Thus, a large aspect of working with the *vrittis* is to use careful and attentive discernment (*viveka* in Sanskrit) to notice if our mental productions (i.e., thoughts, plans, memories, beliefs, attitudes, and perceptions) are tinted or flavored by the *kleshas* and/or *gunas*. *Vrittis* can be helpful or unhelpful, skillful or unskillful, auspicious or inauspicious *depending on* their flavoring by or (relative) freedom from the kleshas and gunas. *Tamas* and *rajas* can greatly affect how the *vrittis* manifest and influence our mind states. When they predominate (over *sattva*), they may interfere with *viveka* (or clear seeing), obscuring our ability to exercise calm discernment about our choices. (Also see the table entitled "*Interaction of the Kleshas and Vrittis*" at the end of this Chapter.)

> Buddhism asserts that there are many stories,
> many viewpoints that unfold in stages.
> Which stage do you inhabit –
> what are the stories you tell yourself?
>
> Stage 1 – I am right, you are wrong;
> Stage 2 – You are right, I am wrong;
> Stage 3 – We are both right;
> Stage 4 – We both just simply are

> In Buddhism, the importance of the vrittis, when flavored by the kleshas (i.e., when made sticky), lies in the fact that they precede suffering.
>
> From this perspective, human suffering starts before anything happens outside of us. Suffering precedes sensations because of the burden of preconceived notions, fixed values, and other mental fabrications or preoccupations that we carry around with us. Sensations and how we perceive or interpret them, both emotionally and mentally, are flavored by the vrittis and the kleshas in a complex interplay of expectations, calcified opinions, and old knowledge.
>
> The trick to relieving suffering is to let go of imputed meaning, that is, to let go of preconceived assumptions, calcified values, fixations on the past or the future, reactive emotions, and the stories and narratives created; to recognize where these thoughts came from (i.e., to identify the root causes); to see them in their context and to recognize that the context has changed; and thus, ultimately to transform them so that we can see reality more accurately as it really is.

Although discussed separately below, all the *vrittis* are intermixed (co-occur at the same time); that is, they generally do not occur as one distinct vrittis at a time. Each *vritti* in and of itself may not be detrimental. At times, a *vritti*, if not flavored by a klesha, may serve a specific and useful purpose or support us in figuring out our world. However, the more a *vritti* is flavored by desire, aversion, ego, fear, or misunderstanding, the more likely it will be to lead us astray or to be counterproductive. *Vrittis* can interact with the kleshas in interesting ways.

Gunas or polyvagal states also affect the *vrittis*. When we are in a state of alert, either feeling a sense of danger or even life threat, how our mind works will be strongly influenced by these reactivities. As we observe our thoughts and stories, it is thus useful to note if we recognize whether they have been flavored or influenced in some way by reactivity to circumstances, emotional tone, or affective predilections that may distort our perceptions.

Pramana or Right Perception

This *vritti* is also translated as right view or verifiable knowledge. It represents accurate perception of ourselves, our reality or circumstance, our relationships, and ourselves. It is a capacity for clear seeing and discernment that we seek to cultivate, strengthen, and reinforce through our integrated yoga practice.
- *Unflavored*: clear perception is where we want to be – we hope to be able to see reality as closely to how it is as possible (see box above); either via direct experience, inference, or testimony
- *Flavored*: we may see our reality clearly and yet are paralyzed or derailed by desire or aversion; thus, we are not responding to what we actually know, but based on the predominant *guna(s)* or *klesha(s)* of the moment

- When we are able to access right view, we can see our misidentifications; we can penetrate our mental constructions to recognize that they are neither truth nor real – we practice the Buddhist principle/joke of *"don't believe everything you think"*
- *Pramana* is associated with beta and, occasionally, gamma brain waves
    - 13 to 20 and 30 to 100 cycles per second, respectively – fast brain waves
- Beta brain waves are predominant when we are awake and alert; during active engagement with our inner or outer world; engaged in clear analysis and lucid thought or conversation
    - beta waves are associated with attention and salience networks; associated with analytical thinking, problem-solving, and clarity of thought
    - beta waves are signal alertness and focus; they are associated with engaged conversations, discourse, or debate
- During high-level cognition, peak performance, and flow, beta brain waves may give way to gamma brain waves above 40 Hz (neural signature of active learning and of meditation), when inspiration, heightened awareness, and deep insight are accessed
    - gamma waves are associated with learning and problem-solving based on inspiration and flashes of insight
    - gamma waves are linked to the understanding of complex ideas and the 'big picture'
    - gamma waves are correlated with the presence of spiritual or transcendent experiences

Viparyaya or Misperception

This *vritti* is about faulty or illogical thinking, about cognitive distortions that affect our view of the world, ourselves, and our relationships, and may be marked by distraction, misunderstanding or confusion, and emotional reactivity.
- *Flavored*: in misperception, we are trapped in opinions, values, ideas, getting lost in rigid perceptions of roles and relationships; we impose our view and skew reality in the direction of our preferences, motives, and mindsets
- *Unflavored*: the helpfulness of not knowing at times lets us dive into situations that we might otherwise not try
- In *viparyaya*, psychological protective mechanisms (also known as psychological defenses) kick in (e.g., projecting, denying, or repressing emotions and thoughts)
- We forget that thoughts are just constructions, and confuse opinions and perceptions as reality – we get lost in thinking that our beliefs and identifications are truths and get carried away by our emotional reactivity driven perhaps by implicit memories and unconscious predictions about what is about to happen (including *gunas*, *vedanas* and *kleshas*)
- *Viparyaya* is associated with high beta brain waves:
    - 21 to 40 cycles per second – very fast (perhaps overactive or reactive) brain waves
    - high beta waves are predominant when we are fully awake and alert; during active engagement with focus on our inner or outer world; while overly or actively engaged in analysis, thought, or conversation; very high beta waves are associated with intense mental activity and possibly with anxiety and overwhelm
    - high beta waves are associated with attention and salience networks, and with analytical thinking, problem-solving, and intense processing; the intensity of thought during high beta waves can lead to hyperarousal, confusion, overload, and misperception

Modern Science Perspective on Perception and Misperception

The way we perceive and mentally process reality is flavored by many influences accumulated over the course of a lifetime and deeply affected by the current-moment context. Perceptions are tangible manifestations of past conditioning as projected onto current experiences and events. They are deeply shaped by past learning, which influences how we think about and emotionally respond (or react) to current events and experiences. In other words, everything in the present has the potential to be flavored by the past – especially if we are not aware of this very subtle (and sometimes not so subtle) influence of prior learning and conditioning. Everything we perceive is a reflection of how we impute meaning based on our history, experiences, and learning opportunities – past and present.

When we are not aware of the influence of past experiences and current contexts on our thoughts and emotions, perceptions (and consequent actions or reactions) in the present are tinged by ingrained reactive patterns (e.g., *gunas* and *kleshas*) rather than being responsive to the reality of the present moment. We always bring our context, our developmental interpersonal matrix and learning, with us into the present moment. Much of the inner limbs of yoga is about becoming aware of these influences of the past and beginning to make more conscious decisions about how to respond in the present.

Perception is the interpretation of sense experiences by recognizing and labeling their distinctive features – as noted above, generally in the context of or via the baggage from past conditioning and experience. The way we perceive and predict things (events, relationships, occurrences, risk levels, and more) is conditioned by our biopsychosociocultural background and specific interpersonal experiences across the lifetime, and especially in childhood. Perceptions are conditioned and flavored by past experiences and by developmental context, along with commensurate *gunas* and *kleshas* that have developed. Perception is heavily biased and conditioned, including by cultural predispositions, social circumstances, biological variables, familial experiences and values, and so on. Because of this, perceptions are full of imputed meaning and do not (perhaps even cannot) reflect any inherent truth – and yet we mistake them as truths. We cling to our viewpoints and confuse our ideas, beliefs, attitudes, opinions, and interpretations with reality.

What this means is that we do not simply experience and perceive – we impute meaning. We layer, on top of each experience, additional meaning that creates a new reality about the current experience or perception. We no longer just see an object, experience a relationship, or have a sensation – we imbue it with meaning. If I feel pain in my back, it means I am getting old. If I have a certain level of comfort in my home, it means security. If a friend does not call me, it means abandonment. If I get a new car, it means status. In other words, things and experiences are imbued with meaning *way beyond* their inherent nature.

Additionally, we create overlays of meaning – we add connotations based on our circumstances (think biopsychosociocultural) and preferences (think learning histories). As we do this, we are totally unaware that we doing it. In each moment of judgment, we think this is the truth, this is reality. Fortunately, once we begin to notice this, we can get better and better at spying our self-referenced interpretations and possible distortions.

A few simple examples can illustrate this point, perhaps seemingly simplistically so, however the implications of these examples are profound when we ponder them for a bit.
- If someone lives in Oregon, rain means "bad" weather. If someone lives in Southern California, rain means "life-saving" weather.
- If I love old cars, I may think of a 1990s VW bug as "vintage"; if I prefer new cars, I may think of it as a "piece of junk".
- If we have liberal politics, we may think of government as an institution in the public service; if we are at the right wing of politics, all we may see are bureaucrats.
- If someone lived through a war, they might consider the nation who warred with theirs as somehow lesser or as aggressive; if someone has only experienced life during peace times, they may not understand the survival instinct reflected in tribalism.
- If we live in an inner city, we may think of a group of young people as a "gang"; if we live in a small town, we may see a group of young people and rejoice in their camaraderie.
- If I had experiences of trauma in childhood, using a strap in yoga class may feel terrifying; if I have had experience of a strap as supporting my asana, I may perceive it as liberating.
- If we value healthy food, we may appreciate a new acquaintance's preoccupation with finding an organic food source; it we live junk food, we may perceive their desire as ridiculous or misguided.
- If someone feels deprived, the success of another may trigger resentment; if someone has a sense of abundance, the good fortune of another may create a deep sense of joy.

To protect ourselves from emotional overwhelm and perceived threats to our identities, roles, emotions, and ways of thinking (i.e., threats to ego), we develop strategies of self-protection (often called defenses, or defense mechanisms, in Western psychology) – ranging from denial, repression, compartmentalization to projection, projective identification, and more. We can draw heavily on psychology to understand these self-protective mechanisms. As more and more connections to the prefrontal cortex slowly come online and become increasingly complex and dispersed, our emerging cognitive complexity allows for increasing executive, cognitive, or top-down control over these reactive and largely unconscious mechanisms. We begin to gain an understanding of the need to decontextualize and reconceptualize our reactive (impulsive) narratives and stories. We begin to see the bigger picture and take a wider perspective on what is transpiring in our and others' lives. We become increasingly capable of shifting perspectives and stepping outside of our own stories and narratives to include those of others. Our minds open up to new possibilities and we begin to realize that sometimes we may just be wrong about our interpretations and less than logical or kind in our reactions.

> "Arrogance is ignorance plus conviction.
> While humility is a permeable filter that absorbs life experience
> and converts it into knowledge and wisdom,
> arrogance is a rubber shield
> that life experience simply bounces off on."
> Tim Urban

Examples of Misperceptions		
Type of Misperception	*Associated Thought, Speech, or Action*	*Resultant Challenges*
Embracing false dichotomies	Attitudes of us versus them, right versus wrong, good versus bad	Creates polarization, can result in dehumanization
Creating rankings	Creating hierarchies based on arbitrary external variables, such as religion, race, culture, educational level, skin color, and more	Means not seeing others or ourselves as we really are, arrogance, feeling better or worse than, sense of entitlement
Living with pretension	Trying to impress, trying to hide certain aspects of ourselves, not being honest	Creates distance and dishonesty, creates separation
Indulging in judgment	Making ourselves feel better by tearing others down and being overly critical	Results in projection, creates separation and dishonesty
Being all-knowing	Having the attitude of already knowing, of knowing better than others	Results in being closed to new learning, alienates others
Showing up with defensiveness	Feeling the need to protect ourselves, feeling attacked or under siege and then reacting from that place	Creates distance, perpetuates hurt by lashing out against others, prevents open communication
One-upping	Needing to feel or be better than others, putting others down to feel better or more secure	Results in hurt feelings, perpetuates emotional distance, creates false hierarchies
Misreading cues	Imposing expectations on experience and interactions that distort what really happened	Leads to misunderstandings, creates interpersonal distance, perpetuates loneliness and isolation
Imposing viewpoints	Interpreting events and relationship from one's own perspective, attitudes, stereotypes, and biases	Leads to misunderstandings, perpetuates lack of mutuality, perpetuates conflict
Being on autopilot	Being inattentive to details, ignoring or not noticing cues in environments or relationships, lacking mindfulness	Leads to misreading situations and people, creates misunderstandings and false recollections
Believing everything we think	Taking our own side in arguments or disagreements, not being able to shift set or view, insisting on being right	Leads to rifts in relationships, keeps conflict alive and limits our capacity to see others realistically
Mistaking memory for reality	Believing that we remember our experiences accurately, living in the past with righteousness	Creates lack of forgiveness, may perpetuate emotional distance, can lead to victimhood or victimization
Getting trapped in roles	Shoehorning oneself or others into certain roles, requiring self or others to play out particular identities in relationships or society	Creates a lack of authenticity for self and others, leads to rigidity in relationships, perpetuates interpersonal patterns and beliefs
Getting stuck in habit	Mistaking ruts as routines, not being able to explore new ways of being, sticking with behavior despite lack of utility	Leads to calcified relationships, creates inattention and mindlessness, keeps us stuck and non-creative
Being mired in various psychological defenses	Getting caught in denial, repression, projection, compartmentalization, dissociation, etc. (Brems, 1999, 2001; Brems & Rasmussen, 2019)	Distorts self-perception and relationship dynamics, impedes wisdom and insight, compassion, kindness, joy, and equanimity

Smriti or Memory

This *vritti* represents our capacity to remember our experiences and our life. It is about recollection, memory, and remembrance and how we utilize this capacity to recall our life. Clearly, memory can have positive or negative reverberations for our capacity to see the world, ourselves, and our relationships as they are.

- *Flavored*: getting trapped in the past, getting lost or stuck in old stories and narratives; reminiscence; getting attached to old identities, memory as a habit or rut – as a narrowing of possibilities
- *Unflavored*: remembrance, mindfulness, time-stamped and place-stamped memory, ability to reflect on past experiences to create change and growth, memory as a helpful guide toward insight
- We forget that the past is no longer real – that our past as we recollect it, is simply a thought in the present moment
- Associated with all brain waves depending on type of memory and stage of memory-related processing (i.e., encoding, consolidation, or retrieval/recall)
    - delta waves are associated with long-term memory consolidation during sleep as it helps with linking and transferring information from the hippocampus to the neocortex
    - theta waves are crucial for encoding (new learning) and retrieval especially of facts and experiences; also involved in spatial memory (such as creating a mental map of a space)
    - alpha waves support encoding as it promotes calm focus and attention, while reducing distraction and thus facilitating recall.
    - beta waves support active thinking and as such is associated with short-term memory and immediate application of knowledge to new situations
    - gamma waves are necessary for working memory and higher-level cognitive processing; it helps with memory integration across various brain areas; it can enhance neural connectivity and as such can be associate with memory as a way to find sudden insight

Modern Science Perspective on Memory

For memories to form, much has to happen. Sensory inputs (e.g., sights, sounds, tastes, and other inner and outer sensory experiences) need to be registered with some level of attention and are often linked with emotion to create the raw materials from which memory is encoded. If there is no sensory input, no attention, and no emotional valence, memories are neither encoded nor stored. *Memory encoding* is the initial process through which sensory inputs are transformed imbued with meaning or emotional valence to make the experience quite literally memorable and salient. Encoding can be visual, auditory, or semantic. The greater the meaning or emotional valence, the more likely it is that we will encode the experience to ready it for storage.

Memory storage follows encoding and refers to the retention of encoded information or material over time. Inputs are temporarily held in short-term memory; they can then be consolidated into long-term memory through processes like rehearsal or association, involving the hippocampus. Memories are stored with time- and place-stamps to support accurate and context-specific recall later. This long-term storage is dispersed across various regions of the brain – it is not like a file folder that holds the complete memory of an experience. Instead, it is a collection of bits and pieces distributed across various networks of the brain that have to work together to create access to the stored information for recall. In other words, *memory recall* is the act of retrieving stored bits and pieces of information from various brain region and coordinating them when needed (i.e., reconstructing the memory of the original inputs). It may be better to think of recall as reconstruction, based on bits and pieces of data distributed across various brain areas, with the hippocampus helping us put together meaning based on prior events and knowledge.

The situation and context in which and the reason why we seek to recall or reconstruct a memory can have a profound impact on how and what we recall. Each time a memory is recalled, it can thus be altered slightly based on current motivation, attitude, mindset, and perspective; external pressures (e.g., timed recall), social context, or relationship influences (e.g., who is present while we reconstruct a given memory); and new learning, concurrent sensory inputs, and other experiences in the meantime (Amen, 2017; Ranganath, 2024). This process allows the brain to continuously refine and rewire – the process of neuroplasticity.

Effective recall often depends on the strength of encoding and the organization of stored information. Memory is never static, being constantly emerging, refined, and changing. In the words of Charan Ranganath (2024), it helps to *"think of memory as less like a photograph and more like a painting. Most paintings typically include some mixture of details that are faithful to the subject, details that are distorted and embellished, and inferences and interpretations that are neither absolutely true or entirely false, but rather a reflection of the artist's perspective"* (p. 75). It is thanks to neuroplasticity that therapeutic interventions can be successful in transforming the impact of our experiences in the past on our way of being in the present (more about this below).

There are various types of memory. One important way to differentiate types is by how long a memory lasts. Short-term memory lasts about 60 seconds and needs to be used immediately. A good example of short-term memory is remembering a phone number long enough to dial it after looking it up. Working memory lasts a few seconds to a few hours. It sticks around long enough to put it to work for a specific purpose. An example of a short version of working memory is solving a complex, multi-portion math problem in your head. A longer-term example is studying for a written test, holding on to the information long enough to perform well. Finally, long-term memory relies on the consolidation of related bits of data across various brain areas for recall within hours to months. Long-lasting memory relies on the same encoding and consolidation process and is defined by lasting up to a lifetime.

Long-term and long-lasting memory comes in many forms, most basically conscious and unconscious. Conscious (or explicit) versions are time- and place-stamped by the hippocampus and include declarative, episodic, and semantic memories. *Declarative* memory involves facts and information, or general knowledge. The *episodic* aspect of such knowledge is about personal felt experiences during and about specific events that are linked to places, times, and emotions (such as recalling your first day of school your first crush, a difficult relationship breakup). *Semantic* memory is about facts and knowledge of your own life (e.g., knowing the date of your partner's birthday) and the world in general, allowing us to learns details about the world we experience and live in, as well as remembering vocabulary and language, board concepts and specific information, and so on. Together, episodic and semantic memories create our *autobiographical* memory – our life stories and narratives, informed both by personal experience and by 'book' and fact learning. Autobiographical memory is central to our perception of self (including in relationship to others) and – by definition – continues to evolve across our lifetime. Our autobiographical memory is conscious and yet also strongly influenced by unconscious memories.

Unconscious long-term memories, also referred to as implicit memory, are not time or date-stamped and are either *procedural* to allow us to complete common tasks without any thought (e.g., the muscle memory we rely on to ride a bike) or *emotional*, such as the unconscious patterns we may have in relationships, automatic reaction to events, emotional reactivities that seem out of proportion to the event that triggers them, and more. Emotional implicit memories are very much related to the kleshas and gunas and have a strong effect on thoughts, interpretations of life events, understanding of new learning and facts, relationship and behavioral habits, and all types of patterns locks (i.e., on the vrittis and samskaras). They are not mediated by the hippocampus and hence have no conscious link to particular events, places, or times (i.e., they do not have time- and place stamps of conscious memory). As alluded to above, different brain waves are important to different aspects of memory. The following table summarizes this information:

Summary of Brain Wave Contributions to Memory		
Brain Waves	**Memory Role**	*Examples*
Delta	Consolidation (deep sleep)	Reinforcing learning during non-REM sleep
Theta	Encoding and retrieval	Learning new information, recalling episodic memories
Alpha	Encoding and recall (calm focus)	Studying, retrieving information in a distraction-free state
Beta	Active recall, working memory	Solving problems, recalling short-term information
Gamma	Integration, long-term storage	Complex learning, forming deep memory connections

Finally, memory – and its functions in learning – is also related to the next vritti of fantasy or imagination. Imagination requires both recollection and prediction. Memory, in many ways, may exist for the very purpose of helping us predict the future. Recalling the past is key to being able to use imagination and to make predictions. We need to have access to all types of memory to interpret the present moment and what it might mean for the future. Of course, we may not always make the right predictions – this is when memory leads to prediction errors, or in yoga language, the vritti of misperception. Our gunas and kleshas affect the nature of our prediction errors, especially as related to implicit memories that function outside our conscious awareness. Further, and as noted above, our level of curiosity and humility may also affect how well we can predict and the accuracy with which we orient to the present moment, use it to encode information to investigate further, and to attempt to ground perceptions and predictions in a larger, more well-informed context.

> "There is no organ in the body that is more designed to change in response to experience than the brain."
> Richard Davidson

Vikalpa or Creativity

This *vritti* represents our imagination, fantasy, creative thinking, future thinking, and daydreaming. It can clearly be used for good or can distort our view of reality. The word derives from *kalpa*, which means imagination; *vikalpa* means crooked or distorted imagination. Memory is necessary for imagination to work. In turn, as modern science shows, imagination is necessary for new learning and curiosity – which, in turn, affect memory. The cycle of interdependence continues.

- *Flavored*: getting trapped in the future, getting lost in daydreams and then not acting; clinging to wishes and desires for particular outcomes of developments
- *Unflavored*: creativity, dreams for the future, impetus for trying new things, creation of change, emergence of new ideas, development of new solutions to old problems
- We forget that the future is not yet real – that our future as we construct it in the mind, is simply a thought in the present moment
- Associated with *theta* and *alpha* waves – slow brain waves
  - 4 to 8 and 8 to 12 cycles per second, respectively
- Theta brain waves are predominant during light sleep, deep relaxation, as well as sub- or unconsciously driven behaviors that have been deeply ingrained and learned so as to unfold routinely
  - associated with daydreaming, visualization, or guided imagery, also with meditation
  - associated with being caught up in a routine or on automatic pilot
  - associated with intuition and lucid dreaming; can help memories rise to the surface to produce creativity and connection or openness toward others and new ideas
  - can support problem-solving skills and enhances new learning
- Alpha brain waves are briefly experienced upon falling asleep and upon waking (the state when insights population into your head when you wake up)
  - associated with deep relaxation accompanied by deep focus
  - associated with non-arousal; with a sense of comfort, harmony, and happiness
  - arises with day dreaming, the default mode network, and free association; invites creativity, brainstorming, and learning
  - habit begins to melt away; creativity emerges during alpha waves
  - flow happens at the intersection of alpha and beta waves – a combination of alert creativity and open receptivity; an openness to novelty and unpredictability

Modern Science Perspective on Imagination

From a scientific perspective, imagination and creativity are complex cognitive processes rooted in a variety of neural mechanisms that are developed from and constantly influenced by our biopsychosociocultural matrix, past experiences, and current motivations. Imagination is defined as the mind's capacity to create new scenarios, images, or ideas based on prior experiences. Imagination is heavily involved in planning, problem-solving, and abstract thinking – just as pointed out above about memory. It allows us to simulate possible future events, understand others' perspectives (theory of mind), and create novel solutions to problems (Schacter & Thakral, 2024). Imagination involves the brain's default mode network (and its connections to the medial prefrontal cortex, posterior cingulate cortex, and angular gyrus); as such, it is particularly active during rest and deliberate introspection (e.g., meditation).

Creativity similarly involves producing ideas, solutions, or creations (including art, literature, music, and more) that are novel and unique, as well as invaluable and constructive. Creativity is essential in both divergent thinking (i.e., generating many ideas) and convergent thinking (narrowing down the options to the most auspicious choice). Like imagination and memory, creativity arises from activity in the default mode network, executive control network for evaluation and refinement, and salience network for switching between these networks. Introspection draws on memory and imagination to create new ideas and then to review them mentally to sort out which are most likely to have merit, value, or meaning.

By now, it likely is becoming clear that there is a constant and crucial interplay between memory, imagination, and creativity. The abilities to imagine something novel or to create something new are firmly rooted in stored experiences and knowledge of the past – that is in memory. Memory provides the raw materials that fuel the brain's capacity to reimagine and recombine existing information into innovative ideas or scenarios; memory is as much prospective as retrospective (Schacter et al., 2008). Imagination draws particularly heavily on episodic memories that yield access to the vivid details of personal experiences. The brain essentially accesses and rearranges fragments of *past* experiences into new possibilities to create thoughts about the *future*, in the context of the *present* moment and its demand characteristics (e.g., such as the problem to be solved or the guided imagery offered during a yoga session). Creativity similarly depends on retrieval of memories in the context of current motivation (e.g., desire to create a piece of art or music or to develop a new scientific hypothesis or theory). New creations are then evaluated by the executive control network for originality and meaning, giving evidence to the idea that creativity transforms prior experience and current intention into something greater than the sum of their respective parts (Addis et al., 2007; Beaty et al., 2018). The richer the fount of experiences and knowledge, the vaster the scope of what can be imagined and created. Exposure to diverse stimuli and the deliberate cultivation of memory can, therefore, enhance creative potential, offering a broader palette of materials for the mind to draw upon. In this way, the past and present continual inform and inspire possibilities for the future, making memory, imagination, and creativity the very fabric of our human capacity for change, growth, transformation, and evolution at a personal and collective level. We will revisit this idea below in the context of transforming reactivity into responsiveness that reflects our access to making new choices rather than being trapped in old habits and pattern locks.

Nidra or Deep Dreamless Sleep

This *vritti* represents the absence of conscious thought or mental fluctuations during deep sleep. It is defined as emptiness or the absence of the other four *vrittis*. It, too, can have positive or negative effects on our perceptions of the world and our experiences.
- *Flavored*: getting trapped in escapism, avoidance, getting lost in spaciness
- *Unflavored*: rejuvenation through deep, dreamless sleep
- Sleep is greatly affected by the gunas and also can help us discern which of the gunas may be primary in our lives:
  - tamas: heavy, dull sleep that leaves us feeling tired and worn out upon awakening
  - rajas: agitated, disturbed, restless sleep that leaves us feeling unrested and perhaps anxiety or agitated upon awakening

- o sattva: deep restful, undisturbed sleep that leaves us feeling bright, light, and refreshed upon awakening
- The nature of our sleep may also give us hints about the nature of mind, or our mind states
- Associated with delta brain waves
  - o 1 to 4 cycles per second
  - o predominant during deepest meditation, unconscious states or detachment from conscious thought (including hypnosis), mental inactivity, and dreamless sleep (active dreaming involves theta waves)
  - o essential to renewal, restoration, regeneration, and healing
  - o linked to the unconscious mind and deep sleep
  - o perceived as highly beneficial to health

Modern Science Perspective on Sleep

Sleep is essentially our brain hard at work during a different state of consciousness. While ancient yoga views sleep as the absence of the other vrittis or mental fluctuations, modern science had demonstrated amply that sleep is not the absence of mental activity. Indeed, sleep is a dynamic process involving four distinct stages of unique mental activity, each contributing in unique ways to health and wellbeing. The four primary sleep stages (defined below) can be categorized into non-REM sleep (comprising three phases of increasing depth) and REM sleep (rapid eye movement sleep). They alternate within cycles of approximately 90 minutes (though this varies over the course of the night, with longer cycles early and shorter ones later during sleep). Ample research points toward ideal circadian cycles for sleep (Panda, 2018), with sleep happening most auspiciously at night, ideally starting between 9 and 11p and lasting for 7.5 to 8 hours for adults, 8 to 10 hours for adolescents, and 9 to 12 hours for younger children.

Deep sleep dominates the early part of the sleep period (which happens most auspiciously at night); REM sleep becomes more frequent later during the sleep period. Each stage of sleep has its own unique brain activity or signature (Ranganath, 2024)

- *Non-REM Stage 1 or Light Sleep*: a transition from wakefulness to sleep, marked by slowed heart rate and relaxed muscles
- *Non-REM Stage 2 Sleep*: a deeper phase where the body temperature drops and brain activity slows, interspersed with bursts of electrical signals called sleep spindles
- *Non-REM Stage 3 or Deep Sleep*: also known as slow-wave sleep (SWS), a phase vital for physical restoration, tissue repair, and immune function
- *REM Sleep*: characterized by vivid dreaming and heightened brain activity, a stage supporting memory consolidation, emotional regulation, and creativity – sometimes called paradoxical sleep because its brainwave signature is similar to the bursts that are seen during waking hours

A multitude of functions have been scientifically associated with sleep in general, and with specific stages in particular. Following is a brief overview of some of the scientific insights into the functions and purposes of sleep. This listing is an overview of major points – it is neither comprehensive nor inclusive; it simply serves as food for thought and motivation to explore more with curiosity.

- *Glymphatic Drainage:* During deep non-REM sleep, the brain activates the glymphatic system, a waste-clearance mechanism that flushes out toxins such as beta-amyloid proteins (linked to Alzheimer's disease). This process, which involves morphological changes in the microglia that allows cerebrospinal fluid to move more freely through the brain (Yang et al., 2024), highlights the restorative and cleansing role of sleep in maintaining cognitive health and preventing neurodegeneration (Jessen et al., 2015). Additional cellular repair processes also occur during deep sleep and thus make sleep important to physical recovery.
- *Memory Consolidation:* Sleep facilitates memory consolidation by processing and organizing information acquired during the day. Non-REM sleep, especially slow-wave sleep, strengthens declarative memory (facts and knowledge), while REM sleep enhances procedural memory (skills and habits). This intricate coordination supports learning, problem-solving, creative thinking, and imagination. The type of memory consolidation that occurs during sleep integrated disparate and vastly distributed bits of data, information, and experience across many parts of the brain enhancing our capacity for context-specific retrieval, seeing the big picture of a situation, and accessing new and wiser ways of seeing the world (Walker, 2018).
- *Hormonal Regulation and Cellular Repair:* Key hormones, including human growth hormone and melatonin, are released during sleep. Melatonin release begins 2 to 3 hours before regular bed time and coordinates the sleep-wake cycle, waxing early and waning by the end of the sleep period. Growth hormone secretion peaks during deep sleep, and metabolic demand decreases during sleep, aiding in tissue repair and muscle growth (Carroll & Prather, 2021; Chennaoui et al., 2021).
- *Immune Function:* Sleep enhances immune function by promoting the production of cytokines, proteins essential for fighting infection and inflammation (Żerek & Sitarek, 2024). Chronic sleep deprivation interrupts this defense system, leading to increased vulnerability to illnesses.
- *Emotional Regulation:* REM sleep is crucial for processing emotions and maintaining psychological resilience. By reinterpreting and integrating emotional experiences during sleep, the brain mitigates stress and enhances emotional stability (Walker, 2018). Sleep deprivation can disrupt this process, increasing susceptibility to mood disorders.

Clearly, prioritizing adequate, high-quality sleep is essential for maintaining health, enhancing performance, and fostering resilience. Unfortunately, sleep disruption, sleep loss, and sleeping disorders are extremely prevalent in the Western world. Sleep quality is highly correlated with mental health, affect (*vedana*), and arousal (*gunas*). Individuals with insomnia have a greater likelihood to have mental or physical illness and individuals with mental or physical illness are very likely to experience insomnia. This is most likely a bidirectional relationship – sometimes insomnia contributes (precipitated or predisposed) to health challenges; sometimes health challenges lead to insomnia. Regardless of the cause-effect relationship, the correlation between the two makes addressing issues related to sleep hygiene a helpful intervention for clients or students with mental or emotional presenting concerns. Sleep deprivation has many potentially serious consequences (Altevogt & Colten, 2006; Walker, 2018), with symptoms increasing with degree of sleep deprivation, including, but not limited to stroke, cardiovascular disease, mood disorder, metabolic illness, and memory impairment.

Science suggests that healthful sleep routines are key to the physical and mental wellbeing that comes from healthful sleep. Following are a few suggestions; a more detailed look is beyond the current scope but encouraged for self-study via relevant readings (Amen, 2017; Panda, 2018; Walker, 2018). Three broad categories are offered below. Yoga has excellent evidence supporting its contribution to all of these, from creating sattvic and healthful sleep environments to moderate and mindful food intake to generally healthful lifestyle habits of supporting ease and wellbeing (Brems, 2024b; Datta et al., 2021; Gupta et al., 2023; Panjwani et al., 2021).

- Sleep environment
  - keep your bedroom dark and quiet
  - lower the temperature in your bedroom – sleep is facilitated by a cool environment
  - choose a mattress that suits your physical needs
  - choose bedding that feels soothing to your skin
  - use blankets/covers that are neither too light, nor too heavy; neither too cool, nor too warm
  - do not keep devices in your bedroom that emit light even when turned off (e.g., LCD alarm clocks, computers, phones, energy vampires)
- Food and drink habits
  - stop eating at least 3 hours before bedtime
  - make your last meal before going to bed a light meal (i.e., dinner may best not be a heavy meal)
  - focus your diet on unprocessed foods
  - make vegetables, nuts and seeds, healthful oils (e.g., olive, avocadoes), and healthful protein sources your primary sources of nutrition
  - avoid sugary foods before bedtime that may spike blood sugar and then drop it quickly
  - avoid alcohol or caffeine close to bedtime – caffeine has a long half-life: for some individuals it may be necessary to avoid caffeine as early as noon
  - ponder if too much water late in the evening disrupts sleep because the need to urinate interrupts sleep – explore how much and how late you can drink water to avoid having to get up
- Daytime and bedtime routines
  - have a regular sleep schedule –go to bed and wake up at the same time each day; do not vary this during the weekend or on non-work days – stay consistent
  - aim for 7-8 hours of sleep for adults (check on recommendations for children and adolescents – they vary by age)
  - minimize naps during the day; if you do power nap, keep it short (less than 30 minutes)
  - do not expose yourself to blue light (e.g., computer or television screens) within an hour of going to bed as this disrupts circadian rhythms
  - engage in relaxing activities before bedtime (e.g., reading, listening to soft music)
  - although exercise earlier in the day promotes sleep, high-intensity exercise right before bed may interfere with falling asleep
  - meditate and clear your mind before going to bed; resolve fights with loved ones if at all possible – do not go to bed angry

> "It is not that something different is seen but that one sees differently."
> Carl Jung

Interaction of the Kleshas and the Vrittis

Pramana Right Perception	**Viparyaya** Misperception	**Vikalpa** Creativity, Imagination	**Smriti** Memory, Recollection
\multicolumn{4}{c}{*Raga = Craving, Clinging*}			
• Enjoying what is in this moment without expectation for repetition • Recognizing craving or clinging and transcending it mindfully • Holding each pleasurable moment loosely – neither craving it, nor detaching from it • Being in the moment • Enjoying the recollection of lovely moments • Remember the past accurately • Getting imaginative about the future • Nurture ideas and plans without clinging • Seeing wiser ways of being	• Clinging to enjoyment that has passed • Creating craving for the afterglow of what was pleasurable before • Longing for what you had before • Not knowing when you have had enough • Losing the pleasure of the moment for wanting it to last longer or forever • Developing catalog consciousness (craving craving itself – looking for things to want) • Getting attached to certain positive outcomes or expecting certain positive conditions • Grasping for more	• Dreaming of future pleasure • Being in the midst of enjoyment and planning for its recurrence ("I want to do this again") instead of being with it right here, right now • Looking for the next strawberry while you are still eating this one • Already reaching for the next moment • Get attached to outcomes of plans made earlier • Always planning for more pleasures to come rather than being with life right here and now • Escaping into fantasy that satisfies desire	• Getting lost in the memory of past pleasures or relationships • Being nostalgic for prior sensations or enjoyable moments "I wish could have this again…" • Craving for the past and not living in the moment • Idealizing the past • Rewriting history as having been more positive than it was • Being nostalgic for the past as better or ideal "those were the days" • Regretting missed pleasure "why didn't I …?" • Escaping into memories to avoid the present
\multicolumn{4}{c}{*Dvesa = Aversion*}			
• Being with resentment, anger, or aversion without getting caught up in them • Tolerating negative affect and investigating it to transcend it • Being with aversion without getting reactive • Recognizing as aversion arises and accepting it, working with it, and letting it go as possible • Recognizing and dealing with past hurts, challenges, trauma	• Clinging to anger, pain, or hurt "carrying the hot coal of anger" • Fighting difficulty or challenge; being reactive • Being resentful or rejecting of sensations or feelings that are less than pleasurable • Avoiding/repressing/ denying current difficult emotions or sensations • Losing present moment awareness by tuning out difficulty or challenge	• Plotting revenge • Planning to get even • Fearing the same challenge in the future • Obsessing, worrying, creating anxiety over anticipated dangers, displeasures, pains • Limiting future behavior based on past experiences "I will never do this again – it was too…" "I can't do this because …" • Planning, shrinking back assuming that more pain is to come • Anticipating the worst, always being	• Getting trapped or caught in ruminations about past slights, pains, hurts, challenges • Carrying forward a hurt from the past, from old relationships or experiences • Regretting or rejecting actions, experiences, or events in the past • Feeling shame for past thoughts, feelings, behaviors or actions • Assuming the past is still present in the current moment – not

| Interaction of the Kleshas and the Vrittis ||||
Pramana Right Perception	*Viparyaya* Misperception	*Vikalpa* Creativity, Imagination	*Smriti* Memory, Recollection
• Being realistic about risk now and in the future – planning to prevent pain without becoming obsessive • Glimpsing a life beyond self-preoccupation	• Increasing physical pain by adding emotional suffering • Dissociating from the now • Clinging to past resentments, to old dislikes or feuds	pessimistic about the future and others • Being resentful if planned outcomes do not seem to materialize • Ignoring possibilities of future pain	being able to transcend and integrate • Denying, yet being stuck in the past • Resenting the past • Holding grudges • Repressing the past
Avidya = Confusion			
• Clear perception not colored by clinging, confusion, or aversion • Accurate perception of experiences and relationships • Correct interpretation of what is in front of us • Clarity about perceptions – undistorted by desire, beliefs, or hatred • Drawing accurate conclusions • Appreciating the past via accurate, clear memories • Accurately drawing on prior learning and experience • Planning for the future with clarity and purpose • Seeing altruistic purpose	• Misinterpreting experiences • Misinterpreting events • Misunderstanding behaviors by others • Jumping to conclusions • Carrying prejudices and prejudgments • Overlooking moments of contentment because they feel neutral • Confusing sense pleasures with joy or contentment • Thinking we are the only one who suffers from aging, death, disease, and accidents • Creating stories to without verification of fact • Believing everything we think	• Mistaking fantasy for reality • Getting lost in imagination without direction or focus • Not knowing how to plan realistically • Confusing thoughts about the future with the present moment • Losing track that future only exists as a thought in the present • Trying to predict the future • Feeling confused or lost when the future does not turn out as envisioned or as planned • Leaning into the future – wanting the next thing • Doing things in order to make something else happen (in-order-to thinking)	• Confusing recollection with the present – losing track that the past exists only as a thought now • Mistaking recollection as reality • Getting lost in memories unable to separate them from the present • Mistaking the past as destiny • Allowing the past to rule the present • Expecting the past to repeat itself and being confused when things turn out differently • Being reactive now due to experience yesterday • Confusing past memory with current experience
Asmita = Ego			
• Seeing the self clearly as interdependent, everchanging, and empty of separate or independent existence • Begin flexible in role identities • Having clarity about relationships and their evolution	• Getting trapped, adhering rigidly to identities we have developed • Misunderstanding roles or personas (our own and others') as the true self • Not being able to shift into new roles as life evolves and new demands emerge	• Wanting to be someone else • Wanting a different identity or life – craving becoming ... • Avoiding facing present self-identities or roles (out of shame, fear, confusion) • Imaging a different kind of self without a	• Rejecting old identities • Feeling shame about past roles, self-identities, or ways of being in the world • Trying to destroy old identities or parts of you • Trying to undo old memories that are no longer consistent

Interaction of the Kleshas and the Vrittis			
Pramana Right Perception	**Viparyaya** Misperception	**Vikalpa** Creativity, Imagination	**Smriti** Memory, Recollection
• Being able to evolve new self-definitions and responsibilities as life evolves • Not clinging to a particular vision of the self or the other • Being open to new experiences and beliefs about roles and relationships • Understanding past roles and responsibilities without regret or clinging – using these understandings to evolve and grow • Envisioning new roles and responsibilities with clarity and purpose • Glimpsing the possibility of a decentered, wiser self • Being able to take others' perspectives • Considering and respecting others' needs and desires • Being open to learning, unlearning, and relearning	• Resenting roles we feel cast into • Striving to uphold expectations placed on us by others • Having particular role expectations of others and feeling let down or confused when they do not conform to these expectations • Assuming roles or identities without clear direction, purpose, or intent • Falling into self-identities that do not feel genuine or authentic • Identifying with the subject of an earlier kosha (body, affect, mind, emotion) • Caring only about our own needs and desires – not those of others • Controlling others because we think we know best • Needing to be right to feel secure	clear plan for how to get there • Telling others what to do and who to be/become • Speaking for others • Fantasizing about different ways of being– different identities, roles, and responsibilities without a clear path on how to achieve them • Getting trapped in imagined or fantasized identities though they do not mesh with actual behaviors and beliefs • Making plans for a way of being (e.g., careers, family planning) that do not match genuine desires for the self as it actually want to be expressed • Grasping for a new identity without the wisdom of evolution toward the next koshas	with who you feel you are now • Getting trapped in old identities or role expectations • Getting trapped in cultural or familial expectations • Accepting roles and responsibilities we belief we "should" assume • Denying self-identities because they feel threatening or unacceptable • Sticking with past self-identities or roles that no longer fit the present • Denying aspects of self out of shame, fear, or confusion • Nostalgia about "old" roles or identities – reviving the past (perhaps coloring it) • Telling others who they used to be • Assuming what others are, need, or want based on dated information
Abhinivesha = Fear of Change			
• Feeling at peace with impermanence • Embracing change, transformation, and growth • Recognizing the shared truth of illness, aging, and death • Openness to change, new relationships, growth, and evolution • Letting life unfold without fear, obsession, or anxiety	• Resisting change, growth, or evolution • Feeling exempted from disease or aging • Feeling invincible or invulnerable • Wanting things to stay the same • Being caught in ruts that no longer serve • Not seeing change in others • Believing in a permanent self or in the permanence of experience	• Fantasizing about things staying as they are • Using imagination to pretend that there is no change, no aging, no illness, no death • Being lost in fantasy to avoid facing change, aging, death, illness • Fantasizing about a happily-ever-after • Resisting the creativity of being and evolving able to	• Being nostalgic for how things used to be • Being lost in remembrance of the good old days • Reimagining the past to create a sense of non-change • Creating a sense of permanence based on memories, especially shared cultural memories • Creating false memories of stability and non-change

Pramana Right Perception	*Viparyaya* Misperception	*Vikalpa* Creativity, Imagination	*Smriti* Memory, Recollection
• Exploring new ways of being in the world with an open mind • Embracing uncertainty • Lacking fear at the moment of death • Glimpsing vijnanamaya kosha and the next stage of development • Moving toward wisdom, transcending samskaras • Opening the heart to the brahma viharas as a means to embrace change	• Using self-protective mechanisms that are no longer functional • Clinging to old beliefs and values • Staying trapped in mental constructions • Not seeing potential for evolution to the next layer or stage of development • Refusing to change in harmony with new realities and circumstances • Misunderstanding change as negative • Perceiving change as dangerous or optional	envision a new way of being • Denying the existential imperative • Striving forcefully for the possibility of a wiser self • Imagining what could be • Craving continued existence • Or to the contrary, craving for an out – craving for non-existence (e.g., due to despair about the present) • Imagining living forever	• Rewriting the past as a way of denying change or growth in self or others • Being stuck in old ways – old habits, old beliefs, old knowledge • Not moving forward by refusing to embrace new truths or new realities • Staying identified with earlier koshas, never glimpsing the next possibility • Using the past as the reason to stay the same

Interaction of the Kleshas and the Vrittis

**Most of our pain is due to a lack of a deeper truth.
The opposite of pain is not pleasure, but clarity.**
Stephen Levine, 2002, Turning Toward the Mystery, p. 99

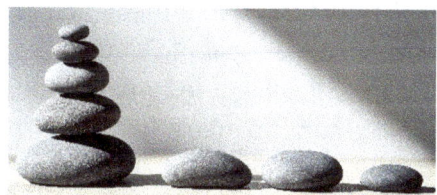

Learn as if you will live forever, live like you will die tomorrow
Mahatma Gandhi

Exercising Reason and Living Our Values

The fact that we explore our beliefs and ideas to identify misperceptions or to caution ourselves not to think that we know better than others, does not mean that there are no bad ideas of beliefs. Andrew Norman, in *Mental Immunity* (2021), gives some helpful guidelines for identifying "bad ideas" or what in yoga we might call inauspicious beliefs. He suggests that we can differentiate good from bad ideas or sound from unsound beliefs by their (potential) consequences and impacts as well as by their provable veracity.

- If an idea or belief has sound scientific evidence (based on quantitative or qualitative research methods), it deserves greater consideration as being a potentially good idea
- If an idea is misleading (i.e., counters evidence that is available based on some rigid belief), it is likely a bad idea
- If an idea leads to harmful consequences for self or others, we must consider the possibility that it is a bad idea

He concludes that "some worry that goodness or badness are 'subjective,' or in the eye of the beholder. This is nonsense. The good-making and bad-making properties of an idea are facts, to be determined by *honest inquiry* [emphasis added] as other facts are. For instance, the harmful effects of incitements to violence may be hard to measure, but they are very read." (2021, p. 41).

Norman (p. 70) also offers six ideas that are warning flags that we may be engaging in "unreason". Namely, if we believe the following ideas for our own or others' beliefs, it is likely that we are not engaging in adequate inquiry to assess whether a belief is potentially harmful, misleading, false, or otherwise problematic.

- Beliefs are private, and no one else's concern.
- We have a right to believe what we like.
- Values are subjective – relative, that is, to a fundamentally arbitrary set of preferences.
- We have no standing to criticize other people's value judgements.
- Basic value commitments are not subject to rational assessment.
- Questioning a person's core commitments is fundamentally intolerant, mean-spirited, or unkind.

The interior practices of yoga invite us to engage in honest inquiry about our and others' beliefs, attitudes, and values. They invite us to assess the veracity and impact of our and others' intentions, thoughts, and actions and to use discernment to let go of beliefs that do not serve the truth or the wellbeing of all.

According to yoga, it is our responsibility to examine our and others' beliefs and perceptions – to reflect upon them and to let go of them, to confront them as we grow and learn. In fact, the very practice of self-inquiry is in line with modern research that suggests that we must constantly learn, unlearn, and relearn to ensure that we maintain critical thinking and logical accuracy.

Mind States

Mind states are created from the impacts of the afflictions (*kleshas*) and fluctuations (*vrittis*) of the mind; *they are the vrittis and kleshas made visible.* They are also influenced by and may reflect the *gunas* – our assessment and response to the environment with regard to safety. Yoga defines five mind states (*kshipta, mudha, vikshipta, ekagra,* and *niruddha,* described below) in the order of degree to which they are affected or tinted by the *vrittis, kleshas,* and *gunas.*

Stabilizing the mind states is a central purpose in yoga practice and helps move us out of distraction, chaos, and ruminations into focused and clear mind states. Thus, yoga teaches us to watch and bear witness to all of our mind states, to recognize that all mind states can arise quickly and transiently or can be pervasive and chronic. Through yoga, we notice which mind states predominate, which come and go, and how long they last. It is important to understand that all of us experience all the mind states and that we can learn to identify, understand, and transform the ones that present challenges. In fact, recognizing our mind states helps us become aware of the importance of investigating what underlies them: *vrittis, kleshas,* and *gunas.* In other words, mind states are a great pathway into better self-understanding.

Kshipta or Disturbed Mind

- Also known as monkey mind or chaotic mind
- Agitated, restless, troubled; chaotic or fickle; mentally scattered; behaviorally frenetic; relationally unpredictable
- Dominated by *rajas* and cycling between extreme states
- Heavily affected by the *kleshas* and *vrittis*
- No access to ease or calm – anxiety, panicked, even delusional
- Confusion reigns and decision-making is impaired

Mudha or Dull Mind

- Also known as cow, donkey, sloth, or slug mind; as well as confused or sinking mind
- Sometimes translated as stupefied (confused, dazed, befuddled, stunned, shocked) mind
- Lethargic, heavy, forgetful, sleepy, sluggish; mentally fatigued, tired; emotionally frozen or shut-down
- Ruminative – obsessively preoccupied with concern or frozen by worry
- Unable to self-motivate or create intention and initiative
- Dominated by *tamas* and lacking vitality; shrinking away from challenge (perhaps due to aversion or fear)
- Heavily affected by the *kleshas* and *vrittis*
- No access to productivity or contentment – sad, depressed, despondent, sinking
- Lack of energy reigns and motivation is impaired
- Cow mind might predominate your mind during the dying process; if we were able to recognize and transform cow mind earlier in life, we might be able to do so during death

Vikshipta or Distracted Mind

- Also known as butterfly mind or restless mind
- Distractable, with attention easily diverted to this or that; partially focused
- Occasional *sattva* arises; until the mind gets distracted and retracts back to tamas or rajas
- Still prone to the *kleshas* and *vrittis*
- Sometimes there is access to stability, but it is easily lost
- Confusion creeps in and concentration can be lost

Ekagra or Pointer Dog or Bird Dog Mind, Bear Mind; One-Pointed Mind

- Focused, fully concentrated, fully attentive – not prone to distraction
- *Sattva* is accessible more regularly and consistently
- *Kleshas* and *vrittis* can be transcended temporarily
- Access to peacefulness, awareness, and clear perceptions
- Intuition awakens and *buddhi* is accessed

Niruddha or Luminous Mind

- Lucid, fully absorbed, stable mind; thoughts are still
- Fluctuations and afflictions have been stilled; *sattva* is present
- *Kleshas* and *vrittis* are still
- Grace reigns
- Ego is transcended and liberation/awakening can occur (*moksha*)

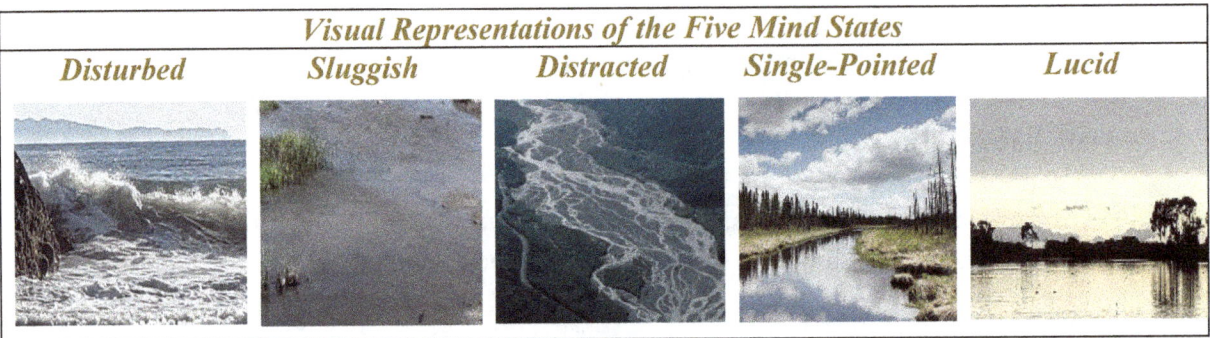

Visual Representations of the Five Mind States
Disturbed | Sluggish | Distracted | Single-Pointed | Lucid

Once we can recognize our mind states and begin to understand their roots in the *gunas*, *kleshas*, and *vrittis*, we can transform the challenges that dysregulate our mind and emotions. For example, if we watch and witness cow or sloth mind, we can cultivate alertness. We can engage with challenge rather than avoiding it; we can reward and seek out interactions and actions through which we can rise to a challenge. If we notice butterfly mind, we can cultivate mindfulness and concentration. We can encourage uni-tasking and stop multi-tasking. We can engage more fully with the present moment.

One way to begin to work with mind states is simply to recognize them. Recognition means not getting caught up in a story about them, which will only add more fuel to the fire of the kleshas and vrittis. We take note with compassion and observe with open-hearted and open-minded curiosity and compassion. We cultivate transitions to mind states of greater ease and do so without judgment, stories, narratives, or expectations. Attuning ourselves to the mind states is an excellent pathway on the road to self-awareness. The mind states are easily observed and creating awareness of them helps us begin to recognize our *gunas*, *kleshas*, and *vrittis*. This recognition paves the way for working with our patterns, habits, and reactivities, allowing us – ultimately – to transform ourselves, our lives, and our relationships.

Notably, even communities can have mind states. Groups can become chaotic, disorganized, dull, or lethargic. Groups can come together toward common goals and luminous purpose. As we learn to read our personal mind states, we can also begin to read the mind states of the various groups to which we belong and with which we interact. This attunement to collective ways of expressing mind states can once again bring yoga off the mat in a way that can foster personal engagement and can create societal change.

For example, if we are working in a group and begin to notice that there is a lot action without any clarity of direction, we can consciously rein in the chaos that is present and help everyone begin to participate in formulating a purpose and a direction for the collaboration. If a group has become complacent and indifferent, we can invite them to refresh their joint interest, become concerned about and engaged in a cause that gives them a clear focus and shared purpose.

The Path Toward Transforming the Vrittis

Vrittis, in combination with *gunas* and *kleshas*, result in habitual ways of responding, experience-based distorted cognitions, conditioned powerful emotions, and harmful habits (called *samskaras*, in Sanskrit). *Samskaras* are patterns and structures in our mental and emotional landscape that self-perpetuate and may or may not be useful, depending on the degree of conditioning, degree of awareness, and degree of coloring by the *kleshas* and *gunas*. Just as with the *kleshas*, the key to working with the *vrittis* is to recognize and learn to let go of our identification with them (more about this below). When *vidya* (as opposed to avidya or all the other *kleshas*) is brought to the *vrittis*, they can become vehicles for growth and change – more about this in the sections on *samskaras* and *karma*.

- We practice mindfulness and concentration so that we can ultimately deconstruct the self as defined by the *vrittis* and *kleshas* – we recognize the impermanence of everything (physical sensation, affect, thoughts, emotions). We begin to notice that all there is, is arising, being, and releasing.
- We work with the *vrittis* by finding their root causes. The mind can only become still if we recognize why it is uneasy to begin with.
- We embrace the notions that yoga – in its definition as the calming of the fluctuations of the mind – in essence asks us to determine the causes of our mental fluctuations so that we might remove them and find peace. In the context of healthcare and self-care, this means that we have a commitment to identifying and treating etiology (causes), not the symptoms, of suffering.
- We recognize our patterns and habits and use our mental capacities of correct perception, imagination, memory, and even sleep to transform these *samskaras*. To do this, it is necessary to understand *samskaras*, or pattern locks, more fully.

Samskaras or Habits, Patterns, and Reactivities

The *gunas*, *kleshas*, and *vrittis* are the root causes that lead to patterns, habits, ruts, grooves, routines, and reactive styles in all the *koshas*. They deeply affect our perceptions and create samskaras – pattern locks that include our habitual and recursive ways of responding, distorted cognitions and cognitive harmful habits (e.g., biases, prejudices), emotional reactivity, and behavioral and relationship patterns. Perceptions of everything we experience within our layers of experience and in our biopsychosociocultural context are neither permanent, nor entirely predictable, nor perfect (i.e., true or accurate; unflavored). They reflect our momentary interpretation of what is happening based on our experiences up to this very point in time. At times, they are reactively (bottom-up) predictable and seemingly permanent; at other times, they can be affected (perhaps made more accurate and changeable) via top-down control. In terms of changing our reactivity and changing our mind, we need to remember that perception is strongly flavored in each and every moment and that it tends to serve us well to explore the accuracy, truth, and malleability of our own and others' perceptions. In other words, it helps to not believe everything that comes to mind.

At the level of *annamaya kosha*, pattern locks overlap with the notion of reflexes. At the level of *pranamaya kosha*, they come in the form of nervous system defaults and affective reactivities. At the level of *manomaya koshas*, *samskaras* take many shapes, such as routines, habits, thought patterns, attitudinal fixedness, belief rigidity, ego identity, relationship patterns, behavioral ruts, and more. At the level of *vijnanamaya kosha*, *samskaras* transform into wise intuition that guides discerning choices while staying open to new possibilities. At this level, the *samskaras* are guided by awareness, wisdom, and the *brahma viharas*.

Development of Samskaras

Ruts, patterns, and habits develop in the brain according to Donald Hebb's (1949) principle of *what fires together, wires together*. Everything we experience, think, say, and do leaves an imprint in our brain – either perpetuating old habits or forging new neural pathways. As we transcend *samskaras*, we promote neuroplasticity and change. As we indulge in habit and reactivity, we perpetuate neural stagnation and narrowing (or fixation) of our perspective and capacity. The more often or repetitively we think a thought or feel an emotion, the more likely it is to arise again and again. The more we engage in certain patterns of behaviors or relationships, the more likely they are to recur. This is habit conditioning that at times even creates morphic resonance – through which we spread our habits and patterns to others.

Clearly, *samskaras* are more than simple habits. They permeate our own lives and penetrate into our collective. They can profoundly shape the culture, values, and practice we engage in and that we encourage and perpetuate in community, in our collective. The responsibility for recognizing and reshaping our *samskaras* thus is not simply individual; it is a collective responsibility that invites growth and transformation toward wholesome change, with clear vision about what serves the greater good.

Samskaras, both individual and collective, are recursive and self-perpetuating patterns of intention, perception, thought, belief systems, actions, and relationships. *Samskaras* in the individual or collective mind lead us to perceive the world based on expectations and predictions rather than reality. *Samskaras* in the mind reverberate into body and vitality (both arousal and affective tone). *Samskaras* in the body are hard-wired into our nervous system and stuck in our tissues; they make themselves felt in our vitality and our mind. In fact, *samskaras* – in any layer of the self – have profound and deep implications for expressions of the other koshas. Their recursive nature creates *vicious and auspicious cycles* of self-perpetuating perceptions, intentions, beliefs, thoughts, and actions.

How do we get into these patterns, habit, ruts, and ideologies? In some ways, we are wired for them. We are embedded, interdependent beings. We need others for survival and we need group memberships and social embeddedness to feel safe in body, energy or affect, and in mind and emotion. It is no evolutionary surprise that we have certain tendencies that support the development of beliefs and the maintenance of these beliefs once we have developed them. We are always in search of explanations and rules of thumb that can guide our behavior. We absorb these from our environment as grow up. The belief systems and structures in our environment will, in many ways, predict when we will believe and how we will believe - with an open, inquisitive mind or with a mind closed to new ideas and ways of knowing.

The human mind does not exactly love doubt. Because of the human tendency to want to understand and to feel as though we already know, we are prone to thinking errors that perpetuate what we already believe. Psychology has identified many biases that have been identified that contribute to our being stuck in certain beliefs or mental patterns, to our tendency to stick our head in the sand to new perspectives, new ideas, to our aversion to ongoing, lifelong learning, unlearning and relearning. Here are four examples:

- *Confirmation bias*: we seek out information that confirms what we already believe; we treat preferentially information and data that supports our pre-existing opinions and attitudes because we want them to be true (e.g., preferential news sources; selective social media feeds; ignoring contradictory sources)
- *Motivated reasoning:* we interpret and use information and data that we are exposed to according to beliefs, biases, and intentions we already have (e.g., we are more likely to dismiss research findings that clashes with our current beliefs, our emotional preferences, or our current behaviors – *"sugar can't be bad for me because ... "*; *"these data are biased"*)
- *Belief persistence*: we stick with a pre-existing personal, social, or societal belief despite evidence to the contrary (e.g., *"I am unlovable"*; *"all purple people are brilliant"*; *"there is no climate change"*)
- *Sunk cost fallacy*: we stick with an action, behavior, or relationship because we have already invested a lot of time or energy in it; we stick with something or someone that clearly is no longer useful or helpful because we do not want to waste the resources we already sand into the relationship or decision (e.g., staying in a bad relationship; keeping a car that is constantly in need of repair; sticking with a bad financial investment)

Because of the human tendency to stay with beliefs combined with our need for social embeddedness, we are prone to simply adopt the beliefs and attitudes that we grow up with – to be loyal to the beliefs that we are fed as our brains mature. Our groups celebrate this loyalty; in fact, some demand it. Others exploit and celebrate loyalty in belief and action, even making it dangerous to disobey or disbelieve. Faith and some political communities may demand complete loyalty to a faith in a supreme power or leader and to certain doctrines without encouraging introspection and conscious choice about one's endorsed faith(s) or values. These faiths and principles are spoken about with complete confidence and become ever more convincing.

Political communities may create social structures that maintain the status quo and perpetuate systems – sometimes even forcing those who dissent into silence or worse. We may see this in our societies as personal bigotry, the unquestioning embrace of all sorts of -isms, and the perpetuation of systemic and institutional forms of discrimination, authority, oppression, inequality, and worse – all in the name of allegiance and loyalty. We may see this in societies or groups that perpetuate ignorance, that demand unquestioning belief, that make it dangerous to dissent, and that limit access to resources that may help people change minds, attitudes, ideas, beliefs, and doctrines. In moments when we hear such confidence and conviction in a speaker (without a trace of doubt or inquiry), it may be helpful to remind ourselves not to confuse confidence with expertise or wisdom. It may be helpful to remember Goethe's admonition that we actually only really 'know' when we *do not* know (enough) because knowledge increases doubt and re-reflection. This also aligns with the idea that as learners we go through four stages of knowing (elucidated more thoroughly in Chapter 6), with unconscious incompetence (or ignorance) often being our starting point. In other words, the more we learn about something, the more we realize how little we know. Knowledge leads to more knowledge; ignorance and blind faith lead to stagnation and unwillingness to change.

Samskaras as Pattern Locks

Samskaras are, in a way, an expression of our biological imperative overriding our existential imperative – our wise and enlightened self. When we are trapped or locked into habitual, recursive, perception-coloring patterns, we stay reactive in that bottom-up sensations and inputs can short-circuit top-down executive control. *Samskaras* can be transmitted across the generations as *epigenetic research* is beginning to document. For example, food choices of grandparents may still be perceived in the turning on or off of particular genes two and more generations later. Trauma in one generation is transmitted and notable in subsequent generations. Recognizing and beginning to work with the samskaras is an important step in gaining more executive control, in moving toward enlightenment, toward inner wisdom.

In the context of *samskaras* and suffering, *kleshas* and *vrittis* function as the second arrow: they turn the human reality of having to face challenge, pain, and stress (i.e., the first arrow of sorrow) into suffering, compounding the initial pain or difficulty with reactivity, emotionality, and lack of understanding. Every identification with a particular kosha and being trapped in particular gunas (or nervous system states) adds to habit power. Together, all of these developmental and personality factors create "wrong view" (*avidya*), often shaped (created and reinforced) by the biopsychosociocultural context in which they arose, developed, were conditioned, were rewarded, and became hardened. In exploring *samskaras*, it can be helpful to remember that identification with particular *kleshas* can lead to calcified ways of being in the world, expressed in the three personality types (greedy/desirous; averse/angry; confused/deluded; see Chapter 4) that then define our intentions, thoughts, speech, and actions.

The *gunas* or polyvagal states in response to the neuroception by our autonomic nervous system of safety versus danger versus life threat also contribute to how we live, relate, and perceive the world. The stronger the influence of *kleshas* and *gunas* (i.e., the more unconsciously they flavor intentions, thoughts, speech, and actions), the more habit driven will be our way of responding to and being in the world – creating very compelling samskaras that create deep ruts. The author of *Think Again* (Grant, 2021) argues that little gets more in the way of new learning, recalibrating our values, and assimilating knowledge skillfully than ego-reactivity, the blind drivenness that comes from our *kleshas*.

Physical, affective (energetic), mental, and emotional fluctuations are not just inside of us. They become *effluents*, so the Buddha says; they flow out of our consciousness into the world. Whatever our emotional or mental vibrations, they will infect the world around us as well. Therefore, if we want to exercise good will (not just toward ourselves, but everyone), we have to learn restraint (or executive control) over both the *experience* and the *expression* of feelings and mental fluctuations, so that they neither harmfully flow out into the world and infect others, nor harmfully stay within us to short-circuit our wellbeing. That is, through yoga, we learn to be discerning about what comes into as well as what flows out of our mind (in the form of speech, actions, and relationship patterns).

Samskaras are in essence a pattern lock and, hence, require a pattern interrupt, a pattern reset to create new neural and cellular pathways. Restraint of the samskaric pattern lock is honed via mindfulness, interoception, and the inner limbs of yoga, starting with pratyahara (Limb 5). The practice of discernment about which inner and outer stimuli, experiences, relationships, and so on are allowed access into our minds (as opposed to arriving at our senses, but not being allowed to *infect* the mind) can help us overcome habitual reactivity or knee jerk reactions. We do not have to let every stimulus past the gates of the senses; whatever we do allow in, has the potential to reverberate in the mind (and hence in our world and relationships) for a long time, infecting us with suffering, with unhelpful or unskillful feelings and thoughts. Mindfulness, attention, concentration, alertness, and meditation serve as a pattern interrupt.

Interestingly, neuroscience has shown that when opinions, attachments, or core beliefs are challenged, this can trigger the amygdala and undermines rational exploration and open-mindedness. We react viscerally and from implicit (self-protective) memory to suggestions that we might be wrong or should change (Grant, 2021). This potential reactivity has implications for how we, as yoga teachers, talk about samskaras and about transcending ideas, opinions, beliefs, and habits in our yoga classes. We do not criticize or attack – instead, we encourage introspection and open-heartedness instead.

Samskaras can be helpful or hurtful. If they are based in *vrittis* strongly flavored or tinted by kleshas or survival patterns of the gunas, they may have been useful at one point but now have become unhelpful, unskillful, or inauspicious. If samskaras are mental shortcuts or habitual patterns that create efficiencies, they are skillful, auspicious, and helpful. For example, we all have routines that support ease of skill execution (e.g., we know how to brush our teeth, ride our bikes, drive our cars). Routines (or rituals) can turn into ruts or grooves, depending on how we use them and how we mindful we are of them. We can make sure that rituals, or useful habits (like a departure list from your work place or a morning ritual of getting ready for the day) stay fresh and auspicious by creating small occasional shifts that prevent them from turning into ruts.

The more refined and unaffected our habits are by the *gunas* and *kleshas*, the more refined, adaptable, changeable in light of new data, and auspicious they can be. If, for example, instead of using a particular ritual or pattern in every instance of being in a relationship, we adapt the ritual or pattern to the specific demand characteristics of the circumstances or interaction, the pattern with its new and adaptive sub-routines, can serve us well. If the *kleshas* or *gunas* guide us unimpeded, however, we cannot adapt the habit or routine to the currently present situational parameters. The *samskara*, or pattern lock, has become afflicted, and hence inauspicious.

Samskaras that are unafflicted by sense pleasures (kleshas) or by gunas can be guided by mature emotions. They will be flavored without bias or judgment by the brahma viharas, the yamas, generosity, and commitment to the wellbeing of all. Such habits are free of affliction and create only auspicious karma. Such patterns are open to new learning; they allows us to learn, unlearn, and relearn – to become flexible, open-minded, and open-hearted; to become fearless in the face of challenging opinions and data and willing to change ourselves and our systems (social, cultural, political, economic, and otherwise)

Samskaras occur in all tangible koshas:
- Samskaras occur *in the embodied self* (physical sensation, physical form, materialism) – these may manifest as attachment to or misidentification with physical habits, ways of moving, ways of pushing through or ignoring pain, ways of over-identifying with physical illness or challenge.
- *Samskaras* occur *in the affective and energetic self* (affective states, energetic states, preferences, cravings) – these may manifest as attachment to or misidentification with affective reactions and states of arousal as if these were the only ways to react/respond to a situation. It is as if our only affective response is the one that is driven by a particular coping style (*guna*) or *kleshas*.
- *Samskaras* occur *in the verbal and social self* (perceptions, mental sensations and formations, emotions) – these show up as attachment to or misidentification with *manomaya kosha* at the levels of *manas* (opinions, labels, attitudes) and *ahamkara* (ego identity), with a visceral amygdala response when these core beliefs or identities are challenged. They are stuck viewpoints that we fail to shift even in light of new data that suggest that our view is incorrect, partial (noting or hanging on to only a piece of the whole story), or distorted by calcified opinions or misperceptions. There is a vicious cycle wherein *samskaras* can affect perceptions, and perceptions (or misperceptions) can reinforce *samskaras*.
- *Samskaras* can also happen *on a societal or collective level* – they are collective, unquestioned beliefs that can be so strong as to be brainwashing. Current day examples of societal *samskaras* are White supremacy, oppression, internalized oppression, and similar calcified patterns of belief and behavior that are systemic and institutionalized to such a degree that they are rarely questioned. To counter societal samskaras, we need to commit to developing social justice habits.
- Other collective *samskaras* may manifest *as generational traumas* (passed down through families or communities) and familial *samskaras* (e.g., particular roles we play in our

families regardless of age; family habits and routines that persist despite being no longer functional or logical or age appropriate).

Samskaras begin to resolve in the more subtle and causal layers of self – though traces can remain. Traces of *samskaras* can remain even in the decentered and wise self (relationships, collective sensations, collective mental formations). This may show up as attachment to or misidentification with *vijnanamaya kosha* and *buddhi*, while still not glimpsing union or oneness (or emptiness of self). It may also be a very subtle identification with the pleasurable aspects of concentration or meditation, making the practice less about transformation and more about engaging in a pleasurable habit. When *samskaras* are transcended (even for a moment), we can access *anandamaya kosha* – we come closer to the truth of empty, interdependent, connected self. Successful work on the samskaras leads us toward insight, compassion, and lovingkindness and ushers in our readiness for moving toward *vijnanamaya kosha*. The challenge, then, is how to work with samskaras to overcome compelling habits and pattern locks in intentions, thoughts, speech, actions, and relationships.

Opening Heart and Mind To Transforming Pattern Locks

The *samskaras*, *kleshas*, and *vrittis* are not overcome by faith or belief, but by mindful and non-judgmental investigation and clear discernment. Mindfulness allows us to notice when we are driven by habit; discernment allows us to investigate the consequences of our pattern locks. Specifically, we use discernment to investigate whether our intentions, thoughts, speech, actions, and relationships are skillful or unskillful, *wholesome* or *unwholesome*.

Work with the *samskaras* helps move us beyond awareness (*samatha*) to insight (*vipassana*) and, ultimately, to compassion (one of the *brahma viharas*, defined below). Work with *samskaras* requires that we can learn and absorb (or assimilate) new information, fitting it into and allowing it to alter and expand our existing knowledge, values, and beliefs. Work with samskaras requires that we transcend reactive and ego-driven mental habits, opening ourselves up to new learning and new ways of being in the world. It does not require blind faith about new information; quite to the contrary, it requires a constant openness to and inquiry about new learning, new ideas, new concepts – a process of evaluating their legitimacy, veracity, and relevance (Grant, 2021). Additionally, changing our mind requires curiosity and humility. Without curiosity, we do not realize that there are other options and we do not feel inspired to pursue them if we do encounter them. Without humility, we get stuck in believing in our being right-ness.

Many frameworks have been proposed and applied for overcoming tenacious adherence to beliefs, opinions, attitudes, biases, and ideas; for disentangling ourselves from authoritarian or doctrinal systems that perpetuate -isms, inequality, and oppression; for taking cognitive responsibility for our ideology and our resultant actions; for resolving moral conflicts that arise from beliefs that do not align with values of collaboration and coexistence (i.e., interdependence and embeddedness). Reason, based on collaborative inquiry and experience-based exploration, can help us begin to recognize our mental shortcuts, emotional biases, cognitive errors, and culturally-skewed ideas and ideals. It can help us engage in rational checks and balances.

A three-step process was reported by Grant (2021) based on work being done in schools to help children begin to reason and develop open, inquisitive minds at an early age. This process teaches children to query the beliefs, 'knowledge', and attitudes with which they have grown up and that they have been exposed to in their biopsychosociocultural context. This is not a query to reject everything – it is a process of double-checking whether a held belief is defensible in the light of evidence.

- The first recommendation in this process is to interrogate, question, and analyze information that is being provided from any source, rather than simply consuming (or swallowing) it hook, line, and sinker.
- The second recommendation involves not being distracted by the rank or reputation of the provider of the information or the popularity of a belief or attitude. Simply asserting something with confidence does not make it true. Just because most people hold a particular attitude, it is not necessarily right. We have many historical examples of humans going wrong because of trusting the wrong leader, however renowned, famous, or infamous, or adhering to the wrong belief, no matter how prevalent.
- The third recommendation for dealing with information and beliefs is to look for the source of any assertion or attitude to which we are exposed or to which we already adhere. Why do we believe what we believe? How do we know it is true? Who told us, how did we learn? Was and is the source reputable?

In this process, we look for evidence and counter-evidence for our beliefs, collecting objective data (outer, measurable evidence). We access subjective (inner, experiential) data to examine our ideas. We test hypotheses to investigate the veracity of our and our group's biases. We collaborate with a wide group of people to draw conclusions. All of these methods (overlapping rather nicely with scientific principles) can be used to challenge our ideational (mental) tenacity (or even rigidity) and/or our faith or loyalty-based views and theories. They can help us challenge predetermined conclusions and cognitions that are self-serving, ideologically-based, or simply ego-protective, akin to Kahan's (2017) concept of identity-protective cognition that short-circuits rationality [and humanity] reflexively to justify beliefs and ideologies.

However, reason alone is not enough. Reason, whether experimentally or experientially based, needs to be embedded in a system of social and cultural values or norms of collaboration, meaning, shared commitments that are wholesome – *not for the select or the few, but for all*. This is where science can go wrong; this is where even simple mindfulness practices can lead to misunderstandings and bad conclusions mired in avidya. Reason must be infused with values of equality, adherence to principles that support the greater good, and altruistic, collective ideals to help us transcend narrow views, inhumane conclusions, and inequitable, even oppressive, ideologies. Reason not grounded in values of compassion, lovingkindness, and collective joy can mislead us profoundly. Mindfulness without value of non-harming, truthfulness, non-stealing, moderation, and generosity can result in selfish goals and even greater *avidya*.

Two frameworks for investigating or working discerningly with the transcendence of the samskaras at an individual level (where this process of honest inquiry must start, though it then also needs to progress to the collective level) come from the Buddhist traditions and have found their way into the yoga world in direct and indirect ways. Both frameworks challenge us to explore the origin of our understandings and opinions to loosen the grip of these beliefs and viewpoints on our consciousness. They encourage us to ask *how* we perceive situations and *why* we perceive them that way; they ask us to explore the true etiology of our viewpoints so that we can transcend them. They do all this in the context of collectively wholesome ethical commitments (think *yama*, *niyama*, and *brahma viharas*) that challenge us to look courageously and honestly at the consequences and reverberations of our intentions, thoughts, speech, and actions *at all times* and *for all beings*, in fact for our entire planet.

> "When we stop seeking the familiarity of samsara,
> when we stop fighting the groundlessness of freedom from imputed meaning,
> emptiness becomes an experience of awe, of the infinite, of limitless space."
> Pema Chodron, 2021, p. 95

RAIN Framework of Honest and Ethical Inquiry

This framework involves the process of **RAIN** (not necessarily used that directly in yoga, but helpful to know about; most yoga classes do not progress beyond the R and A of this acronym). RAIN (Kornfield, 2009) is a way of investigating the mind that employs inquiry along with self-compassion and the release of attachment or clinging.

- **R**ecognizing – becoming aware of when we get trapped in the *gunas*, *vrittis*, and *kleshas* (and their intersections)
- **A**llowing – looking openly at how this creates suffering in body, energy, affect, and mind
- **I**nquiring/Investigating – engaging in calm, mindful, concentrated inquiry that looks for the causes of this suffering, looking at the causes dispassionately; investigating how what we bring to an experience (i.e., our perceptions, attitudes, cravings) affects how we respond; looking deeply into how our perception of what is happening can change our experience of it; exploring the flavoring added to our actions, speech, and thought by our gunas, kleshas and vrittis. In this step, we are peeling back the layers of the onion – looking at how the outer actions are reflections of deeper habits, afflictions, and coping strategies learned earlier in life.
- **N**on-identification/Nurturing – ultimately transcending the causes by creating new ways of understanding what is happening; even small shifts in how we respond to our habits can transform maladaptive ruts into adaptive and auspicious rituals

For a Western-based framework of honest, values-based inquiry see *Mental Immunity* (Norman, 2021) pp. 347-351.

Awareness-Based Framework of Honest and Ethical Inquiry

This framework involves working with awareness (which, of course, is also needed in practicing RAIN). It is premised on the idea that samskaras are created when we cling to our experience of body, breath, and mind (in all its manifestations, including perception, recognition, and memory; volition, intention, and motivation; emotion, ways of being in relationship, ego, and self-identity; identification with certain communities, families, or cultures; as well as consciousness). Clinging to or identifying with the layers of self is the challenge; mindfulness of these layers of self – without attachment – is the solution. Mindful awareness coupled with insight clears *avidya* and leads to clarity of perception.

- Through mindful awareness and cultivation of insight, we recognize that all layers of self are impermanent – from the microscopic to the macroscopic. We note that all experiences, whether arising from body, breath/energy, or mind, come and go – they arise and they fall away. We can begin to recognize this arising and passing away and from this gain insight into how to prevent ourselves from clinging to them. We key into the constancy of change.
- Through mindful awareness, we recognize the emptiness of self – we recognize that our layers do not define us.
- We are not our body, we are not our breath, we are not our thoughts, we are not our emotions, we are not our roles or relationships, we are not our believes or values.
- None of these fabrications makes up who we are, we are not identified with them. We realize that *self* is just a concept – like weather or a rainbow or a stellar constellation in the sky: made of individual components each of which in tun is just a concept.
- We deconstruct the idea that *self* as real. It is simply a co-construction, a temporary interdependent co-arising of experience.

The process for achieving this clarity means that we transform our layers of experience into objects of mindful awareness and exploration, rather than objects of clinging. We observe them to become aware that there is nothing to cling to. This process of transforming the layers of experience from objects of clinging to objects of mindfulness includes the following steps:
- Awareness of when we get trapped in the *vrittis*, *kleshas* (and their intersections), and *gunas*
- Awareness of the *vrittis'*, *kleshas'*, or *gunas'* absence
- Awareness of the conditions and objects that bring about the *kleshas* or *vrittis*
- Awareness of conditions that help *kleshas*, *gunas*, or *vrittis* abate
- Awareness of conditions that prevent *gunas*, *kleshas*, or *vrittis* from emerging in the future (e.g., patience, maitri)

This process of awareness, analysis, and introspection prepares us for the next step toward creating wisdom, namely, the work with karma or the law of cause and effect. Working with karma moves us toward dissolving reactivity and prepares us for discernment, insight, and openhearted embrace of mature emotionality that serves the greater good.

> "A hallmark of wisdom is knowing when it's time
> to abandon some of your most treasured tools –
> and some of the most cherished parts of your identity"
> Adam Grant, 2021, p. 12

Karma or The Law of Cause and Effect

Our work with the *samskaras* is necessary to begin to affect the direction, meaning, and reverberations of our life on the greater collective. It is crucial to the operationalization of *karma*, the law of cause and effect. Working with the law of cause and effect is the process of turning reactivity into discerning wisdom and responsiveness. Working with *samskaras* and *karma* demands that we begin to deeply understand the impact we have on the world, to recognize and acknowledge that our intentions, thoughts, speech, actions, and relationships have consequences. These consequences can shape our own life and the lives of others in wholesome or unwholesome ways. The more familiar we are with our habits and patterns locks, reactivities, affective proclivities, and calcified opinions, the more capable we become to exert executive control to move from reactivity to responsiveness. This is crucial to creating a life that moves us and our biopsychosociocultural context toward compassion, kindness, joy, and equanimity.

Karma results from how our intentions, thoughts, speech, and action reverberate into the greater web of life. It is a reflection of the consequences of our actions and of our impacts on everyone and everything around us. The law of causes and consequences clarifies that we are the authors of our actions, habits, and intentions <u>as well as</u> their consequences. Since we are the agents of our actions and consequences, we can choose to break unhelpful habits (*samskaras*) in all layers of experience to change the impacts for self and others. Through exploring our impacts and making new and discerning choices to change our actions to create new consequences, we create neuroplasticity and more auspicious consequences.

Our intentions, thoughts, speech, and actions can take three forms:
- *Auspicious:* These are wholesome actions (broadly viewed as thought, speech, behavior, relationship patterns, and other actions) arising from ethical and honorable intention with auspicious consequences for self and other. Such auspicious action leads to long-term happiness, not short-term pleasure for the individual and the collective. It concerns itself not only with wholesome personal effects but also positive and healthful impacts and consequences for others (wishing others good *karma*; wishing others the joy of finding the yogic path; wishing others the powers of discernment and agency). Wholesome or positive action is not to be confused with obedience or passivity – positive action may mean standing up forcefully for what is in the best interest of all (i.e., has the most auspicious outcome for the wellbeing of the collective or others involved in a given interaction).
- *Inauspicious:* These are unwholesome actions with negative or dishonorable intentions and/or detrimental consequences for self and others. Such actions typically are caught up in and emerge from unhelpful *samskaras* (flavored by *gunas* and *kleshas*, resulting in negative expressions of *vrittis*) that we engage in habitually and without discernment or executive control – or with executive control, but without being informed by ethical values and commitment and without reflecting engagement of the *brahma viharas*. They harm both the perpetrator and the recipients of the action and are often easily detectable as action with poor outcomes and detrimental consequences.
- *Mixed*: These are actions arising from mixed intentions and/or with mixed consequences for individuals or collectives that are affected; while some individuals involved in the chain of event benefit and feel positive effects, others are affected in shameful ways that are harming them or their communities. Mixed actions can be tough to discern, especially if the individual taking the action had a positive or desired outcome, suggesting the action was wholesome. Individuals creating mixed *karma* may overlook the negative consequences that arose for others, the collective, or even the planet and delude themselves that their action was wholesome, when in effect it had an unwholesome outcome that was hidden from view (perhaps of their biased perceptions, lack of understanding, or lack of clear vision).

Inauspicious karma is the effect or impact of the samskaras unchecked. Auspicious karma is the effect or impact of the samskaras transcended.

As we apply yoga skills to the transformation of the *samskaras*, we begin to transform our and others' life and their effects by creating a pause between stimulus and response, between cause and effect. We take a moment to remember our grounding *sankalpas* and values and to consciously seek to engender positive impacts and auspicious consequences – for everyone – of our perceptions, intentions, and action. With this, we engage the law of *karma*, the law of reaping and sowing the outcomes of our intentions, thoughts, speech, actions, and relationships. *Karma* refers to recognizing that engaging in any and all actions (all the way from intention to thought, speech, behavior, relationships, and impact) results in individual and collective consequences and impacts that have profound ripple effects beyond our own lives.

When negative consequences arise from our intentions, thoughts, speech, and actions, they were most likely affected by the *vrittis*, *gunas*, and *kleshas*. Resultant *samskaras* are still controlling our individual and collective lives and standing in the way of finding wisdom and clarity. The accumulation of negative consequences (inauspicious *karma*) is the effect of these causes. Transformation requires that we become more conscious and conscientious agents or owners of our intentions, thoughts, speech, actions, and impacts (or consequences); that we exercise freedom of choice with discernment and compassion. It is in that sense that karma is the law of cause and effect. It is in that sense that *karma* is created in each and every moment.
When we commit to breaking the habit power of *samskaras* and to creating auspicious causes and effects for ourselves and others, we carefully consider the potential individual and collective consequences or impacts of each action, speech, thought, and intention before we engage in them to make a more informed choices about how to proceed. This way of making decisions and initiating actions is a top-down process in the brain, with full awareness of bottom-up inputs.

Discerning choices in the moment between stimulus and response leads to a transformation of our perceptions, relationships, ways of being in the world, and impact on others. Learning to work discerningly with cause and effect, means that we begin to cultivate skillful and wholesome action, speech, thought, and intention and let go of unskillful or unwholesome action, speech, thought, and intention. Pondering *karma* in this way teaches or reminds us that *we are the authors and owners of our actions and habits, as well as the heir of their consequences*. We recognize that we can exercise choice in every single moment to break inauspicious and unwholesome habits and to change the long-term impacts on ourselves and our collective.

> **Between stimulus and response there is a space.**
> **In that space is our power to choose our response.**
> **In our response lies our growth and our freedom.**
> (attributed to) Victor Frankl

Karma viewed in this way is a belief in the power of action, the power of agency. It acknowledges that all of us have the capacity and wiring for both wholesome and unwholesome actions, speech, thoughts, and intentions. It suggests that we can and need to learn to exercise discernment and intelligent control of the mind, transcending blind faith, fixed beliefs, stagnant attitudes, and willful ignorance. Living with awareness of cause and effect becomes essentially about exercising our freedom of choice in each and every moment to change our life course, to change our impact on the world, to respond differently from how we responded or reacted in the past. We take a pause between stimulus and response and infuse this pause with awareness, virtue, and concentration to make new choices with new outcomes or impacts that are more wholesome and helpful for ourselves and our communities. Auspicious and discerning decision-making in the present moment results in *personal and collective* growth and freedom.

Tools for Auspicious Choices in Each Moment

Notably, neuroplasticity is agnostic, or value-neutral. If we engage the mind in habitually negative, non-productive ways, we create neuroplasticity that is unhelpful. Awareness of karma and changing our habits and patterns in positive and auspicious ways creates neuroplasticity that serves us. When we stay mired in habit, we do not create new neural pathways; instead, we sacrifice neuroplasticity for neural stagnation. As soon as we step out of habit, we embrace neuroplasticity, forging new pathways in the brain and creating a new reality in our brain physiology.

When we commit to skillfulness, choice is exercised to embrace behavioral and relational expressions with the most auspicious and wholesome consequences or impacts on self and others, with both valued equally. The freedom to choose is ours in that wisdom-infused pause between stimulus we are encountering and that discerning choice that we are making that will shape and guide our response. Several yogic practices help us in this moment of decision-making or choosing our next action. These practices range from the values clarification that began with the ethical and lifestyle practices of yoga (the *yamas* and *niyamas*) to the *brahma viharas*, and are deeply supported and honed by the inner practices of concentration and meditation.

> "Ethics is not like any ordinary science.
> It must arise from the deepest understanding of human qualities,
> and such understanding comes only
> when one undertakes the journey of discovery personally.
> An ethic that is built exclusively on intellectual ideas
> and is not buttressed at every point by virtue, genuine wisdom, and
> compassion has no solid foundation."
> Matthieu Ricard, Happiness, 2003, p. 250

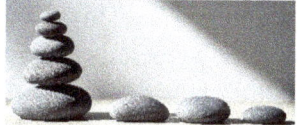

Concentration and Awareness

We engage in the inner limbs (or interior practices) of yoga to hone our mind so that we begin to be able to gain more executive and top-down control over the *kleshas, vrittis,* and *gunas*. This leads to the capacity for discernment in how we perceive, react and respond to, and affect the world. It leads to the capacity to notice our impact regardless of the intentions that guided our decisions and to learn from our impact to create more change in the future. This level of mindfulness is an essential and necessary ingredient toward personal and collective transformation.

Discernment and Wisdom

We begin to use our bodily, verbal, and mental fabrications in new and discerning ways that lead to skillful responses rather than habitual ones. We learn to see our fabrications or fluctuations with clarity and mindfulness to transform our response to the world in a way that creates auspicious or no *karma*. We are open to noticing and hearing feedback and advice from others about the impact of our actions (including intention, thought, speech, and relationships) and to begin to consider unanticipated consequences in future decision-making. We look to the past, recognizing that although we cannot change it, we can learn from it and uncouple from its (perceived) power over us. We look to the future to imagine different choices and outcomes and recognize the life-changing possibilities of heeding the advice from others. We become empowered by knowledge and the recognition that we can change, grow, and transform – creating mind sets of high expectations and credibility (Grant, 2023; Yeager & Dweck, 2020).

Wisdom thus acquired leads to greater willingness to take responsibility for how we affect the world regardless of our initial intention. We stop hiding behind positive intentions if our actions lead to inauspicious or harmful consequences. We cultivate openness to feedback from others and ourselves to engage in ongoing explorations of how the *gunas*, *kleshas*, and *vrittis* may show up in subtle ways. For example, we may recognize that we can even be attached to our perception of our intention. We become open to the possibility that we misjudged our potential impact because we were (seemingly) well-intentioned. We stop hiding behind defensiveness in light of such unintended impact, no longer denying the harm we did by pointing to good intentions. We own our responsibility in creating ripple effects into our relationships, into our world. We apologize and regroup; we learn and respond differently next time.

Virtue and Positive Intention

Working with awareness and discernment is necessary to the cultivation of positive or auspicious consequences of our actions. However, awareness and discernment, although necessary ingredients in the pause between stimulus and response, are not sufficient in and of themselves. They need to be based in the goodness of your own heart (a concept that foreshadows the need for the development of the brahma viharas). The deliberation in the pause between stimulus and response needs to include a commitment to virtue that results in right intention, right effort, right concentration, right mindfulness, and right action. This means action needs to be grounded in the yogic path that includes all eight limbs, but especially the yamas and niyamas, as well as the brahma viharas. Virtue needs to guide our agency – especially agency in arenas of influence where we can have powerful impacts, both good or bad.

Deliberation that is not based in the ethics of the yamas and the maturity of the brahma viharas may not lead to auspicious action. In other words, mindfulness and cognitive alertness are not sufficient. Only action guided by awareness, deliberation, <u>and</u> virtue has the potential for positive impact and consequences. We have to exercise virtue (including a sense of justice, irreproachableness, honor, integrity, dignity, decency, and mature ethics) to have virtuous impact. Virtue is yet another essential ingredient in the pause between stimulus and response. At time, it may be a sufficient ingredient to result in positive action.

Generosity

Virtue includes generosity, not only the yamas and brahma viharas. Generosity thus defined includes not just material generosity but also useful and meaningful gifts of time, energy, respect, compassion, love, equanimity. Generous gifts are given spontaneously (not because of some event or outer urging that tells you so) to make other happy, with respect, without expecting reciprocity, without regret, with happiness while giving, and in ways non-harming to the self and the recipient.

Brahma Viharas

The most important capacities we can develop to influence wholesome choices in the gap between stimulus and response are the *brahma viharas*. The four *brahma viharas* (*upekṣā, maitri, karuna,* and *mudita*, described below) reflect the compassionate wisdom of *vijnanamaya kosha*. They are sometimes referred to as the wholesome, unflavored *vrittis* (*vrittis* free of attachment, aversion, ego, fear, and confusion). Mindfulness and remembrance now meet virtue and create a loving, compassionate, joyful and peaceful way of seeing one's self, others, and the world. The *brahma viharas* are the developmental outcome of increasing neurological integration and relational maturity. They depend on the functional capacity of the prefrontal cortex, on top-down control without becoming cold or analytical. They combine clarity of thought with openness of heart. They are grounded in the principles of the *yamas* from a perspective of *providing for* the wellbeing of others, *rather than being the recipient* of care from others.

> **Adherence to the brahma viharas has profound impact on our thoughts, speech, and actions. The Buddha applied the ability to be equanimous (unaffected), compassionate, kind, and joyful to speech, by reminding us to make sure that speech, and consequently thoughts and actions, is:**
>
> - Timely – not untimely
> - True – not untrue
> - Gentle – not harsh
> - Kind – not hateful
> - Connected to intentions of doing good – not intentions of doing harm or hatred
>
> **In other words, the cultivation of the brahma viharas leads us to be skillful – not unskillful – in intention, thought, speech, action, and relationships. It leads to auspicious karma.**

Cultivation of the *brahma viharas* is grounded in the attainment of compassionate wisdom, *jnana* (as in *vijnanamaya kosha*) and virtue (as guided by the *yamas*). Wisdom in this sense is defined as looking out for the benefit and welfare of others and oneself and knowing how to transcend or transform the causes of suffering (i.e., thoughts and emotions) and their personal and collective outcomes or impacts. Transforming the causes of suffering means not just simply restraining them (which would just drive your thoughts or emotions underground without resolving anything), but learning how to think thoughts and experience emotions that serve us personally and that serve others and how not to think thoughts or experience emotions that do not serve.

This capacity implies that we can sit with whatever arises (i.e., cultivate awareness), analyze it (i.e., use discernment), understand it (i.e., cultivate insight), and transform it (also see RAIN above). Such virtuous, compassionate wisdom is very practical – it means seeing (recognizing) and solving (transcending) problems. We discern the difference between a symptom and a cause; once we have identified a cause for a symptom, we can work on a plan to move toward a solution (which really means working the eight-limbed path).

This capacity not only gives us access into our mind (thoughts and emotions), but also transforms our actions – actions then become wise and skillful and are in service of personal and others' benefit and welfare. We transcend selfishness, recognize negativity bias, and recognize abundance and joy in our lives (within our given biopsychosociocultural context). We become open-hearted and connected without expectation. We become responsive, not reactive, both emotionally and mentally.

> **No deed is good if you regret it.**
> **Buddha (in the Dhamma Pada)**

The mature emotions (also known as the abodes of the heart; *vihara* being the Sanskrit word for "inn") are grounded in and directed by a commitment to compassion and virtue, including the *yamas* and generosity. As such, they are deliberately and lovingly thoughtful or discerning. They reflect awareness of and commitment to an underlying set of values that guide action to increase the auspiciousness of resultant action. The *brahma viharas* are not synonymous with being "nice"; they are value-based and principled mature emotional responses to our experiences in the world and in relationship. For example, sometimes the most compassionate response to something or someone may be a response of challenging assumptions or pointing out the inauspiciousness of a particular behavior. *Brahma viharas* are best understood via several considerations: their defining features, far enemies (polar opposite emotion or mental fluctuation), near enemies (emotions or mental fluctuations that can easily be mistaken as the *brahma vihara* as defined but with profoundly different intentions and impacts), and antidotes (emotions and mental fluctuations we can cultivate to create more ease with a particular *brahma vihara* and to counter their far enemies).

Upekṣā or Equanimity

Equanimity is the fruit of wisdom that allows for balance, responsiveness, imperturbability, and a peaceful mind. It is the superpower of mindfully being present with whatever is arising with peacefulness and without reactivity, without coloring (i.e., not being deceived or disturbed by) from the kleshas (i.e., without grasping, aversion, or confusion). Equanimity is the seed of (and is reciprocally supported by) the other three *brahma viharas* because it makes compassion, kindness, and appreciative and altruistic joy truly boundless. Equanimity embraces everyone without prejudice or bias, holding all things equally – with peace, tranquility, and open-hearted engagement. Equanimity leads to purpose, to engage action on behalf of the betterment of society. It is anything but passive. It is the profound capacity to stay balanced and connected to our essence in the midst of upheaval, challenge, and suffering.

Definition: Equanimity can best be defined as peace (neither pain nor pleasure), tranquility, imperturbability, and calm composure in light of personal or others' joy or suffering. It is the ability to access emotional and cognitive balance that supports positive action on behalf of self and others. It reflects a balance of mind based on recognizing truth; non-reactivity coupled with responsiveness; meeting the unexpected with patience and mental composure; and impartiality with a lack of bias or prejudice based in seeing clearly. Equanimity is one of the three feeling tones (pain, pleasure, equanimity) and, as such, it is another tool on the path to moksha, or freedom. Equanimity requires patience: being with, holding space, and trusting that things will unfold auspiciously. Equanimity, thus defined, is the embodiment of resilience – the capacity to maintain faith, remembering our strength, trusting the process, patiently learning from experience, and always seeing opportunities for growth.

Equanimity is based in wisdom and arises when the *kleshas* have been transformed. Equanimity brings with it a way of being in the world that is without attachment and hence without expectation. This allows us to be completely engaged with life as it is. We can engage in our actions with an open heart without being driven by attachment to a particular outcome – we act without expecting reward. In this sense, the patience of equanimity invites generosity, truthfulness, resolve and commitment, and patient yet diligent effort.

Equanimity is also based in the transformation of the *gunas* and the continuous accessibility of a sattvic (or ventral vagal) state in the nervous system. Being around equanimous, imperturbable people is very co-regulating for the nervous system into a ventral vagal space. Similarly, being around non-equanimous people can be dysregulating for the nervous system as we absorb their *tamas* or *rajas*.

- *Central features*: clarity of thought, removal or clearing of distraction, and peace of mind (a mind that neither hungers for something nor shrinks away from something); "the heart that is ready for anything" (gratitude to Tara Brach who used this phrase in a talk)
- *Near enemy*: equanimity is not detachment, indifference, apathy, neutrality, emotional distance, or lack of initiative; these are common misunderstandings or misidentifications of equanimity; equanimity is fierce and clear in its commitment to the grounding virtues of serving the collective wellbeing – not indifferent, distant, or detached
- *Far enemy*: the opposite of equanimity is craving, clinging, grasping, coldness, prejudice, bias, or taking sides in an uninformed way
- *Antidote*: When the far enemies of equanimity show up, we can practice lovingkindness to help us move back into equanimity

Upeksa: "The heart that is peaceful and ready for anything"

Maitri or Lovingkindness

Lovingkindness is an opening of the heart that helps us remain loving and kind with one another and with oneself regardless of the circumstances. Lovingkindness encompasses warmth, forgiveness, respect, service, and humility (Ferrucci, 2007). It requires a deep understanding of others and their difficulties and suffering. It includes the clarity of the principle of the universality of suffering that arises from the conditioned states of humans. Lovingkindness does not discriminate or waver.

Definition: lovingkindness, friendliness, benevolence, and goodwill toward all sentient beings, including one's self; unconditional love
- *Central features:* an opening of the heart that helps us remain loving and kind with one another and with oneself regardless of the circumstances; lovingkindness encompassing of warmth, forgiveness, respect, service, and humility – without becoming a martyr or masochist; understanding of the universality of suffering
- *Near enemy*: lovingkindness in not selfish love, selfish affection, conditional love, possessiveness, or sentimental attachment; these are common misunderstandings or misidentifications of *maitri*; lovingkindness is unconditional and non-judgmental – not selfish or flavored by the *kleshas*
- *Far enemy*: the opposite of *maitri* is ill will, hatred, anger, revulsion, loathing; lack of understanding of the universality of suffering
- *Antidote*: When the far enemies of lovingkindness show up, we can practice compassion to help us move back into *maitri*

Maitri: "The heart that is openly loving toward everyone"

Karuna or Compassion

Compassion is the capacity to connect with others' and one's own humanity; it is the transcendence of selfishness and the "antidote for anger" (Hanh, 2011). It is the desire to end suffering along with the willingness to take action to do so. It embodies the bodhicitta ideal of Buddhism – the ideal of enlightened individuals who have dedicated their life to the awakening of others, even if it means that they themselves have to stick around in difficult circumstances. It is grounded in the profound recognition that humans lives in interdependence and that experiences co-arise, are co-constructed, and can be co-regulated. Compassion includes the commitment to contribute to a positive and supportive collective that brings happiness to all, not a select few; as such, compassion leads directly to proactive helpfulness and (pro)social engagement.

Definition: wish and willingness to end suffering for all sentient beings, including one's self; heartfelt, unselfish helpfulness and support
- *Central features:* the capacity to connect with others' and one's own humanity; the transcendence of selfishness; the antidote for anger and hatred; the desire to end suffering along with the willingness to take action to do so
- *Near enemy*: compassion is not pity, grief, or co-suffering; these are common misunderstandings or misidentifications of compassion; compassion is helpful and proactive – not stifling or fearful
- *Far enemy*: the opposite of *karuna* is cruelty, malice, spite, malevolence, evil, wickedness; lack of understanding of interconnection and interdependence
- *Antidote*: When the far enemies of compassion show up, we can practice altruistic joy to help us move back into *karuna*

Karuna: "The heart that seeks the end of suffering for all"

Mudita or Altruistic and Appreciative Joy

Altruistic and appreciative joy reflect the recognition of abundance in one's life (which does not simply refer to material abundance but abundance in other forms, such as social connectedness and health); the ability to provide for one's own emotional needs without external validation; and the capacity to rejoice in the good things happening to other people. Joy is appreciative when we experience it on our own behalf and feel a deep gratitude for the gifts we have been given, whether they are accomplishments, achievements, love of others, good fortune, or others. Joy is altruistic when we feel it on behalf of others – truly rejoicing in their good fortune, accomplishments, gifts, and so forth – without jealousy, envy, or hypocrisy. Like *karuna*, joy is grounded in the clarity of human connection; suffering can only be healed in the collective. Joy, especially altruistic joy, can only be truly achieved if abundance and equal access to gifts, achievements, accomplishments, and good fortune is achieved for everyone.

Definition: altruistic or appreciative joy; empathic joy or rejoicing; rejoicing or delight in one's own and others' accomplishments and good fortune; appreciation for what is given to others and one's self.

- *Central features:* recognition of abundance; ability to provide for one's own emotional needs; clarity about interconnection and the consequent happiness of shared joy
- *Near enemy*: altruistic joy is not comparison, insincere joy, or hypocrisy; it is not tinged by exhilaration, exuberance, intoxication, addiction to a dopamine rush, victorious enjoyment; these are common misunderstandings or misidentifications of *mudita*; altruistic joy is gentle and collective – not addictive or self-referenced
- *Far enemy*: the opposite of *mudita* is jealousy, envy, resentment, greed, bitterness, aversion
- *Antidote*: when the far enemies of altruistic joy show up, we can practice equanimity to help us move back into *mudita*

Mudita: "The heart that is joyful for everyone"

To summarize and highlight their importance and centrality in the practice of yoga, the application of the *brahma viharas* – lovingkindness, compassion, altruistic and appreciative joy, and equanimity – nurtures personal wellbeing and collective harmony. On a personal level, these qualities of the heart cultivate inner peace, emotional resilience, and a deeper connection to others, reducing personal suffering and embracing the need to live with purpose that serves a greater good. Collectively, when practiced in relationships and communities, the brahma viharas dissolve barriers of division, encourage mutual understanding, invite open-mindedness and open-heartedness, and create an environment of mutual support and commitment to ethical and virtuous living. As the virtues of the *brahma viharas* ripple outward, they have the potential to transform societies, fostering cultures of kindness, inclusivity, and wisdom that benefit all beings. The deep embrace of these qualities is the essence of yoga psychology. It is the key to a yogic practice that is a lifestyle of respect and honor – for each human being, for all collectives, and for our shared, fragile planet. Bringing the *brahma vihara*s to bear is our existential imperative and allows us to transform and transcend our biological, affective, and emotional urges. Bringing the *brahma viharas* to bear allows us to embrace our own humanity, to imagine humanity in others, and to create societies that nurture freedom and wellbeing for all.

> **The Buddha's Ranking of Praiseworthy People (as per Thanissaro Bikkhu)**
>
> 1. Those who work for the benefit and welfare of others and themselves
> 2. Those who work for the benefit of themselves
> 3. Those who work for the benefit of others
>
> This ranking shows that we need to take care of and know our own mind and have control over our own mind before we can truly work for the benefit of others; if we do not understand our own mind (thoughts and emotions), we may define a benefit for others that may not be so.

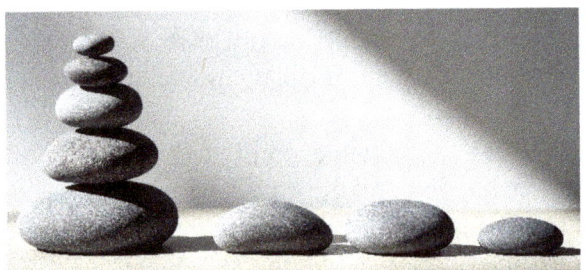

Application of Yoga Psychology to Yoga Services

Now that we have journeyed through yoga psychology, the time has come to begin a very deliberate application of these principles to the teaching, clinical practice, and therapeutic use of yoga. Yoga teaching and therapeutic yoga in healthcare cannot be separated from yoga psychology. It is essential for a successful and compassionate yoga professional to understand yoga psychology and to let it inform all decisions and actions with students or clients who are seeking out yoga interventions to improve their experience of self, other, and life in general.

Given the fact that yoga psychology is the foundation of competent teaching, Section 2 operationalizes yoga psychology principles and practice for the context of teaching classes, especially those that are therapeutic in nature, and therapeutic yoga service delivery. It offers yoga psychology-based guidance about creating intention in teaching, creating developmentally sound sequences of yoga sessions (whether in a context of teaching or healthcare), and elucidates teaching principles that translate psychology into action. Section 2 addresses the complex decision-making yoga professionals face in how best to guide students to an integrated holistic practice of yoga. It provides guidance for decisions about touch, relationship-building, managing tough classroom or therapy office situation, grounded in yogic wisdom, yogic ethics, and modern science insight and professional codes of conduct.

Section 2: Integrated Holistic Yoga Pedagogy and Practice Principles

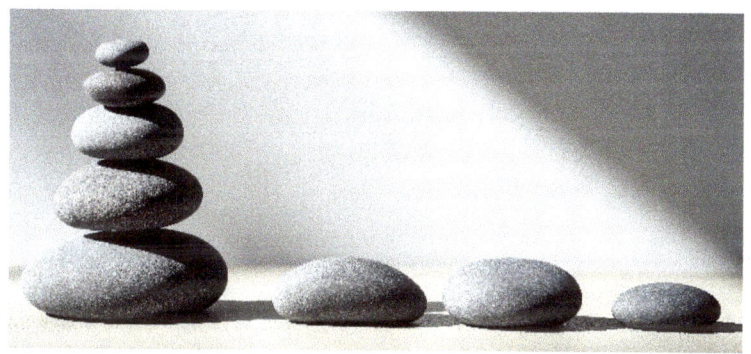

Section 2 Introduction

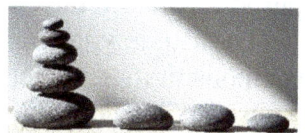

Yoga Pedagogy and Practice Principles Overview

Successful teaching relies on a multitude of variables, including creating physical and psychological holding environments through successful communication skills, adherence to the yamas and niyamas, and careful attention to individual student needs, always carefully weighing the needs of the individual against the safety of the group. Analysis of how to create a physical, emotional, and psychological teaching space that honors the needs of all students or clients through discerning choices about space, atmosphere, safety, and privacy is key to compassionate teaching. Such preparation and commitment requires respectful time management, etiquette, priorities, and boundaries; careful attention to group and power dynamics; and diversity-sensitive and informed verbal and non-verbal communication, including language and word choices, actions and behaviors, and teaching principles.

To teach yoga successfully and to deliver sensitive and tailored yoga-based clinical services it is important for yoga professionals to explore personal teaching styles and to consider how personal style may interact with student traits and needs. Not all yoga professionals and clients are compatible; not all yoga students thrive with the same style of yoga or teaching style and not all clients benefit from the same approach to yoga-based therapeutics. Yoga professionals take responsibility for recognizing when there is a match or mismatch between provider and students or clients. At times, certain individuals may need to be directed to other teachers if a teacher's style and student's needs are not congruent or compatible; same is true for clients and clinicians. Providers are responsible for ascertaining that assistants and substitutes are aligned with the advertised teaching style, intention, and qualities.

Yoga professionals can be most helpful to students or clients if they have engaged in personal exploration of how non-violence, honesty, and a keen sense of abundance are needed to make ethically challenging and responsible decisions. They are clear about personality traits, biases, and preferences they bring to the classroom. This capacity is greatly supported by a disciplined practice of yoga (Limb 2), commitment to truthfulness (Limb 1), deep mindfulness, inward practice, and compassion (cultivated by Limbs 5, 6, and 7). Presence versus absence of these qualities may greatly enhance or detract from the teachings or services and can strong affect the provider-client relationships. Awareness of personal qualities, including strength, weaknesses, and biases, is essential to truthful, safe, and committed teaching and yoga-based therapeutics.

Once a thoughtful environment has been established in which to provide yoga services and personal self-exploration has created awareness, wisdom, and compassion, the work of preparing and delivering services can begin in earnest. One of the first priorities is understanding and committing to wise and compassionate class design that reflects thoughtful and tailored sequencing of the yoga-based offering. Auspicious sequencing integrates the creation of a theme and/or intention, attention to the integration of all eight limbs, and development of a class arc that expresses the theme or intention and the integrative function of a complete yoga class. Integration of all limbs and a greater purpose result in the creation of a class of balance, beauty, and joy. In demonstrating, observing, and assisting, yoga professionals pay keen attention to these principles – embodying them in demonstrations, searching for them in observation, giving feedback about them in response to an observation, and using them to assist and redirect.

Well-sequenced classes or yoga-based therapeutics are rounded out by appropriate teacher demonstrations and mutual provider-client observation. Important demonstration considerations have to do with decisions about which version of a shape to demonstrate, the purpose of the demonstration (with care not to let ego of the yoga professional result in extreme or 'showy' versions of postures), and the needs and skills of the students or clients in the room. All interactions between provider and client are guided by in-the-moment observation of the students or clients, their skill level, striving, and capacity for self-regulation and self-guided adaptation and modification. Based on their understanding of the client or students, yoga professionals offer choices and options in every practice, teaching students and clients from the very beginning that they (the clients, not the providers) are in charge of the chosen expression of any proffered practice. All options, whether modifications, adaptations, or alternatives rely on ample and appropriate use of yoga props.

Safety in yoga therapeutics arises not only from proper demonstration and the offering of modifications, adaptations, and props. It also arises from the appropriate choice of verbal or physical supports or guidance. The safest defaults are verbal supports offered to the entire class or group based on in-the-moment observation. Supports are not offered randomly, but address a specific and noted need in the moment either by one or several individuals. Thus, supports are always predicated on providers' observational skills, client needs, and informed choices about the least intrusive level of intervention to support students or clients toward more healthful alignment, more balanced breath, less dysregulated presentation, or emotional balance. Supports are offered with safe biomechanics, clear intentions, enhanced healthfulness of the embodied practice, and increased stability in body, breath, and mind.

Finally, yoga therapeutics necessitate adherence to ethical, and legal professional and business practices. Such guidelines reflect the ethical and lifestyle principles of integrated holistic yoga and emphasize adherence to the Yoga Alliance (YA) and the International Association of Yoga Therapists (IAYT) Codes of Conduct, Scopes of Practice, and commitments to equity, inclusion, and accessibility. Yoga professionals ideally engage with ethics principles and practice values in a self-reflective manner and review all relevant documents for the yoga school in which they are enrolled, YA, IAYT, and other organizations that may be relevant to their extant scope of practice (e.g., ethics and laws related to the healthcare practice into which they hope to integrate yoga therapeutics).

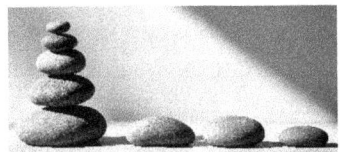

Yoga Pedagogy and Practice Principles Learning Objectives

1. Be able to create a physical, emotional, and psychological teaching space that honors the needs of all students or clients through
   a. discerning choices about space, atmosphere, safety, and privacy
   b. respectful time management, etiquette, priorities, and boundaries
   c. careful attention to group and power dynamics
   d. diversity-sensitive and informed verbal and non-verbal communication, including language and word choices, actions and behaviors, and teaching principles

2. Understand and successfully apply personal teaching styles and teaching styles of co-teachers, assistants, and substitutes with attention to
   a. delivering clear information about class offerings
   b. detailed preparation for class
   c. skillfulness about addressing special needs of individual students or clients

3. Understand clients' learning process and adapt teaching styles and principles as needed to
   a. assure all students or clients can find ways of learning
   b. offer multiple modalities in each class that speak to different learners
   c. recognize when intervention or referral may be needed to help a student succeed

4. Identify, apply, integrate, and transform personal yoga professional qualities that affect teaching style and relationships with students or clients through
   a. awareness of the impact of interpersonal style
   b. cultural and diversity-sensitive skillfulness in interactions
   c. adherence to yoga ethical principles

5. Identify and apply principles of demonstration, observation, assisting, and modifying, through understanding and applying all of the following:
   a. sequencing for safety and meaning
   b. skillfulness regarding demonstration through choices that honor student needs and maximize safety
   c. skillful observation that recognizes student needs and leads to appropriate choices and actions for assists, adjustments, and modifications
   d. skillful choices about use of props, pose variations, and pose adaptations tailored to class themes and student needs

6. Understand and apply guidelines related to the business and legal aspects of providing yoga services by
   a. being knowledgeable about Yoga Alliance policies and ethics
   b. securing appropriate licenses, credentials, permits, insurance, and similar legal details
   c. understanding legal liability, ethics, and scope of practice
   d. securing appropriate consent and liability paperwork from students or clients
   e. using appropriate marketing, referral, disclosure, and advertising

Yoga Pedagogy and Practice Principles Recommended Readings

Bondy, D. (2020). *Yoga where you are*. Shambhala.
Farhi, D. (2006). *Teaching yoga: Exploring the teacher-student relationship*. Shambhala.
Feuerstein, G. (2013). *The psychology of yoga: Integrating eastern and western approaches for understanding the mind*. Shambala.
Heyman, J. (2021). *Yoga revolution: Building a practice of courage and compassion*. Shambhala.
Lasater, J. H. (2021). *Teaching yoga with intention*. Shambhala.
Rountree, S. (2020). *The professional yoga teacher's handbook*. Bloomsbury.
Rountree, S., & DeSiato, A. (2019). *Teaching yoga beyond the poses*. North Atlantic Books.
Stephens, M. (2011). *Teaching yoga: Essential foundations and techniques*. North Atlantic.

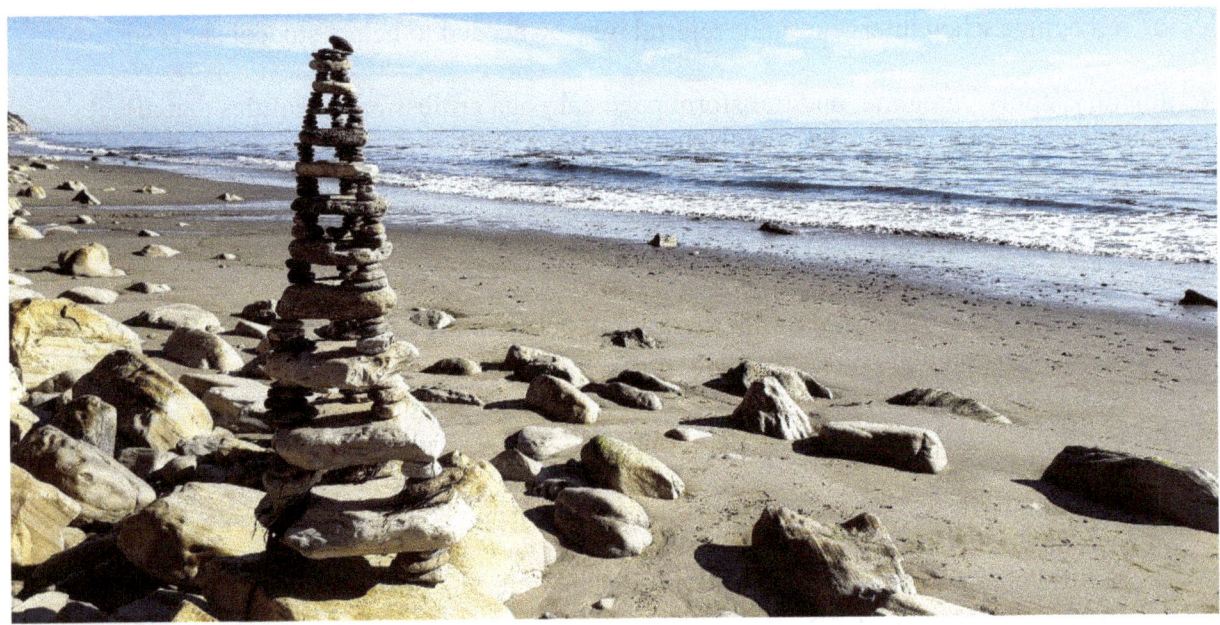

Chapter 6: Yoga Services Based in Integrated Holistic Yoga Psychology

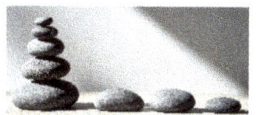

Covered in detail in the Yoga Psychology section, the principles of integrated holistic yoga (IHY) deserve a brief review before diving into the nuances of teaching therapeutic yoga from an integrated holistic perspective. All pedagogy and practice recommendations offered in this section are firmly grounded in the five characteristics of integrated holistic yoga. They operationalize and put into teaching practice the following five integrated holistic yoga principles:

- *Intentionality* – promising to making the world a better place; living with intention; committing to basic ethical values and practices
- *Accessibility* – creating affiliation, solidarity, and belonging; promoting social justice, engaged action, and personal as well collective empowerment
- *Beneficence* – creating access to the health and mental health benefits of yoga via several mechanisms of change; pledging first to do no harm
- *Wholeness* – addressing the layered experiences of consciousness, biopsychosociocultural context, interconnection, and community in all their complexity
- *Integration* – embracing the eight traditional practices (aka limbs) of yoga, four ways to glean a deeper understanding of our students or clients, interweaving of science and soul, and interdependence and coregulation

Yoga Pedagogy as Rooted in Integrated Holistic Yoga Psychology

Intentionality is reflected throughout all yoga teaching and service, and most concretely in the commitment to teaching with intention and purpose on the part of the teacher. Each practice is carefully sequenced and developed with a clear purpose and meaning in mind. Students or clients are further invited into creating their own intentionality for each practice via intention-setting practices early in each class or session.

Accessibility is attended to at all times when teaching yoga or providing yoga-based clinical services from an IHY paradigm. Accessibility becomes most concrete in the careful planning of sequences that are tailored to the people in front of us, the capacity to change plans on the fly depending on observations, and being prepared to use props, offer variations, create adaptations, and engage in accessible and compassionate demonstration. Accessibility is reflected in the environments in which we teach and practice, the attitudes we bring to our teaching and service, and relationship-building skills of the yoga professional.

Beneficence is always at the heart of any yoga offering. First and foremost, as yoga professionals, we commit to doing no harm. Practically, this means we are well-prepared for teaching or service, for meeting our students or clients where they are, and offering carefully-designed sequences that serve a clearly beneficent purpose and are open and honest about possible risks, challenges, and contraindications. Beneficence also translates into a commitment to ethical principles, ongoing learning, and seeking consultation and supervision when we encounter challenges while teaching that move us beyond our current level of learning or capacity to remain resilient and present.

Wholism refers to the reality that each class clearly invites all koshas or layers of human experience into the practice. Nothing is left out – body, vitality, mind, wisdom, and joy are deeply honored and always attended to. Wholism consider the interaction of all living beings to create an environment and experience for all layers of experience. Wholistic practices do not focus on specific components or features, instead they are dedicated to the understanding, wellbeing, and support of the entire human experience and system in all its multidimensional complexities. No *kosha* is ignored; none is left out. Teaching and learning approaches that embrace wholism integrate all human traits, teaching and attending to the physical, energetic, mental, emotional, behavioral, relational, and psychological aspects of all who are coming together for the purpose of learning and practice. Wholistic yoga services are offered from a place of personal and collective responsibility, accountability, duty, wellbeing, welfare, security, health, and happiness.

Integration is the commitment to integrating all eight limbs of yoga at all times – preferably explicitly and always at least implicitly. Teaching pedagogy as a whole embraces this commitment to the integrated practice of yoga. It draws on all limbs of yoga to offer the most intentional, beneficial, accessible, and wholistic practice possible. To recap, ancient or traditional yoga consists of eight sets of ancient practices called limbs of yoga (Hartranft, 2003; Iyengar, 2006), grouped into four categories based on modern research (Gard et al., 2014; Ward et al., 2014). *Values and Lifestyle Practices* of yoga direct practitioners toward ethical (yama) and intentional (niyama) living informed by purposeful values and meaningful life goals. *Physical Practices* (*asana*) transform the practitioner's anatomy and physiology, and support accurate sensory perception of the body from the inside out and of the environment from the outside in. *Breathing Practices* (*pranayama*) stimulate the parasympathetic nervous system, allowing access to a calm, relaxed state from which to become adaptively responsive to inner and outer life demands, achieving systemic homeostasis in body and mind as well as social connection. *Interior Practices* (*pratyahara, dharana,* and *dhyana*) draw the practitioner into self-exploration, personal insight, and interpersonal transformation, leading to the shedding of maladaptive habits, reactivity, and stereotypes while opening space for new choices, adaptive responsiveness, compassion, and resilience in body, emotions, mind, and relationships.

The practices offered via integrated holistic yoga (IHY) are enormously beneficial to practitioners and have been so for millennia. Modern sciences are finally catching up to this recognition that yoga – as an integrated practice, not a single-minded postural practice – has profound impacts on human wellbeing. The general pedagogy and practice principles in this section of the book thus deal with all limbs and most explicitly draw on yoga ethics (Limb 1: *Yamas*) and yogic lifestyle commitments (Limb 2: *Niyamas*). Specific yoga practices (such as *asana, pranayama,* and contemplative practices; covered in later volumes in the series) continue to draw on Limbs 1 and 2, as these first two limbs, in combination with the brahma viharas, are the very foundations of all yoga offerings. The table that follows provides a very brief summary of the alignment between IHY psychology and IHY pedagogy.

Sample Yoga Practice Principles within the IHY Categories

- *Wholism* (i.e., koshas, biopsychosociocultural context)
  o Embrace the complexity of human life and growth while resting in the simplicity of a well-designed practice
  o Avoid reductionism that hones in on a single or a couple of aspects of the individual who is coming to the practice of yoga without honoring their full history, experience, and complexity
  o See the entirety of each individual regardless of presenting concern, context, or relationship – honor clients' biopsychosociocultural context, embeddedness, and interdependence
  o Attend to all layers of self – body, vitality and affect, mind and emotions, intuition and wisdom, joy and connection

- *Integration* (i.e., eight limbs and other practices)
  o Honor all limbs of yoga explicitly or implicitly
  o Attend to the interconnection of the various yoga practices
  o Integrate modern science with ancient wisdom
  o Do not teach any single yoga practice (especially asana) in isolation of the others
  o Infuse the ethical and lifestyle practice of yoga into all offerings
  o Link the practices of yoga on the mat to life skills off the mat

- *Intention*
  o Have clear meaning and purpose for each class
  o Carry a theme throughout the class
  o Invite clients' personal intentions and derivation of meaning for the practice
  o Guide clients to take yoga of the mat and into life with clarity and purpose
  o Invite a dedication of merit and a take-away from the practice at the end of class
  o Choose language, demonstration, and offered practices with clarity of intention and impact

- *Accessibility*
  o Offer a yoga practice that is inclusive, respectful, equitable, and inviting to everyone, regardless of background and current biopsychosociocultural context
  o Explicitly invite and treasure students' and clients' freedom of choice, empowerment, and agency
  o Use, demonstrate, encourage, and normalize (destigmatize) props and supports
  o Be thoughtful in how practices are demonstrated and portrayed, including in marketing and social media contexts
  o Use cues that communicate commitment to safety, inclusion, and understanding for all
  o Create an atmosphere of consent

- *Beneficence*
  o Discuss potential positive outcomes of particular practices
  o Be realistic and honest about what yoga can and cannot do
  o Address risks and contraindications
  o Share knowledge about research evidence for helpful outcomes of a yoga practice
  o Collect feedback about the impact of offerings and convey openness to constructive criticism and input from clients
  o Commit to lifelong learning to ensure that offered practices are optimal for the clientele being served
  o Stay committed to doing no harm – teach in line with the *yamas*, *niyamas*, and *brahma viharas*

Yoga ethics (*yamas*) and lifestyle commitments (*niyamas*) further guide yoga professionals to ensure that they develop and maintain a strong commitment to creating communities of equity, diversity, inclusion, justice, beneficence, intention, accessibility, and complexity – as well as integrated holistic yoga practices of intentionality, accessibility, beneficence, complexity, and integration. These approaches clearly translate yoga psychology into therapeutic yoga teaching and services. Through operationalizing the essential aspects of yoga psychology shared in Section 1, yoga pedagogy embraces and reflects deliberate intentions, thoughts, actions, and relationships cultivated by yoga professional to embody their unequivocal commitment to integrated holistic yoga principles. The following topics are covered below as examples of the clear expressions and operationalization of integrated holistic yoga psychology in general, with particular consideration of the yamas and niyamas in particular:

- Environments of safety
- Provider qualities
- Teaching or yoga service delivery styles
- Teaching and therapeutics with intention
- Teaching and therapeutic yoga sequencing
- Teaching and therapeutic practice principles
- Strategies for student and client guidance
- Foundational ethics and professional commitments
- Scope of practice and types of yoga services

Environments of Safety, Accessibility, and Ongoing Consent

A supportive and therapeutic environment honors the *yamas* and *niyamas*, while being attuned to student or client needs in terms of their developmental levels as related to the koshas. It is an environment that creates a deliberate and committed atmosphere of consent and collaboration. Successful integrated holistic teaching, especially in the context of *therapeutic* yoga, depends on the creation of a psychological holding environment that conveys compassion, kindheartedness, accessibility, equality, and inclusions. It is an environment that offers clarity about procedures and rules, establishment of boundaries and priorities, management of group dynamics, respect for each student or client, and insight about individual versus group needs in the classroom.

Clarity and Consistency in Logistical Procedures, Structure, and Rules

Safety- and Respect-Related Etiquette

To create a positive and respectful classroom or therapeutic environment, several key guidelines and expectations are helpful. First, safety and respect are fundamental in a therapeutic yoga context, and this includes clear procedures to minimize distractions. Interruptions during class are requested to be kept to a minimum, with protocols being established for events such as silent entry and exit, notifying the teacher if a student needs to leave early, and taking bathroom breaks at auspicious times for the student body overall (if possible). Students or clients are requested to maintain common courtesies, such as curbing the use of phones or other electronic devices, avoiding offensive language and rude behavior, to foster a welcoming and inclusive atmosphere for all. In terms of learning engagement, students or clients may need help to understand how and when to ask questions during class to ensure the learning process remains smooth and respectful for everyone. Additional expectations, such as adhering to suitable dress codes and maintaining ethical and legal behavior, are also useful and clearly communicated in a matter-of-fact manner. Finally, it is helpful to define boundaries for student-teacher interactions outside of class or session to ensure professional and respectful conduct at all times and prevent surprises.

Class Structures and Logistics

To establish a consistent and structured classroom environment, it is propitious to maintain predictable patterns across the various aspects of each class or session. Language and prosody are best used with consistency and predictability, as well as in a manner that reflects compassion and kindness, helping students become familiar with and able to adapt for themselves the preferred tone and style of communication. Sessions serve students or clients well (in terms of calming nervous systems with predictability) if they follow a structured and predictable sequence of events to create a reliable flow of activities. Lighting levels are adjusted consistently based on time of day and natural light availability, providing a comfortable and steady atmosphere. Noise and sound management is best kept equally predictable, whether through the use of white noise machines or clear guidelines about how the teacher will handle noise from students, such as chatter or snoring. Additionally, the use of assistants and substitutes teachers follows a uniform approach, ensuring that these individuals are properly integrated into the class while maintaining and asserting the lead teacher's responsibility over roles and relationships vis-à-vis each other and their clients. Establishing routines and rituals helps create a sense of safety and predictability in the classroom or office. Moreover, consistency usefully extends to preferences about after-class availability, ensuring clients know when and how they can access support. Lastly, a commitment to ongoing consent procedures, particularly regarding touch and level of guidance in teaching, is crucial for maintaining respectful, compassionate, and safe learning environments.

Time Management Commitments

Effective time management is essential for both classroom sequencing and overall classroom management. Classes ideally are structured with clear focus on time-management skills, ensuring that each phase of a session (e.g., centering, warm-up, peak pose, cool-down, and meditation) is appropriately and predictably timed. This level of consistency enhances session flow and reflects commitment to professionalism by demonstrating respect for clients' time and by establishing and adhering to clear boundaries. Practical time-management tools, such as using a clock that is clearly visible to the instructor and utilizing time-sensitive cues for transitions, can help maintain session rhythm. It is as important for students or clients to adhere to time management rules as it is for providers, including adhering to guidelines for late arrival or early departure and about minimizing disruptions. If possible, instructors ideally allocate a defined amount of time to address clients' questions and concerns, ensuring a student-teacher relationship that is compassionate and kind, while also being boundaried and disciplined.

Clarity in Personal Boundaries and Priorities

It is helpful to optimize opportunities for emotional support and safety for clients. This can be accomplished via the following suggestions (though this is not an inclusive listing):

- Attend to positive relationship development between instructor and students
- Be aware of and do not abuse power dynamics between provider and client
- Stress the importance of mindfulness of and attunement to others and self
- Maintain equanimity (i.e., optimize capacity to stay in a ventral vagal space) in times of challenge, stress, or crisis through teacher or clinician preparedness
- Have an emotional safety plan for distressed clients (and your own debrief thereafter)
- Maintain awareness of and effectively resolve transference and countertransference
- Stay attuned to participants, especially their level of arousal as related to their polyvagal state; this is not to say students will never "dysregulate" – they will; the key is to help them reregulate and to become attuned to their capacity to do so
- Stay attentionally connected to your students as much as possible – noting their physical and energetic responses
- Stay responsible for the conduct of any assistants used and establish clarity about their role vis-à-vis the primary yoga professional and session participants

Explicit respect needs to be expressed for each individual, even those who present challenges to teachers, providers, or other participants. This does not mean that no boundaries are set; quite the opposite. It means that there is clarity in communication and relationships that supports the wellbeing of all people in the room. The following suggestions may be helpful:

- Listen attentively and respectfully to students or clients
- Respect others' points of view, beliefs, and culture
- Speak truthfully, politely, and directly to participants
- Strive for the most compassionate and kind ways of providing information, including performance feedback, to students or clients as well as assistants
- Strive to accommodate diverse learning styles in communicating with clients
- Be skillful in addressing specific and emerging needs of individuals
- Be self-aware and discerning about tone of voice (e.g., non-commanding, clearly audible, warm, inviting, modulated to present-moment occurrences)
- Be self-aware and discerning about choice of language (e.g., gender-sensitive, trauma sensitive, invitational, respectful of individual choices)
- Do not allow personal beliefs and values to adversely influence the relationship with students or clients
- Do not impose personal beliefs on students or clients

Throughout the teaching period and beyond, it is key to promote student or client self-empowerment, autonomy, and agency. Yoga is about helping people grow and evolve in a positive and self-guided manner. Inviting clients to make their own decision and experience their own power is crucial to communicating that each student is invited to make their own choices, while still honoring and attending to the needs of others. The following suggestions are offered to create such an atmosphere of empowerment and agency:

- Know all students or clients to some degree – introduce yourself to new students or clients, including those presenting unexpectedly or unannounced
- Support participant autonomy (e.g., vis-à-vis touch/no-touch, use of props, selection of mat location in class) always giving choices, making invitation, and avoiding directives

- Support and encourage student self-rule about variations and adaptations, inviting them to sense inward into all their layers of experience to make decisions and choices that are supportive of how they are showing up in any given moment
- Balance individual client needs and desires with group needs, weighing a single student's choices against their potential impact on the group
- Use strategies that reduce the oft-perceived power of the instructor over the student, such as making auspicious language choices, giving consideration to mat placement (e.g., teaching in a circle), adjusting pacing, and making auspicious choices about demonstrations, cuing, and assisting (more about this below) – being invitational and surrendering power to the student (as appropriate to maintain safety and respect in the classroom)

When there is a need to do so, it is key to prioritize client needs ahead of provider needs (unless such action would result in offensive, unethical, dangerous, or similarly undesirable interactions or actions). Some of the following points are worthy of consideration in making decisions about prioritizing whose needs are key in the classroom in a specific situation or moment:
- Maintain boundaried relationships with students or clients
- Stay responsive and try not to be reactive toward students or clients
- Remain defenseless and open-hearted, especially vis-à-vis input or feedback from clients
- Maintain your own nervous system regulation, trying to optimize staying in your ventral vagal space
- Hold the space and the relationship and remember that teaching yoga is about students' needs, not teachers' needs or desires – do not overly self-disclose
- Listen and help students or clients feel seen, heard, and understood
- Debrief and consult as needed, especially after challenging situations occurred in a class or with a student

Management of group dynamics is best handled with kindness, compassion, and clarity. To be clear, a laissez-faire approach does not meet this definition. Compassion and clarity need to be applied to all participants and teachers. This may require weighing options and choices about how to handle specific events, actions, or interactions. Following are some helpful considerations:
- Recognize and know how to manage power dynamics – both with individuals as well as with the group overall
- Understand and know how to use strategies for handling disruptive, intrusive, noisy, … students or clients
- Understand and know how to use strategies for handling injury or crisis in class
- Create clarity about strategies for co-teaching – clarifying the role of co-teachers and assistants in class
- Special considerations in clinical settings re teacher confidentiality
- Special considerations in clinical settings re confidentiality across students or clients

Yoga professionals encounter many types of students or clients, settings, and situations. It is helpful for the provider to remember that it is important to be knowledgeable about and to honor needs of individuals who may present with special concerns or characteristics. The following considerations list a few helpful suggestions and skills.

- Awareness of personal biases and how they may perpetuate barriers to practice for certain students or populations
- Awareness of how power dynamics may affect certain types of clients, especially those with trauma histories or the experience of racism, sexism, and other prejudice, bias, oppression, or stereotypes
- Basic knowledge of trauma-informed yoga principles (also see (Justice et al., 2019)
- Skillful use of inclusive and inviting language
- Conscious decisions about use versus non-use of Sanskrit
- Skillful use of props to encourage variation and adaptation
- Recognition of the need for referral or interprofessional collaboration on behalf of certain students or clients
- Understanding of yoga principles targeted to special populations, if the teacher expects to work with these types of students or clients; for example:
    - trauma-informed yoga
    - yoga for veterans or first responders
    - yoga for athletes or bigger bodies
    - yoga at various developmental periods (e.g., older adults, children, adolescents)
    - yoga for specific physical conditions (e.g., pregnancy, back care, cancer, chronic pain, balance)
    - yoga for specific emotional conditions (e.g., anxiety, stress management, resilience, depression)

Provider Qualities for Client Empowerment and Safety

In addition to being properly trained and working within an appropriate scope of practice, teachers need to cultivate awareness of personality traits, biases, and preferences they bring into the classroom and have clear intentions and plans about their classroom management style. These capacities are greatly supported by teachers' disciplined practice of yoga (Limb 2), commitment to ethical practice (Limb 1), and deep mindfulness, inward practice, and compassion (as cultivated by Limbs 5, 6, and 7). Presence versus absence of these qualities can greatly enhance or detract from the teachings and have a strong impact on the teacher-student relationship.

Clearly, personal insight about strengths, weaknesses, and biases is crucial to teacher development. Yoga providers can lead students or clients only as far as they themselves have progressed. Thus, teachers need self-awareness about their own koshic development to know from which kosha they function most typically and habitually. The most successful providers have attained the capacity to function in vijnanamaya kosha and have a strong desire to embody the brahma viharas.

Awareness of personal qualities is essential to truthful, safe, and committed teaching and service. It may make the difference between ethical and successful work versus work that is unsafe for clients. Auspicious personal qualities and teaching practices create meaningful student-teacher relationships and environments that are both psychologically and physically arranged to optimize cues and opportunities for safety. They support practice accessibility through a deep appreciation for students' or clients' empowerment, self-agency, and resilience. Although a few personal and interpersonal qualities are discussed below, this listing is not to be meant all-inclusive. There are many other qualities and biopsychosociocultural influences on the client-provider relationship. Thus, ongoing mindfulness, vigilance, and humility are essential to being an open-hearted and open-minded yoga teacher.

"Teachers instruct, rouse, urge, and encourage"
Quote from a dharma talk by Thanissaro Bikkhu

Personal Alignment with Yogic Principles

Yoga professionals need to make sure that their intentions, thoughts, speech, actions, and relationship reflect their profound personal alignment with yogic principles, especially as outlined in the yamas, niyamas, and brahma viharas. Teachers are role-models and actions speak louder than words. The following are recommendations for yoga professionals' commitments and conduct:
- Living in tune with the yamas (peaceful, truthful, joyful with a sense of abundance, moderate in the use of life energy, generous) – these principles of ethical living and virtue in thought, speech, action, behavior, and relationships are to be applied in personal contexts as well within systems, institutions, work relationships, and healthcare systems
- Living in tune with the niyamas (clean and pure, content and calm, disciplined, introspective, and devoted to a greater purpose or cause)
- Embodying and modeling mindfulness, patience, and non-judgment
- Being willing to seek consultation and supervision as needed if pushed outside one's scope of practice or realm of teaching comfort by the needs of a client or clients
- Being self-aware and able to admit lack of knowledge, to acknowledge and repair mistakes, or address and transcend personal limitations
- Demonstrating integrity and self-awareness
- Being trusting and trustworthy by adhering to codes of conduct, ethics, and laws
- Committing to authenticity and genuineness; showing up with non-pretentiousness and humility
- Engaging in appropriate self-care to ascertain healthful functioning as a teacher or clinician and seeking out help when signs of stress or burnout emerge

Cultural Skillfulness and Sensitivity

Yoga professionals need to commit time, energy, and honesty to cultivating cultural skillfulness and sensitivity. Here are a few descriptions of how such cultural appropriateness can be learned, expressed, and maintained.
- Deep understanding of the biopsychosociocultural context and its impact on development and developmental opportunities; relationships and power structures; experiences and opportunities in the world; exposure to trauma, racial and other bias, and oppression
- Deep understanding of the biopsychosociocultural model and its impact on systems and the perpetuation of White supremacy and systemic, as well as institutionalized, racism
- Awareness of the impact and manifestation of personal biases, prejudice, and privilege

- Understanding and embracing difference with a strong commitment to diversity, equity, and inclusion
- Knowledge, awareness, and skills relevant to cultural differences and diversity, lived and applied with sensitivity and humility
- Open-mindedness about values, behaviors, and approaches to life
- Restraint from imposing personal values, standards, or beliefs
- Openness about personal characteristics of diversity, such as gender identity, race, culture, religion, age, levels of ability, socioeconomic factors, educational opportunities, and more
- Non-offensive, nonsexist, non-ageist, nonracist, or otherwise biased or disrespectful language
- Ability to discern both intention *and* impact of actions, speech, and even thought
- Ability to apologize and make amends for microaggressions or missteps – along with non-defensiveness and humility
- Willingness to have challenging conversations with others – students, peers, supervisors, the general public – whenever bias, oppression, and other diversity and equity issues emerge
- Willingness to seek cultural consultation
- If White, active solidarity and advocacy that elevates Black, indigenous, and people of color; shrinking back from speaking for groups with different diversity characteristics other than one's own; and active commitment to expose, counter, and repair systems of White supremacy

Interpersonally Relevant Traits for Relationship-Building

There are innumerable traits that support positive relationships between providers and clients. Here are a few examples – note that this is not an all-inclusive listing, just food for thought:
- Being interpersonally attuned via empathy, kindness, compassion, and mindful awareness of personal impact on students and co-teachers/assistants
- Being interpersonally perceptive with an ability to listen attentively and fully, read nonverbal communication, and be respectful
- Being able to joyfully celebrate the success of students and progress of clients
- Embodying and demonstrating calmness, groundedness, and equanimity in general and especially under pressure and during challenge
- Reducing interpersonal power differentials to communicate clearly that students or clients are in charge of their bodies, are invited to exercise self-agency, have the power to say "no", and have the power to make choices they deem auspicious for themselves

Qualities with Impact on Teaching Style, Management Style, and Optimizing Safety

Alluded to already in the contents above, it is key for yoga professionals to cultivate skills and qualities that optimize safety, reflect appropriate management of challenging situations and day-to-day interaction, and result in a teaching style that is inviting, invitational, and respectful. The following traits are useful in a yoga professional in these regards:
- Capacity to set limits and offer safe boundaries to students or clients to who may create challenge, stress, or dangers for others or themselves
- Openness to new ideas, new discoveries, new ways of learning and teaching – life-long learning, unlearning, and relearning

- Self-awareness and discernment about tone of voice (e.g., non-commanding, clearly audible, warm, inviting, modulated to present-moment occurrences, prosody)
- Self-awareness and discernment about choice of language (e.g., gender-sensitive, trauma sensitive, invitational, respectful of individual choices) and communication skills in general
- Self-awareness and discernment about interpersonal behaviors, relationships, and ways of approaching and being with participants, staff, and co-workers (e.g., respectful, kind, compassionate, emotionally regulated, capable of emotional connection, thoughtful about interactions)
- Willingness for ongoing continuing education and specialization
- Engagement in self-care that supports the provider's own physical, energetic, mental, emotional, and communal health
- Role-modeling taking care of personal needs, of drawing successfully on personal resources, and of knowing when to be appropriately assertive to protect one's own integrity and values

Additional Aspects of Creating Safety in Healthcare, Clinical, and Residential Settings

A few other topics that are worthwhile pondering and addressing include the following. This is by no means a complete listing, but it serves to direct yoga professionals' attention to the importance and responsibilities that are inherent in their teaching or clinical role.
- Privacy matters
- Confidentiality concerns
- Interfacing with other staff in the environment regarding yoga class attendance
- Understanding the limits and boundaries of information exchange with other staff about yoga clients or students
- Referral procedures to and from yoga teachers or healthcare practitioners

Teaching or Yoga Service Delivery Styles

Successful yoga services presuppose that the yoga professional has made a firm commitment to bring to bear the *yamas* and *niyamas* in a variety of practical ways. It requires that yoga professionals have made conscious and ethically-guided decisions about class management and teaching styles (via svadhyaya and more) as adapted to the populations represented in their classes. Providers are most successful and least likely to do harm if they abide by the *yamas*, *niyamas*, and *brahma viharas*, and recognize the needs and skill levels of their students or clients to tailor service delivery style to them. If a provider has only one particular teaching style, that style needs to be clear to potential students or clients so that they may self-select based on their own preference.

Styles and Types

Not all students or clients thrive with the same style of yoga and they need help understanding this reality. At times, certain individuals may need to be directed to other yoga professionals if the provider's style and the client's needs are not congruent or compatible. Teachers are responsible for ascertaining that teaching assistants and substitute teachers are aligned with the teacher's advertised teaching style, intention, and qualities. Clearly, non-violence, honesty, and a keen sense of abundance are needed by the teacher to make such ethically challenging and responsible decisions.

Clear information for clients about yoga service delivery styles and methods is crucial and can be ensured via the following:
- Advertise personal style and intention
- Help clients understand there are many different styles of yoga teaching and therapeutics
- Create awareness of the interaction between each client's unique learning process and each provider's personal delivery style
- Encourage clients to "provider shop" until a good student-teacher or client-clinician match has been identified
- Consider offering a free (or discounted) first session so clients can make informed choices

Clear information about type of classes and experiences offered by the yoga professional is essential for clients to make auspicious choices for themselves. The following information will support their agency in decision-making:
- Class or session sizes and number of providers and assistants in the class
- Class or session level and faithfulness to the advertised level
- Cohort sessions versus walk-in classes
- Commercial yoga that is primarily asana- or fitness-focused
- Commercial yoga that is eight-limbs-based
- Commercial yoga that is adaptable to special needs with certain parameters
- Therapeutic yoga classes that are adapted to enhance one to two therapeutic themes, are clinic or hospital-based, and have a clear target group of students
- Yoga therapeutics offered in a particular clinical, healthcare, or community health setting
- One-on-one or one-on-two yoga therapy

Clear information about a particular style or styles of yoga to be offered can be helpful for some students. Possible styles may include, but are not limited to, the following:
- Hatha yoga
- Kundalini yoga
- Yin yoga
- Vinyasa yoga
- Restorative yoga
- Raja yoga
- Therapeutic yoga
- Integrated holistic yoga

Clear information about the intention of the experiences offered by the yoga professional supports healthful choices for clients. The following descriptions or information may be useful:
- SNS-stimulating classes (vinyasa, hot yoga, power yoga, ashtanga, Bikram)
- PSNS-focused calming classes (restorative, yin, nidra, gentle flow)
- Factors that contribute to class intention, such as attention on:
    - breath versus less time for/focus on mindful breathing
    - alignment versus flow
    - mindfulness versus athleticism
    - slow pace versus fast pace
    - strengthening versus balance of all potential physical impacts
    - therapeutics versus exercise

Preparedness

Preparedness for each class or session along with ability for intentional adjustment and revision is essential to teaching in a manner that is wholesome, integrated, holistic, and respectful of students. Coming to sessions unprepared and making up practices 'on the fly' can short-change participants and may be a form of stealing. Some suggestions for prior preparation include the following, but certainly providers can go far beyond these basics in getting ready for sessions.

- Make a plan for each session in alignment with principles set forth later in this section and each of the specific practice chapters; for example:
  - have a clear intention for each session
  - have a defined session plan with flexibility to modify as needed
  - feel centered and ready to teach or provide therapeutics
  - stay mindful of yourself, including your vitality and breath
  - be mentally and physically ready to teach or provide therapeutics
  - be prepared to assert etiquette and boundary guidelines
- Be mentally, emotionally, energetically, and physically prepared for the types of people being recruited into the session – this will lead to the capacity to be fully present in all koshas, to respond to the demands of each moment, to feeling centered and present, and to being able to offer an environment and context that optimizes the potential for safety, promotes collaboration, and supports engagement and mutuality
- Be knowledgeable about and prepared for the type and level of practices being taught with the capacity to meet all participants where they are in the moment
- Have clarity before starting the session about how to offer adaptations and variations for each included practice based on student or client presentations
- Be prepared to change a lesson plan because of unexpected circumstances (such as historical events, client presentation, provider challenges, and more)
- Be prepared to seek consultation and supervision for teaching or other service challenges
- Be prepared to seek therapeutic supports in case of personal difficulties or challenges that affect teaching or service delivery

Prioritizing Accessibility, Diversity, Equity, and Social Justice

Successful yoga offerings rely on multiple variables, not the least of which is attention to the physical and organizational environments and larger community in which yoga takes place. Environment does not simply reflect the physical space, but also the ambience and "feel" of a yoga space. Important environmental and organizational factors need to be considered, including space and policy considerations, creation of a conducive physical and organizational atmosphere, and optimization of opportunities to experience safety and containment. Environment and organization need to reflect and honor the yamas and niyamas to set the stage for a truly holistic yoga practice. They need to give evidence to openness, humility, inclusivity, and diversity as well as reflecting the promotion of student empowerment, self-efficacy, and agency. A few listings of specific environmental and organizational features follow. They are not complete but serve to invite thoughtfulness and creativity.

Optimization and Embrace of Accessibility, Diversity, Equity, and Inclusion

- Location and transportation options available in neighborhood
- Location and physical accessibility within the building (e.g., ADA compliance)
- Creating a welcoming atmosphere that creates emotional and psychological accessibility
    - full representation of human experience (e.g., race, gender, age, ability, mobility, etc.)
    - intentional inclusive, non-culturally appropriating décor
    - intentional and thoughtful clothing of staff and teachers
    - non-binary merchandise (if a store is on the premises)
    - availability of non-binary bathrooms and changing rooms
    - intentional cues that request feedback and input about systems improvements to promote emotional and psychological accessibility
- Culture of diversity, equity, and inclusivity vis-à-vis:
    - religion and religious or spiritual expression (e.g., non-denominational, non-appropriative, non-colonizing)
    - language that is inclusive, accessible, non-appropriative, non-colonizing, non-prescriptive, and empowering with conscious choices about use or non-use of Sanskrit
    - availability of non-English speaking teachers and classes
    - vibe of the space (e.g., no guru vibe, no new age vibe, no cliquery)
    - respectful and heartfelt acknowledgement of yoga's historical roots – expressing cultural appreciation rather than cultural appropriation
    - clarity about the setting's commitment to fostering open dialogue, positive and active listening to diverse voices
    - openness to feedback about how to improve regarding diversity, equity, and inclusion
- Practical matters related to diversity, equity, inclusion, and access:
    - time schedule diversity
    - affordability and financial options (e.g., sliding scale, work exchange)
    - prop availability (maybe show substitutions with common household items)
    - range of classes with appropriate descriptors (find alternative labels to "beginner" or "advanced" – maybe focusing on content more so than 'skill level')
    - diversity among teaching staff
- Financial supports to promote inclusion and diversity

Optimization of Safety via Conducive Environmental Features

- Careful consideration and choices related to environment features
    - lighting (e.g., dimmable/adjustable; not too dark in eve)
    - colors (e.g., not overly bright or upregulating)
    - smells (e.g., fragrance free)
    - sound (e.g., surrounding sound levels; use of sound in the room – such as music)
    - temperature
    - air exchange/circulation (including the sounds from such systems)
    - ease of access to props in the room
- Size and shape of the physical space to accommodate different layouts for teaching (e.g., rows versus circles)

- - Let students or clients choose their own spot
  - Invite students or clients to assemble their own props
- Maintenance of safety-conscious student-teacher ratios
- Maintenance of high levels of teacher, substitute teacher, and teaching assistant training and qualifications (also see scope of practice below)
- Careful consideration of space features that convey thoughtfulness and signal safety:
  - maximize and optimize the degree of privacy and confidentiality
  - assure the availability of emergency exits
  - make conscious decision about how to deal with windows and/or window coverings
- Creation of safe and supportive containment in the room
  - select an appropriate class size for space
  - choose wisely how to use versus or not use mirrors
  - select accessible and comfortable floor coverings
  - minimize clutter and maximize ease with which the space can be navigated

Creation of Procedural Clarity and Embrace of a Strong Code of Conduct

- Clear statement of mission, vision, goals, and values, including a clear statement to "*do no harm*" and to strive for inclusivity, equity, and accessibility for all
- Appropriate labeling of class level to inform students or clients accurately about level of preparation and intention for each class
- Proper teacher preparation and qualification (including teachers, substitute teachers, and teaching assistants) and accurate descriptions of teacher or clinician yoga credentials
- Clear lines of responsibility for teachers, subs, assistants, and other staff
- Maintaining proper functioning and cleanliness of the environment
  - lighting
  - cleaning schedule
  - maintenance of mats and props
  - awareness of noise and other intrusions
- Clear mechanism for collecting and welcoming feedback, input, questions, and more
- Clear set of policies and procedures, including but not limited to:
  - cost and refund policies
  - grievance policies
  - attendance policies
  - application policies
  - anti-retaliation policies
- Clear code of conduct for teachers, staff, and participants, including but not limited to:
  - antiharassment policies
  - sexual misconduct policies
  - active embrace of equity and inclusion
  - clarity about and adherence to scope of practice
  - clear communication of respect in the student-teacher relationship
  - honesty and forthrightness in all communication, in clinician honoring privacy and confidentiality
  - clarity about informed consent related to touch

- Compliance with applicable laws and public health codes
  - insurance verification
  - ADA compliance
  - health and safety considerations
  - ethical pay of teachers

Marketing, Social Media, and Public Relations

Although it may seem somewhat unrelated, how teachers and schools interact with marketing and social media matters greatly. All public relations need to reflect a commitment to safety and explicit values, including social justice, to support the kind of safety and welcoming in the environment that supports yoga teaching in healthcare settings. The following issues can be attended to in this context:

- Honesty in all advertising and public communication – making no false, deceptive, fraudulent, or ethical claims or statements
- Media messaging that reflects commitment to diversity, equity, and inclusion in language and images
- Clarity about fees, policies, and similar practical matters
- Making no unjustifiable claims about the positive effects, historical context, or scientific basis of yoga
- Judicious use of social media
- Up-to-date website
- Informational events that allow potential students or clients to meet teachers without having to make a financial investment or commitment
- An authentic brand that reflects yogic values and a genuine commitment to them
- Commitment to reflecting ethics, professional practice, and integrated holistic yoga principles in all services and public interactions

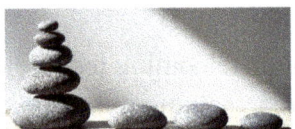

Stages of Learning

As individuals learn how to become a yoga teacher or yoga professional, it is helpful to remember the stages of learning any new skill. Understanding this model of development supports self-compassion and self-inquiry in the process of becoming a yoga teacher or clinician. It reminds us to move into ongoing openness to new learning as time progresses, and to continue to engage in introspection about one's teaching skills as they unfold across time. It also reminds us of our ethical commitment to being the most compassionate and well-informed teacher or clinician possible in each moment.

If we understand the following stages, we will be more open to being honest (*satya*) with ourselves and our students or clients about what we can and cannot (yet) provide or offer in a manner that is beneficial (*ahimsa*) and kind.

Stage 1: Unconscious Incompetence

Teachers might do the most harm during this stage of their development: they do not (yet) realize what they do not know about yoga and often think they know more than they do. They may teach with conviction and bluster, explaining what they do not actually understand or have mastered – whether related to yoga philosophy, psychology, alignment, Sanskrit, history, or more. This inaccurate self-assessment of knowledge is one aspect of a cognitive bias called the *Dunning-Kruger effect* wherein an individual overestimates their own level of knowledge and expertise because of a lack of knowledge of the very area of expertise they think they already possess.

Stage 2: Conscious Incompetence

This is a tough time for every teacher: the teacher has now learned enough to recognize their own lack of knowledge in all aspects relevant to teaching yoga. They are now painfully aware when their knowledge does not suffice to lead a class skillfully or to answer a student's specific question knowledgably. It is a much safer stage for clients as the yoga professional now answers with humility, is motivated to learn more, recognizes the limits of their scope of practice, and seeks out more knowledge and learning. This is where many yoga trainees start their yoga teacher or yoga therapeutics training. It is a great place from which to start as it invites openness to new learning and humility about what is and is not yet known to the learner.

Stage 3: Conscious Competence

This is a time of great motivation and enormous growth: teachers at this stage spend a significant amount of time prepping and learning. It is a time of applying a growing store of knowledge and wisdom in expanding creativity and accessibility. This is the stage that any yoga teacher training program hopes to reach with its teacher trainees. Trainees who have not reached this stage may not be ready to take the teacher's mat without additional supervision, guidance, or mentorship.

Stage 4: Unconscious Competence

This is can be a time of joy or disconnect for the provider: if the provider continues to track level of knowledge and offers services in an accessible way, joy ensues for provider and participant. If such yoga professionals – in their own competence – begin to misread or misjudge the competence and knowledge of their clients, their offerings may become inaccessible and incomprehensible to participants. This is the second aspect of the Dunning-Kruger effect – now instead of incorrectly assessing their own level of competence, providers mis-calculate their students' or clients' level of knowledge or competence. This oversight or misunderstanding can express itself in inaccessible language, postures, breath, or meditation practices, or in offering practices that are not yet appropriate for the students in a particular class.

Knowing where we are on this continuum of learning and skill development creates humility; openness; willingness to learn, unlearn, and relearn; and a desire to connect with students and other teachers to collect feedback about one's own teaching and services. As new skills are learned (e.g., to expand scope of practice), these stages are likely revisited again and again.

Next Steps

Once we understand these basic principles of preparing the environment and ourselves, as yoga teachers or clinicians, we are ready to begin to ponder teaching principles and pedagogy. We will begin this journey with an exploration of how to plan and sequence yoga sessions and series and how to teach with keen attention to many pedagogical and philosophical principles. We will revisit many of the points that were introduced in Chapter 6 – from a slightly different perspective, namely from a perspective of putting these principles and preparations into applied action.

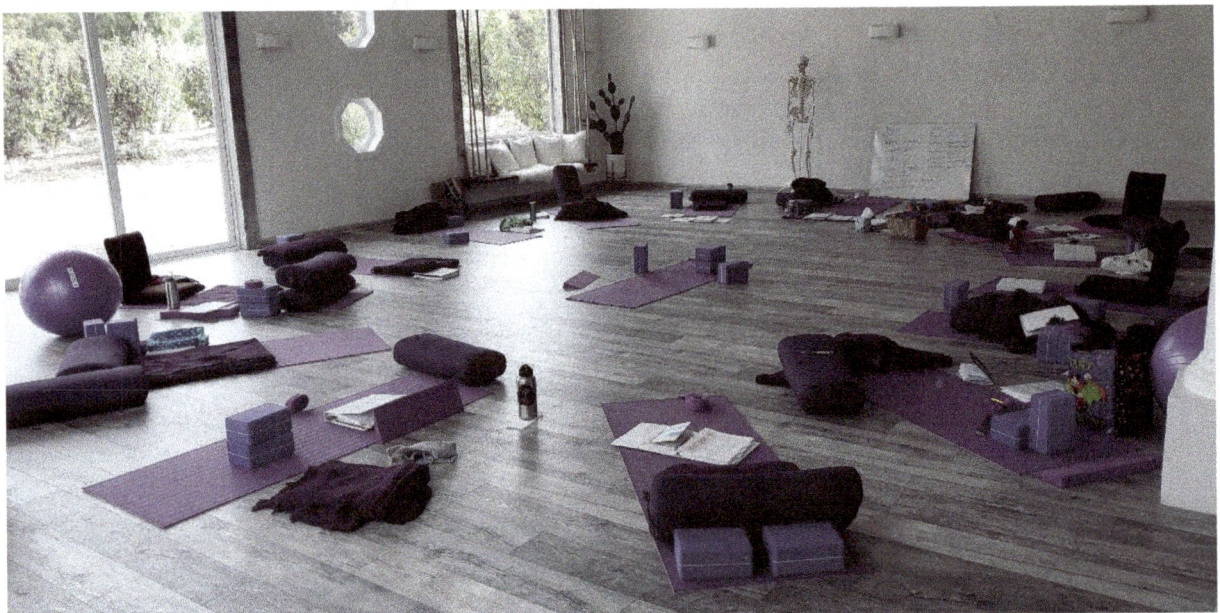

Chapter 7: Principles of Sequencing and Teaching with Intention

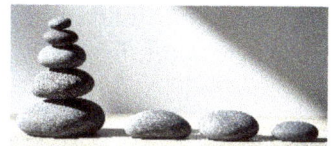

Integrated holistic yoga teachers remember that physical posture is only the tiniest tip of the yoga iceberg – the real work happens energetically, emotionally, and mentally. We understand and are in the physical world first and hence we grow and evolve from there. Yoga teaches us to understand, acknowledge and inhabit our bodies – not deny, repress, or dissociate from them. We learn to understand the physical and how to rest in equanimity regardless of what happens in the body. Alongside the work with the body, we work with breath and energy, mind and emotions, and ultimately, we move toward samadhi or enlightenment, awakening to a new level of consciousness.

Working from an integrated and holistic paradigm of teaching yoga avoids reductionism and embraces holism (which really should be spelled *wholism* as this is really what it reflects). It embraces the complexity of human life and growth while resting in the simplicity of a well-designed practice. Just like a spiderweb, a yoga class is the weaving together of many intricate strands with great attention and purpose. The result is a complex structure that is beautiful to behold in its seeming simplicity.

What does reductionism look like? Reductionism hones in on a single or a couple of aspects of yoga without honoring its full history and complexity. It may hone in on the physical aspect of the practice. It may hone in on images of yoga that make it look exclusive to certain populations; it may restrict access through materialism. It may exclude and frighten as opposed to including and inviting. The opposite of reductionism is wholism, the honoring of complexity, critical analysis, and thoughtfulness as guides to teaching. From this paradigm, providers offer services based on principles applied and tailored to the specific individuals and circumstances of the current teachings or therapeutics, informed by the intention for the practice overall as well as each practice component.

Teaching with Intention

What does wholism look like? Wholism is a spiderweb of complexity that integrates many interrelated and interactive elements that influence one another and arise codependently. Holistic integrated teaching acknowledges that yoga is multi-faceted, firmly grounded in the eight limbs and not reducible to a single practice, while being accessible to all. It is grounded in the developmental notion of the koshas and embraces the whole of its practitioners and their biopsychosociocultural circumstances. It is firmly grounded in a clear intention for each practice and its components. The notion of intentionality is integral to yoga philosophy and is called *sankalpa* in Sanskrit and was covered in Chapter 1. To honor the intentionality of a holistic teaching practice, SANKALPA also is the acronym for the various components of the holistic teaching spiderweb promoted in this book.

Elements of the Sankalpa Teaching Spiderweb

Holistic yoga services attend to a multitude of variables that all influence how well a yoga professional transmits the wholeness of yoga and how well they translate the practice for all participants. It invites the provider to understand the deeper dimensions of yoga and to unfold – for their clients and themselves – the healing power inherent in these various dimensions. The model presented below is a work in progress. No doubt, there are other dimension to which we attend. Do not let yourself be limited (or intimidated) by the model – embrace it as a place from which to start and from which to unfold your own interpretation of what constitutes integration and wholism in yoga and in yoga instruction.

To honor integration and wholism, yoga professionals attend to and weave together – at minimum – the teaching elements described below as they conceive, develop, implement, tailor, and refine classes. Attention to each component is explicit in the conception and development stage of a session. All elements are present in its implementation though some may remain implicit. In other words, explicit voicing of all elements is not necessary, though entirely possible. Implicitly, all elements are present in the teacher's mind and awareness.

In a spider web, any string you pull affects the rest of the web. Similarly, teaching or offering yoga therapeutics in a holistic and integrated way means attending to the multitude of variables that affect the teachings and how these variables interact with one another in shaping the experience of the yoga practice. The smallest change in one strategy, element, or component of the spiderweb will have resonance in all aspects of the class and teacher-student relationship. An optimal approach to this way of teaching is to understand and apply the principles that are offered here and let them guide your instructions in a flexible and tailored, adapted and accessible way.

Instead of offering canned or rote instructions that are always the same for a particular practice, competent teachers let instructions be guided by the context and clients with whom the principles are applied. In other words, teachers use critical thinking to decide on what to say and how to say it. They let themselves be guided by intention and wisdom and invite students to integrate instructions with equal measure of wisdom and discernment. Clients always have choices and options about how to receive and apply instructions. They are not passive recipients of directives or orders, but active and empowered agents of their own choices about how to move, breathe, and practice. As mentioned, the components of the spiderweb honor the intentionality of holistic integrated teaching by forming the acronym **SANKALPA**:

S = student variables
A = aim or intention
N = new learning
K = koshas
A = applied psychology
L = limbs of yoga
P = pedagogy or practice principles
A = affiliation

Visual Representation of the Complexity of Integrated Holistic Teaching – SANKALPA or Teaching with Intention

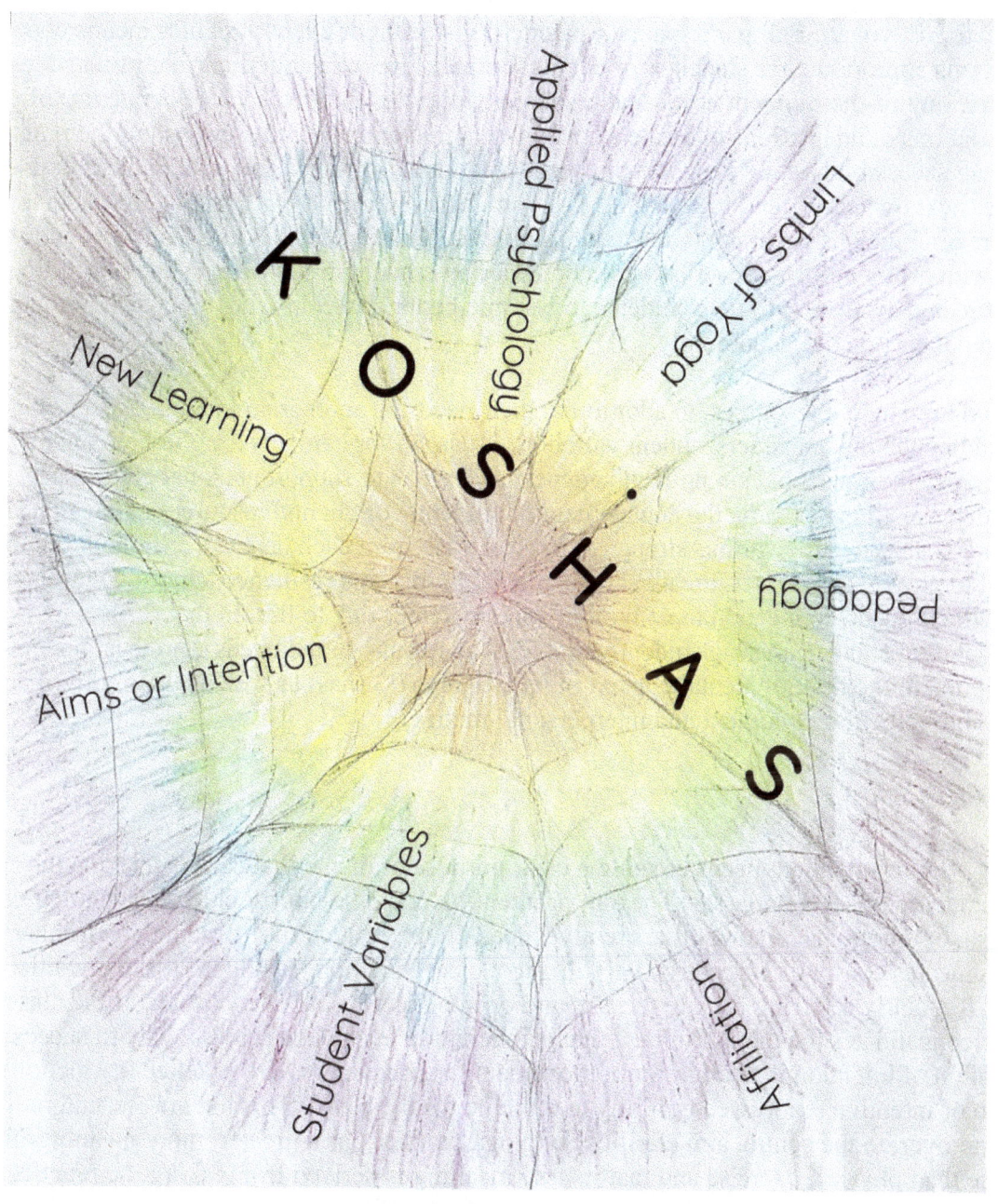

Red	= Annamaya kosha
Orange	= Pranamaya kosha
Yellow	= Manomaya koshas at manas
Green	= Manomaya koshas at ahamkara
Blue	= Manomaya kosha at buddhi
Purple	= Vijnanamaya kosha
Grey	= Anandamaya kosha

Student or Client Variables

Recognizing client needs and resources is at the heart of creating and supporting accessibility of the practice of yoga for all participants. Considering student or client variables means choosing yoga forms appropriate for students' or clients' bodies, level of vitality, current mind state, and other relevant in-the-moment needs and resources. It invites the free and deliberate use of props and variations or adaptations to create a student-centered and tailored approach to the practice. To create accessibility at all koshas – physical, emotional, mental, relational, and cultural – requires acknowledging and recognizing that there is no single way to practice. Instead, as teachers or clinicians we honor, and attend to individual needs, while balancing these individual needs with group needs and wellbeing. In considering student needs we also cue mindfulness, attention, and awareness to help students to become better at recognizing their own needs and adjusting their practice accordingly.

The cuing of student resources, in addition to their needs, is another an integral aspect of accessible yoga that considers student variables. It can be very empowering to help clients begin to recognize their personal strength and agency, as well as to support personal choice and fortitude or resilience. Cuing the engagement of students' or clients' resources can lean heavily on cuing koshas and the various strengths that can arise from each layer of self, including but not limited to physical resources, breath access, mental agility and resilience, emotional attunement and wellbeing, and connection to community and a greater link to life. In that sense, understanding and considering student variables – as resources and needs – are best understood and applied in the developmental context of participants (koshas) as well as their current and past biopsychosociocultural context and interpersonal matrix.

Aim or Intention

Having Aim or intention means creating a clear purpose or theme that carries through the entire class or an arc of several classes. The aim or intention could be philosophical, psychological, physical, or emotional, among other creative ideas. In the context of the theme, the teacher communicates clarity of purpose by verbalizing a clear intention (sankalpa) for the practice at its outset. Regularly referring back to the aim and/or intention during every aspect of the class further consolidates the thoughtfulness that is inherent in each yoga session. Key to successful integration of intention is to align form, movement, breath, and inward practice instructions with the aim or intention (expressed typically as a theme for the class). This integration and return, over and over, to the central aim clarifies that yoga practice has a greater, more meaningful purpose than physical exercise and that its true meaning is derived from taking the practice off the mat into life. Intentions can be shared or collective (offered by the teacher or clinician to the group), as well as deeply personal and individual (invited by the teacher of each student at the outset and the end of the practice). Intentions and dedications offered in this way can become a personal or collective point of concentration on and off the mat.

New Learning

Teachers ground their offered practice in neuroscience and other research and commit themselves to ongoing new learning that can inform all teaching. Weaving in research findings as relevant and appropriate to intention, students or clients, and class level facilitates understanding of the practice and transfers knowledge, experience, and enjoyment from the mat into life. For example, it can be enlightening for students or client when teachers explicitly tie the aim or theme of the class to science related to brain changes, polyvagal theory, impacts on physiology, impact on nervous system regulation, effects on pain, support for trauma recovery, and more. Using science and research as a guide further helps teachers offer a practice that maintains safety and reduces potential for harm. The same is true for using new learning about anatomy and physiology to inform anatomical sequencing that honors neuromuscular integration, dynamic stretching principles, and kinesiology, as grounded in research and biomechanics. Similarly, new learning will help clinician continue to refine their offerings related to the anatomical, physiological, and psychological aspects of breathing. Teachers can state new learning or specific research findings explicitly or leave them implicit depending on context.

The principle of lifelong learning also enters yoga providers' practice through personal commitment to being curious and perhaps even becoming a researcher, collecting impact and outcome data from students or clients (Brems, 2023). Both qualitative and quantitative research methods are appropriate, especially given that even historically yogis have collected personal data and experience to ground their practice. By being committed to personal new learning, teachers and clinicians offer ongoing opportunities of new learning to students or clients.

Koshas

The most crucial aspect of the spiderweb is to ground every practice in all koshas – the layers of self or layers of experience. It is key to recognize and explicitly acknowledge that the koshas are the backdrop for students' or clients' entire lives, experiences, and growth. To do so competently, yoga providers need to be fully familiar with the koshas as a modern developmental concept as well as a yoga concept that is deeply historical. Based on this knowledge, teachers can then introduce, define, redefine, and integrate the koshas as appropriate and facilitate their students' or clients' transfer of learning about the koshas to daily life. It is helpful to name at least all the tangible koshas or layers of self in each class, inviting clients into a relationship with their body, breath, and mind. Whether directly or indirectly, it is also key to address wisdom and intuition as well as the seeds of bliss or joy. (For a review of the koshas, please refer back to Section 1.)

Applied Psychology

Using applied psychology means giving the offered practice a greater context and purpose by integrating yoga psychology concepts and their application to a householder yogi's life (e.g., yamas, niyamas, gunas, kleshas, vrittis, mind states, brahma viharas, karma, and more). Aspects of yoga psychology may be related to the aim or intention of the class and introduced throughout a session as appropriate and relevant (you do not have to overdo this; in any one class, limit this to what is reasonable within the frame of the class intention and length). Applied psychology also helps teachers create intentional and appropriately boundaried relationships with students or clients, applying psychological principles of reflective listening, attentiveness to participants in all their layers, along with personal boundaries and ethics (see *Affiliation* below).

Limbs of Yoga

Attending to all eight limbs of yoga in each class is a given in the context of integrated holistic yoga. To the degree that it is feasible and efficient, yoga professionals attend to ethics, discipline and purpose, physical form and movement, breath, introspection, concentration, meditation, and joy or union. They remember and make use of the reality that at least to some degree the eight limbs align with the koshas and thus represent a means of speaking to each kosha implicitly and explicitly. The eight limbs also align with the greater arc (i.e., sequencing) of each yoga class, which implicitly or explicitly acknowledges ethics, commitment, movement, breath, sense withdrawal, concentration, and meditation – in in the service of enlightenment, joy, and wisdom. The eight limbs also enter each class through the explicit example set by the teacher who lives in accordance with and commits to these eight limbs in personal and professional contexts. Ethics are carried into all classes via the teachers' or clinician's implicit commitment to the lifestyle limbs of yoga.

As appropriate, the ethical principles of Limb 1 can be voiced directly, especially given the profound commitment of healthcare-oriented yoga professionals to work and live with *ahimsa* and *satya* at all times. The first limb of yoga also keeps us, as teachers and clinicians, grounded in appropriate ethical and boundaried relationships with our students that honor and respect clients' rights, invite agency, and empower personal choice.

Pedagogy

For each chosen practice, drawn from any of the limbs, it is necessary to apply and tailor sound practice and teaching principles. Yoga professionals become skilled in and use applicable practice and teaching principles for each type of yoga practice: values, posture, breathing, and introspective practices. General pedagogical principles are the overarching purpose of Section 2 of this Volume in the series; practice-specific pedagogy and practice principles for each specific practice limb of yoga (i.e., *asana*, *pranayama*, interior practices) are the topics of Volumes 2 (*asana*) and 3 (breathing and inner practice) in the series. Learning practice and teaching principles is an ongoing and never-ending process. We constantly learn new facts about human bodies, emotions, minds, and resilience. Yoga teachers who are committed to using practice principles auspiciously stay connected to new science as it emerges and continuously refine and evolve their teaching skills (see *New Learning* above). They engage in ongoing continuing education, use their own experience, and learn from their students or clients to stay up-to-date, connected to modern science, creative in their delivery of classes, and humble. They do not get stuck in canned or rote instructions that presume that all participants have the same needs or wants.

Affiliation and Safety

Yoga teaching and therapeutics are grounded in the provider-participant relationship first and foremost. As noted above, the *yamas* and applied psychology help set the stage for a positive, boundaried, and ethical relationship that reflect the respective roles and vulnerabilities of all relationship partners. Setting up environments of physical and psychological safety are key to positive relationship building and have been covered at the outset of Section 2. Maintaining ethics, working within one's scope of practice, and committing to equity and access are also foundational to auspicious relationships and are covered in the code of conduct. Key to building positive and respectful affiliation and safety is the capacity to listen, to empathize, and to tailor practices to students or clients as they show up in each moment. It requires self-reflection and self-awareness in the part of the teacher to prevent personal biases and prejudices from entering relationships in an unconscious or inauspicious way.

Personal traits of teachers were covered above. Last, but definitely not least, safety and affiliation rely on the capacity of teachers to attune to their students or clients at multiple levels. This requires observation skills with attention to participants' bodies (annamaya koshas); energy, affect, and arousal (pranamaya koshas); narratives, attitudes, beliefs, and emotions (manomaya koshas); and intuition and self-agency as well as their embeddedness in a greater social, cultural, and familial context.

In Buddhist psychology, there are four prerequisites for healing and enlightenment. Serving with intention helps us invite our clients to embrace and embody these four principles.

1. *Cultivate relationships that motivate growth, invite self-transformation, and lead us into clarity*: We are encouraged to associate with others, especially teachers, who are ahead of us developmentally, who inspire us to do better. Growth happens in mutual relationships; it is stunted by relationships that hinder development.
2. *Open up to nurturance for a clear and open mind, to teachings that invite discernment*: We are encouraged to pursue the dharma, yoga psychology, teachings about generosity, ethics, mindfulness, compassion, noble truths, and the eight-fold path. Growth happens when heart and mind are open to hear, read, experience, and absorb the teachings. Repeated exposure and absorption of teachings is important just as we have to eat again and again.
3. *Commit to wise work with the mind to arrive at full understanding and recognition of causes*: We are encouraged to experience and feel what we feel, not simply to create mindfulness but to develop insight and wisdom. Growth happens from understanding of how we get stuck and create suffering. Such clarity guides us to new responsiveness and transforms reactivity.
4. *Transform wisdom into wise action, always seeking the practical application of the learning.* We are encouraged to let insight transform into intentions, speech, and actions that are unaffected by attachment, aversion, and delusion. Growth happens as we learn to:
   - Transform thought patterns beliefs ... we rethink and relearn
   - Act ethically and from a clear set of altruistic values ... we are compassionate!
   - Live mindfully and practice (yoga, meditation) with quietude and simplicity (ease) ... practice with passion (effort)
   - Respond to the way things actually are, seeing the world beyond our expectations ... we open our hearts and minds!

Sequencing for Safety and Meaning

Auspicious Session Sequencing

Sequencing a session (whether a class or yoga-based therapeutic service) integrates the creation of a theme or intention, attention to all eight limbs, and development of a class arc that expresses integrated holistic yoga principles. This focus results in the creation of balance, beauty, and joy. In cuing, demonstrating, observing, and assisting, the yoga provider pays attention and stays connected to IHY principles – embodying them in language, cuing choices, and demonstrations; bringing them to bear in observation; giving feedback in line with them in response to observation; and using them to assist, support, and redirect. Sequencing creates an arc toward a single or multiple peak poses while creating meaning that goes beyond the physical. It deeply reflects all integrated holistic principles, emphasizing the layers of human experience, clear intention, careful design to ensure accessibility, and clarity about the potential benefits of the practice. Sequencing that embraces the integrated holistic paradigm deeply honors the principle of first doing no harm.

The suggested outline provided below helps ensure that a session, whether a class or yoga-based therapeutics, is integrated, wholistic, intentional, accessible, and beneficial. It embeds the practice in a context of meaning, intention, and purpose. Some of the pieces can be moved around into a slightly different order; however, all are included and honored in an intentional and respectful manner. Specifics vary based on population served, session context (e.g., healthcare, studio, gym, residential treatment), and intention of the yoga professional on behalf of the clients. On-the-fly adjustment and deviation may be necessitated by how clients present, based on what is happening in the environment, and in line with interpersonal dynamics that emerge spontaneously during the practice (e.g., between teacher and student, among participants). As teachers and clinicians, we plan carefully and then stay on our toes to be able to pivot and deviate from our careful plans based on the reality of each and every moment. We stay closely connected to our students or clients and honor their needs most of all.

Suggested Outline of a Yoga Session
- Opening comments
  - welcome and setting the stage (especially if new students or clients are present)
  - introduce props that may be needed
- Conditioned stimulus for mindfulness
- Presentation of the theme and intention for the class (could choose to call this a *dharma talk* or *psychoeducation* depending on setting)
  - grounded in an explicit aspect of yoga psychology, context, clientele, and/or neuroscience
  - carried through the rest of the session – explicitly and implicitly
  - in a multi-session sequence, refer back and tie theme(s) together across sessions
- Opening Centering and/or Breathing practices
  - attention or awareness
  - observation
  - practice a particular type of breathwork (if appropriate)
  - return to observation
- Intention setting for the students or clients (sankalpa)

- Form and movement practice
  - warm-up forms and movements
  - preparatory forms and movements
  - peak posture(s) and/or peak breathwork
  - counter or relief practices
  - cool-down and calming practice
- Inner practices
  - resting / relaxation posture
  - guided meditation or concentration
  - touch on body, breath, mind, intuition, bliss
  - silence (length determined by perceived needs and risks presented by students or clients)
  - intentional reentry (e.g., return to senses, return to koshas, transition to a seat)
- Closing comments
  - tie back to the class theme or intention
  - link mat work to daily life; perhaps dedicate merit
- Expression of gratitude

Using this suggested outline, each practice is planned with discernment about session intention and composition. This means minimally attending to all of the following aspects of planning a sequence or series:

- Have a clear intention for the session overall and each chosen form, breath, or inner practice
- Know your teaching or therapeutic service space and plan for a deliberate layout of mats (e.g., rows, circles) and related logistics
- Assess if all needed props are available and (re)plan accordingly
- Prepare to demonstrate the most accessible and beneficial versions of each planned practice from across all eight limbs
- Decide on and remain open about compassionate and accessible variations and adaptations that can be used on the fly
- Know the risks, contraindications, and benefits for each offered practice
- Think through language, cuing, and interactional choices (e.g., touch choices) ahead of class or session time
- Know and be facile with appropriate verbal and physical adjustments for all planned practices, using them wisely (read the relevant materials below before trying this out)
- Have proper cuing prepared in your mind (or notes) for transitions from shape to shape, breath to breath, practice to practice – not just a general idea, but specific notions about how to cue students or clients from each preceding to the subsequent practice
- Have a clear sense of cuing for each practice that is to be offered, aligning cuing with physical, vital, emotional, mental, and other aspects of the participants as well as with the intention for the session overall

Although careful planning is definitely essential and follows these basic principles and suggested outline, yoga professionals remain open and flexible to adapt to in-the-moment demands and do not become overly attached to their plan when in-person experiences clearly suggest a pivot. However, this pivot really does need to be necessary given the context – it is not based in a random desire or unexplored intuition. It is based on current assessment and deep knowledge about how to deliver the wisest, most aware, and most compassionate practice.

Sequence-Planning with Intention

Creating careful anatomically, energetically, emotionally, and cognitively accessible sequencing reflects optimal preparation of body, breath, and mind for the peak pose(s) and allows for proper recovery and cool down of all individuals who participate in the practice. It is combined with the overall intention for the session and never independent of its deeper purpose. Opening centering, warming up, preparing, peaking, and cooling down, and closing the session follow one another in such a logical flow that participants feel completely prepared for each aspect of the practice in all of their koshas. Their body, energy and breath, mind and emotions, and intuition and wisdom are all on board for the offerings contained in the practice and feel in alignment with one another.

To achieve such integration and wholism, yoga professionals start their sequence-planning with at least two things in mind: *session intention* (or theme) and selected *physical peak pose(s) or practice* (e.g., a particular focus on asana or pranayama). Intention and peak expression of the practice cannot be separate from one another; they deeply inform one another and therefore are best chosen in tandem. Sometimes, the peak practice is identified and then a commensurate intention is created (more likely in the context of teaching a class). At other times, there may be a deeper intention and the peak practice grows out of this purpose of meaning (more likely in the context of yoga therapeutics). Regardless of which is primary, the two end up being carefully coordinated and synergistic.

For example, a desired peak practice experience that involves forward folds may be more auspiciously linked with an intention of looking inward and creating self-awareness. A peak pose that is a wide-open backbend may be more appropriately linked to an intention related to cultivating an open heart. Similarly, a therapeutic goal of fostering peacefulness and emotional balance may be linked with a gentle standing balance asana practice culminating in alternate nostril breathing. The discussion that follows is written with the *intention* as primary and the peak practice as aligned with the intention. Again, this order can be reversed as appropriate to context. It can be just as helpful to make the *practice* primary and let the intention follow. The key is that the sequence is developed with purpose and clarity of directions. IHY teachers and clinicians prepare for sessions – generally speaking, *they do not wing it*.

Considerations in Choosing a Class Intention or Theme

Intentionality occurs on two levels. First, the teacher or clinician has clarity about the intention and purpose of each session as well as across time, if sessions are embedded in a greater overall series. A series can be defined as *a set of sessions*, carefully sequenced and framed around a particular topic that runs for a particular length of time (e.g., the Yoga for Health and Resilience 10-series offered by YogaX; Brems, 2015); or *an ongoing series* of classes that occur indefinitely or for a specified period of weeks, tailored to a particular kind of students (e.g., the oncology series offered free and online via the Santa Barbara Breast Cancer Resource Center). Whether planning a session or a series, the clinician or teacher had a clearly expressed intention for the series overall as well as for each individual session, whether part of a series or not. The second level of intentionality invites students or clients to develop a personal intention in each session and/or purpose or meaning for a series of sessions that unfold across time. This is done via an explicit invitation, early in a given session, offering students the opportunity to reflect on their own intention for a class. This is invited as choice of students defining their intention via a simple word (e.g., peacefulness, compassion), phrase (e.g., may find freedom, may all be happy), a felt sense that is non- or trans-verbal, or as an alignment with the offered collective intention.

In our current context of using intention for sequencing and planning, focus is on the *teacher or clinician* creating intentionality for series and/or session(s). In framing an intentions, clinicians carefully consider the greater context of whether a session is offered as a one-time event, a regular event with drop-in students, or a series of sessions for a cohort of students that remains the same for the entirety of the series.

Intentionality from both perspectives (*for individual sessions or for entire series*) includes the following considerations:
- Ground intention in the needs of population that is to be served by the session or series
- Understand why students or clients are seeking out a yoga class and what challenges they may bring along
- Understand the goals or shared reason for the students or clients who will be in the session or series
- Let the intention be aligned with the context of what is possible in the environment in which the session unfolds, considering issues such as noise level, prop availability, confidentiality, size of space, number of students, and so on
- Ensure that the intention is one that increases opportunity for psychological and emotional safety and that the intention does no harm or does not feel coercive
- Create an intention that can be carried and cued across all levels of experience (i.e., that honors all koshas)
- Create an intention that allows for expression through all eight limbs of yoga (e.g., asana, pranayama, concentration)
- Choose an intention is aligned with research findings (i.e., avoid intentions that are based in questionable assertions or misinformation)
- *If planning a series*: create an intention and purpose that spans across the entire series (ideally, decide beforehand how many sessions will comprise the series)
  o slowly and deliberately, over the course of several sessions, move clients or students toward their goals and the shared intention for the series overall
  o ensure that the intention for the series is grounded in beneficence and remains accessible
  o develop each session within the series in line with the overall intention and purpose – honor the gradual unfolding of the overall intention with aligned sub-intentions in each session in the series
  o still allow students to set their own intention in each session
- *If offering a single session*: create an intention and purpose that guides the session with meaning, clarity, beneficence, and accessibility
  o let knowledge of the students who will take the session guide the intention considering the likely needs, challenges, contraindications, and other personal and biopsychosociocultural variables that may play a role in what is or is not accessible and beneficial for the likely group represented in the session
  o ensure that the intention can be realized given the context and setting for the session – considering environmental and safety factors that may need to be accommodated

Considerations in Choosing Peak Practices

The peak shape or movement is carefully coordinated with the intention for the session that is being planned, also considering whether the session is part of a series that allows for development across time. Needs and resources of the students or clients to whom the class is tailored are carefully considered alongside the intention when the peak shape or movement is chosen. In other words, it helps to have a sense of who the class it targeted to and to choose wisely based on what is known about their (likely or anticipated) experiences in all koshas. The following considerations will serve well in choosing and sequencing for the peak shape or movement:

- Have clarity about variations that are possible and healthful for the peak shape and the shapes leading up to it – variations are individually tailored expressions of the peak shape that are not presented as lesser than the stereotypical expression of the peak shape; variations are compassionate and kind, not of less value or meaning
- Be knowledgeable about respectful and compassionate practice adaptations that may be offered, tailored to the clientele and environment in which the session
- Have clarity about how to offer and use available props to create an accessible practice for all participants – do not commit to a peak that requires resources that are not available in the environment or within the capacity of the students who are anticipated to attend
- Be thoughtful about how to demonstrate peak shape(s) in an inviting and creative manner – do not habitually demonstrated stereotypic variation (often and inauspiciously called the *full expression of a shape*); instead choose variations that are accessible to the majority of the individuals in the class or session and emphasize that the optimal expression of a shape is the one that best serves a student's experiences in all layers
- Know the risks and benefits of offered practices and name contraindications – voice such cautions as a matter compassionate action, not as a way of instilling fragility mind sets, fear, or anxiety
- Do not force the lesson plan, instead be prepared to adapt, delete, and substitute on the fly – generally speaking, and counterintuitive for many teacher, it is the peak pose that is the best pose to delete if time runs out and the full sequence as planned cannot be offered

Considerations in Planning Session Opening

Once clarity has been developed for the intention and peak shape, actual session planning can begin. The first stage is to plan the opening of the session. This is the phase of the practice that welcomes students to the mat, grounds and centers them into the present moment, and orients them to what is ahead. This plan may differ greatly depending on whether students have been together for a while and/or have an existing relationship with the teacher, or whether most students are new to the practice, teacher, or cohort. Teachers plan ahead for new students and how to greet them, if a class is open to drop-ins or new joiners for a cohort class/series.

Regardless of whether new clients need to be integrated, regular opening practices that are planned for this phase of a session include the following possibilities and sequencing; however, some rearrangement of order and emphasis is invited depending on context.

- Offer opening comments that welcome everyone and that set the stage for the practice (especially if new students or clients are present); introduce the props that may be helpful and give students time to gather them if they did not do so already
- Present the collective theme and intention for the class – this could be framed as a dharma talk or as psychoeducation, depending on setting and context; the theme or intentions might be grounded in an explicit aspect of yoga psychology, a particular context, a specific clientele, or modern neuroscience
- Offer an opening centering and/or conditioned stimulus for mindfulness – this invitation into the present moment can be a powerful practice of attuning students into all layers of experience
- Invite personal and deliberate intention setting for the practice (see *Student-Level Intention* above)

Considerations in Planning Breathwork

Since the class being planned is an IHY class, breathing practices are fully incorporated throughout the session. Careful planning is necessary to blend chosen breathing practices with session intention and chosen peak shape(s). Generally speaking, optimal functional breathing is invited throughout the practice – from beginning to end. This means that there are consistent reminders about breathing gently (*not deeply*), quietly (no – the breath should not be heard…), smoothly, through the nose, and via the diaphragm (Brems, 2024b). If no other breathwork is offered in a session beyond optimal functional and resiliently adaptive breathing, the goal of pranayama integration has been attained. A few additional planning and sequencing recommendations follow. It is highly recommended to pay careful attention to this suggested sequencing, as it tends to be most auspicious to the majority of students. It is not necessary to offer complex breathing practices in every class. Instead, it is more helpful to cultivate healthful breathing over time as many clients arrive in yoga classes with dysregulated breathing patterns.

- Cultivate attention or awareness of the breath, deliberately attuning how breath is emerging naturally in the moment and instilling curiosity about how the four phases of the breath (i.e., inhalation, pause at the top, exhalation, pause at the bottom, exhalation) are showing up
- Invite observation of a particular aspect of the breath (e.g., texture, sound, volume, rate)
- Offer a particular type of breathwork that serves a clear purpose aligned with session intention and peak shape – this step can be skipped as attuned breathing alone can suffice and represents a powerful breathing practice for many students
- Return to observation and attunement through the session
- Continue cuing optimal functional breathing, especially nasal breathing and quiet breathing

Considerations in Planning Warm-Up and Preparation Poses

The next step in the planning and sequencing process is to define a path to the optimal experience of the peak shape *in all koshas*, not just in the anatomical or physical sense. The peak shape needs to feel like a natural and logical outcome of the practices that preceded it. The lead-up practices carefully prime all layers of experience for the peak shape, attending to preparation for body and sensory experience, energy and affect, thoughts and emotions, actions and relationship, and wisdom and intuition. Following are a few helpful hints about how to plan the preparation and warm-up phase of the practice:

- Warm the body and invite blood flow by gently and intentionally engaging muscles
- Commit to the intentional inclusion of the six movements of the spine, making choices that are natural and logical for the chosen peak practice and individuals who are present
  - flexion, extension – perhaps also adding axial extension
  - lateral flexion to the right; lateral flexion to the left
  - right rotation and left rotation
- Be intentional and purposeful about each choice of movement and posture – it needs to lead the student somewhere, either physically/anatomically, energetically/emotionally, or mentally/ideationally
- Prepare all koshas for the peak shape or movement – remember not simply to teach to the body; very deliberately and explicitly include all layers of experience in the preparation
  - anatomically progress toward the peak pose: ground what needs to be grounded, open what needs to be opened, strengthen what needs to be strong, stabilize what needs to be stabilized for the peak
  - choose dynamic stretching that progressively increases range of motion and ease through repetition in different muscular engagements and approaches
  - integrate strength and balance through out
  - energetically progress toward the peak pose by choosing breathing patterns and practices that can be maintained or reengaged throughout the practice and that facilitate the peak posture – invite awareness of breath, vitality, energy, and affective responses or reactivities
  - mentally and emotionally progress toward the peak pose – the peak should not be an emotional surprise, but more of an *aha* moment; pay attention to narratives and mind stories along the path of the full session
  - engage the mind with information, awareness and attunement; invite awareness of emotional responses to the practice as it unfolds
  - leave lots of space for tuning in mentally and emotionally and remind students regularly not to tune out
  - relax the nervous system and invite a ventral vagal state of social engagement and connection – create a sense of community, collaboration, and co-regulation

Considerations in Planning and Offering Counter- and Recovery Procedures

This aspect of planning a sequence refers to neutralizing any extreme effects of a particular shape or practice – if necessary, anatomically (not usually an issue unless offering an extreme set of postures), energetically, mentally, and emotionally. In integrated holistic yoga, extra attention to planning countering may not be necessary as the very definition of IHY is to maintain awareness, attunement, and resilience. Ion other words, in IHY ongoing rebalancing of the nervous system is part and parcel of the practice. A better way to frame this aspect of sequencing may be as a deliberate facilitation of neuromuscular and psychological integration, with a consistent return to a ventral vagal state throughout the session. It does not mean integrating (anatomical) counter poses throughout; instead, it means not destabilizing clients with extreme physical demands. If countering is desirable because of a particular choice of sequencing or shape, do not counter so often that preparation for a particular anatomical or psychological intention is lost. An example of such inauspicious countering is the common practice to insert forward folds regularly after each backbend in a heart-opening series. This countering can dilute the opening in the front body and the strengthening in the back body, as well as the cultivation of willingly moving into emotional and psychological openness and vulnerability. In such a practice, it would be better to choose less demanding backbends and allow them to penetrate all layers of experience in a safe and appropriate manner.

Considerations in Planning Cool-Down and Release

As a practice winds down after the peak shape, it is good common practice to deliberately plan for (re)grounding the nervous system. Ideally, students are helped to access a ventral vagal presence and connection toward the end of the practice, as they are invited to return to balance in all layers of experience. A sequencing recommendation for this phase follows, but other possibilities exist:

- Cool the body, reduce heart rate, and relax muscles
- Calm the breath and energetic state – support a sattvic experience of contentment and help students recalibrate their energy budget
- Calm mind and ease emotions to invite psychological responsiveness – attempt to leave students in a state of empowerment and agency, rather then vulnerability or fragility (unless another choice is wise for a particular student, as may occur in a mental health-focused clinical session that integrates yoga therapeutics)
- Connect to wisdom and joy with compassion, intention, and community
- Stay with or reconnect to the class theme as well as individual intentions
- Prepare for inner practice and savasana in all layers of experience

Considerations in Planning Inner Practice, Meditation, and Savasana

The final active phase plans for deliberate movement into inner practices. It may begin or end with a plan for a guided imagery, guided meditation, intentional concentration practice, or similar inner work. It includes a planned and deliberate period of savasana, a premier practice of pratyahara. A suggestion for planning and sequencing this inner work is offered here, but other inner practice sequencing options exist:

- Invite students to find a resting shape that is conducive to turning inward with ease (savasana is the classic shape for this part of the practice, but not always the best choice – be willing to offer alternatives and to help students find an easeful position for their physicality, energy, and psychology)
- Settle the body into the present moment and release it to the earth
- Settle the breath and release it to the flow of lifeforce that is all around us, that connects us to one another
- Settle the mind by letting be whatever shows up without attachment or aversion, without trying to define or understand – invite acceptance; surrender thoughts and emotions to inner wisdom, trusting that the wise self will return the student to what is needed once off the mat
- Offer an inner practice, concentration, meditation, or imagery that recaptures the collective theme and intention – make a clear connection to foster integration into vijnanamaya kosha
- Move deliberately into savasana by
    - offering *silence*
    - suggesting *darkness* (e.g., eye pillow, dimming lights)

- reminding students or clients about *warmth* (e.g., cover up with a blanket, put on a sweater and socks)
  - <u>not</u> talking during savasana (this is not the time for the teacher to speak – not even to read favorite quotes or poems; those can happen after savasana, not during)
- Move deliberately out of savasana with a predictable sequence of movements that help students find an upright seat

Considerations for Planning Practice Closure

Teachers often forget to plan enough time for the closing of the session and rush students from savasana to a seat to saying goodbye. It is psychologically and emotionally more supportive to allow students to make a deliberate journey from inner work and savasana to a seated closing that invites them back into contact with the outer world and into community. Thus, sessions best close with a planned, mindful, and deliberate journey out of savasana, a guided re-entry into outer and inner awareness, and a process for finding a seat to meet for the closing. Once seated, students can be invited to process the practice consciously to facilitate generalization of the benefits accrued in the practice to life off the mat. The following practices are a possible flow of offered experiences once students are back in a seated position:

- Welcome students back to a seat and into the present moment
- Ask students to make note of a positive take-away from class (e.g., something interesting, helpful, new, captivating, meaningful), inviting them to let that take-away integrate into all koshas (e.g., integrate into their tissues, their energy, their nervous system, their neural pathways)
- Invite a reconnection to the personal or collective intention, perhaps integrating that intention with the take-away
- Combine intention and take-away to create a dedication of merit and offer a process for doing so (e.g., with an inhalation draw that dedication into your own heart; with an exhalation send it silently into your community of choice)

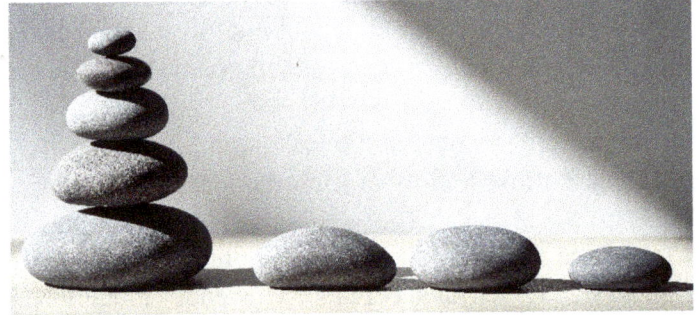

Chapter 8: Principles for Teaching with Integration and Wholism

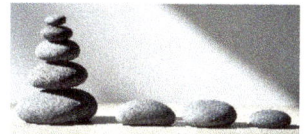

All practice principles offered in this chapter are applied in the context of all koshas and limbs, consistent with the integrated holistic yoga paradigm. Whether we practice or cue safety, ease and effort, nonattachment, or grounding, expansion, and stabilization – we are always in the practice and in our teaching with all layers of experience and open-hearted presence.

A practice with safety and meaning very explicitly integrates optimized opportunities for safety in all teaching methods, regardless of which limb is most prevalent. All interactions and instructions are offered with compassion and wisdom, without scaring students or clients or inducing a sense of fragility. Humans are resilient; we do not want to discourage exploration and growth. As humans, we must expand beyond our comfort zone eventually – however, we do not want to push too far, too fast. We encourage students or clients to play at their physical, energetic, emotional, mental, and psychological edges to slowly expand these boundaries (or bandwidths) or to pull back if there is a tendency to overdo. Sometimes, the comfort zone that needs expanding is not the body – it may be emotional or mental attachment or aversion that needs more resilience. In such cases, expanding the comfort zone may mean accepting that it is more healthful to do physically less, rather than more. Sometimes this means exploring emotional limits, expanding opinions, or loosening a belief.

Principles that Create Opportunities for Safety and Self-Agency

Honoring Yoga Ethics, Commitments, and Intentions

Yoga teachers honor safety by working within yogic principles of ethics (yamas and brahma viharas) and lifestyle commitments (niyamas) to provide a transformative and integrated asana practice (Farhi, 2006). Especially if we, as teachers, are working in mental healthcare or behavioral health, we remember that teaching yoga is not primarily about the body, but more importantly about energetic wellness, emotional resilience, and mental health and wellbeing (Brems, 2020). The integration of psychoethical attention is essential to an integrated holistic yoga practice. It reflects our clear understanding that all of us, without exclusion or exception, are integrated into the same web of life. We are part of an interdependent and dynamic process wherein every intention, thought, speech, decision, and action has causes and consequences. This wisdom needs to permeate our teaching.

Wisdom, awareness, and compassion coexist in our practice, teaching, and life. They intermingle and co-depend. This means that work on the mat and daily life are grounded in ethics and compassionate values that guide us to take responsibility for our own life, other people, our environment, and our relationships. Moment-by-moment, action-by-action, and decision-by-decision, we cultivate awareness and compassion, generosity, lovingkindness, patience, moderation, joy, and more. This constant commitment to the yamas, niyamas, and brahma

viharas is deeply integrated into our teaching, including our sequencing choices, demonstrations, cuing, and offerings.
- We honor the yamas by working with the discernment of non-violence, truthfulness, abundance, moderation, and non-grasping for a deeper pose.
- We integrate the niyamas by inviting purity in the work, discipline, introspection, contentment, and devotion to a purpose beyond physical exercise.
- We honor the brahma viharas by teaching with compassion, lovingkindness, altruistic joy, and equanimity.
- We consistently ground and reground our teachings in the philosophical, anatomical, physiological, energetic, mental, emotional, behavioral, and relational intentions for the practice.
- We work with patience, consistency, and regularity to create an environment that optimizes opportunity for students or clients to feel safe and supported, as well as optimally challenged and encouraged to broaden their window of tolerance, enhance resilience, and increase dedication to personal growth and transformation.
- We cultivate a sense of personal responsibility for our teaching and practice – we live and teach with the realization that we may become a role model and expert for our students or clients, whether we see ourselves in that way or not.

Fred von Allmen (von Allmen & Seifarth, 2007), a renowned European Buddhist meditation teacher, offers a framework for teaching and practicing meditation that can be beautifully applied to the teaching and practice of yoga. He suggests that as teachers and practitioners, every time we step up to practice and at all moments of our life, we do so with a commitment to honor a wholesome beginning, a wholesome middle, and a wholesome end.

- *Wholesomeness at the Beginning*: set an intention for the action to follow that reflects compassion, wisdom, and altruistic motivation
- *Wholesomeness in the Middle*: bring awareness, attention, gratitude, appreciation, compassion and other ethical and altruistic commitments to each action, whether on the yoga mat or in life – infuse each asana, pranayama, or interior action with this attitude of honoring and integrating the wholesome
- *Wholesomeness at the End*: once an action has been brought to completion (e.g., at the end of a yoga or meditation practice or at the end of a life event) dedicate merit by offering the benefit from the action or practice to the greater good

This process deeply invites and honors the setting of intentions, development of clear aims, and the integration of a theme throughout the practice. As teachers, we are encouraged and serve our students or clients well if we:
- Create a clear understanding of the intention for the class or series of classes
- Develop key words and phrases that capture this theme at its essence
- Apply or offer these key words and phrases in all contexts of the class to make sure the theme is:
    - discussed in depth or breadth as desired in the opening talk
    - integrated into the core of the opening centering
    - woven into breathing instructions

- incorporated into the cuing of asana – key words are especially great here
  - intertwined with movement into stillness at end of class – could become the theme of the meditation, concentration, or guided imagery
  - recapitulated in the closing comments

Healthful Physical, Vital, and Cognitive/Emotional Boundaries in all Koshas

We honor students' or clients' and personal safety by working within healthful physical, affective, and mental boundaries and wise application of body and breath mechanics (Lasater, 2021), especially when working in healthcare and mental healthcare settings, where we will encounter greater vulnerability in students or clients. Minimally, as integrated holistic yoga teachers, we attend to the following cautions, all of which are addressed in more detail below. We teach in a way that helps everyone:

- Maintain healthful range of motion to protect muscles, ligaments, and joints
- Understand and make healthful use of extant physical reflexes
- Coordinate movement with breath
- Learn how to differentiate discomfort from pain
- Honor and understand pain signals
- Understand and apply trauma-informed yoga principles
- Practice with attunement, mindfulness, and awareness

Throughout our work, we invite students or clients to work at their edges of physical, energetic, mental, emotional, behavioral, and relational comfort (Lasater, 2020, 2021). We invite students or clients to:

- Safely work at the edges or boundaries of physical flexibility, honoring the needs of annamaya koshas while investigating resilience and areas of possible new opening and strengthening
- Safely work at the edges of arousal and affect tolerance, using breath and energy awareness to explore the possibilities for widening bandwidth and the window of tolerance – neither trying too hard nor too little
- Safely work with the edges of mental comfort and discomfort, exploring thoughts and emotions and the capacity to accept, tolerate, or work with them as challenge arises – neither overstressing nor shrinking away
- In all koshas, recognize and differentiate between the maximum edge, intermediate edge, and minimum edge (White, 2007)

We continuously demonstrate, use, and cue discernment for student supports that increase the likelihood of physical safety. We suggest that everyone, providers and participants:

- Use props freely, especially in demonstrations
- Avail ourselves of choices, variations, option, and alternatives
- Invite, never demand or direct and generally defer to clients' judgment about their own body, breath, energy, and mind
- Be thoughtful about which shapes and movements to demonstrate and which variation to choose – beware of showing off
- Default to verbal adjustment cues whenever possible

- Never use physical adjustment with force or without explicit and ongoing collection of informed consent
- Consider touch/no-touch cue cards on mats regarding physical touch and additionally use ongoing collection of informed consent

Scaffolding across the Koshas

A scaffolded practice creates balance, integrity, and beauty across all koshas. It considers the reality that the koshas are developmental, that each student may have access to each kosha in a different way, and that students or clients evolve developmentally and thus have changing needs across time. A scaffolded practice weaves all koshas into the session to provide opportunity for all students or clients to find an access point that resonates with their needs, be it physical, energetic, mental, emotional, behavioral, or relational. Following are ideas for cuing that may help yoga providers learn how to engage in this deliberate interweaving of the koshas throughout their teaching. The hope is that these ideas create additional ideas for each individual clinician or teacher, leading to repertoire of cues that can be seamlessly integrate in all yoga therapeutics.

Physical scaffolding considerations and cuing suggestions for mindfulness-based movement (Schmalzl et al., 2014) *(annamaya kosha and beyond)*:
- Work with physical needs and resources
- Attend to the inner body more so than the outer body
- Draw on props and variations
- Use tailored demonstration
- Encourage balancing the gunas and recognizing their nervous system impacts
- Encourage balancing the autonomic nervous system

Energetic scaffolding and cuing considerations for optimal functional breathing (Brems, 2024b) *(pranamaya kosha and beyond)*:
- Start with attention or awareness; from there move to observation; then a specific practice; return to observation → natural to controlled
- Work with vital needs, energy budgets, and affective resources
- Draw on props and variations in breathwork
- Use tailored demonstration or breathing practice
- Invite tailored attunement or control
- Work with kleshas at all levels of the koshas
- Encourage tuning into attachments, aversions, confusions, fears

Mental and emotional scaffolding and cuing considerations for turning inward (*manomaya koshas and beyond*):
- Find mental stillness and mindfulness
- Attend to and guard the senses – draw inward
- Become increasingly aware of gunas and kleshas and how they flavor the mind
- Notice the vrittis and mind states
- Recognize and then make informed choices about habits

- Recognize that past actions have led to present circumstances and that present actions will lead to future circumstances
- Become aware of and cultivate gaps in thought, behavior, and action
- Live mindfully and open-heartedly to make conscious choices about present actions and future implications
- Find an open heart and open mind
- Live open-mindedly to allow new, prosocial and pro-self, behaviors, emotions, and relationships to emerge
- Create altruistic purpose out of new insights and choices

Relational scaffolding and cuing considerations for finding union (Borghardt, 2016) (*vijnanamaya and anandamaya koshas*):
- Create and seize opportunities for concentration and single-pointed focus
- Embrace a state of integration and oneness (or samadhi – the 8th limb of yoga)
- Notice and transform distractions
- Express samadhi by radiating lovingkindness, joy, compassion, and equanimity;
- Find mindful non(-self)-judgment and self-acceptance
- Serving the benefit of others as part of the regular flow of day-to-day life

Balancing Effort and Ease

This key teaching strategy of balancing effort and ease within each practice as well as in daily life helps participants understand what they need physically, energetically, mentally, emotionally, behaviorally, even relationally – that is, in all koshas (Iyengar, 2006). When we, as teachers, cue effort and ease, we invite students or clients to tune inward, so that they may experience and understand themselves from the inside out. Using the principle of combining effort and ease, we invite participants to develop strength and pliability in all limbs of practice; to work at their edges in body, breath, mind, and emotion to invite balance and integration, resilience and wholism that honor everything that shows up on the mat and in life while also exploring and remaining open to new possibilities. Effort and ease are manifest in body, breath, and mind; they can each show up in many different voices in our head, which can make for a quite lively discussion or an all-out fight.

Effort and ease are each on a continuum from *too much* to *not enough.* We need each in optimal amounts and the two need to be balanced with one another. Balancing effort (*sthira*) with ease (*sukha*) leads to a wholesome body with wholesome energy, and a wholesome mind. Kaminoff (2021) offers the simile of a cell membrane: it has to be strong, yet permeable. In the same way, our bodies are at their healthiest when they are strong yet flexible; our breath is optimal when it is full, yet soft; our mind is at its most resilient when it is persistent, yet open; our emotions guide us clearly when they are defined, yet fluidly evolving.

sthiram-sukham asanam
Patanjali's Yoga Sutra *2.46*

Sthiram – Commitment to Working the Path

Sthira – well-translated as effort or steadiness – represents the commitment to work toward a greater purpose, to create a practice and a life with meaning. It invites a commitment to staying aware and present, to be awake to what unfolds, and to return to this presence of awareness over and over and over with consistent effort and engagement. We cannot relax our way to wisdom – we have to absorb ourselves in committed and ongoing work to apply yogic values, to remain clear and focused in our motivations, and to remember that each moment is important. Sthira invites us to work at our edges of comfort in all koshas, as well as to set firm boundaries that protect us while leaving us room for growth and transformation. Balanced effort encourages committed action infused with fire, endurance, and heart. It brings our entire being into the moment with dedication and steadfastness. Sthira brings stability, steadiness, and strength to our life and practice, helping us persevere (without being perseverative or dogged) during difficulty and continue despite obstacles.

Sthira brings alertness, attentiveness, and preparedness to our practice, without creating tension or strain. In other words, sthira exists on a continuum of *not enough* to *too mu*ch and finding just the right amount, the middle way, is key. Tension and strain result if sthira is taken to an extreme (and not balanced with sukha) and thus becomes rigid, bossy, unbending, inflexible, dictatorial, unyielding, always right, perseverative, obsessive, or stubborn. Not enough effort, on the other hand, becomes bored, sluggish, unfocused, and indifferent. From the practice of too much effort arises the caution to temper sthira with sukha (and, of course, vice versa).

Sukham – Commitment to Staying Playful and Serene

Sukha – well-translated as ease or delight – represents the commitment to stay playful and compassionate amidst effort. It invites a serene, equanimous, and calm resting in awareness of all experiences in each moment. We cannot force or muscle our way to enlightenment either – we stay light-hearted, open-minded, and easeful to find wisdom, compassion, and awareness without becoming attached to the fruits of our labor. Sukha brings sweetness, gentleness, space, a sense of humor, and pliability to our practice and our life. Sukha allows us to work at our edges with kindness, love, compassion, flexibility, and gentleness. It supports actions on our own and others' behalf that is kind, open, resilient, sweet, and adaptable. It supports plasticity and change, flexibility and honesty, tenderness and understanding.

Sukha brings sweetness, relaxation, serenity, and comfort into our practice, yet without creating dullness or laxity. Lika sthira, sukha is on a continuum from *too much* to *not enough*. Dullness, meekness, and laxity can result if sukha is taken to an extreme (and not balanced with sthira). Too much sukha becomes careless, monotonous, lifeless, lethargic, sluggish, weary, or slothful. Not enough sukha lacks heart, engagement, and caring. Thus, as noted above, arises the importance of tempering too much sukha with sthira.

Balancing Sthira and Sukha

Balanced effort and ease (aka stability and comfort, aka challenge and support, aka kindness and discipline) bring compassionate and skillful intensity to your practice. Such balance invites transformation as growth is most likely, in fact may depend upon, both comfort and difficulty in the form of supportive challenge or challenging support. One without the other, relaxation without commitment, or effort without surrender, will not lead to the wholesome and integrated evolution and transformation facilitated by the combination of both. Effort by itself can be harsh, even judgmental; ease by itself does not challenge us sufficiently to move beyond our current physical, energetic, mental, emotional, behavioral, and relational edges. It is important to note that while the balance and integration of effort and ease is highlighted in the *Yoga Sutras by Patanjali* (Hartranft, 2003) in the context of *asana* (Sutra 2.46), it applies to all yogic practices on and off the mat and across all koshas.

> "..., asana must embody steadiness (*sthira*) and ease (*sukha*) not only in an active, external sense, as in selecting a posture and support best suited to profound stillness, but also in an interiorized, receptive way.
>
> Moment by moment we must allow our awareness of embodiment to deepen, even as each new wave of sensation buffets our attention and threatens to unmoor it from its fixation in the present."
> *Hartranft, 2003, p. 38; commentary about Yoga Sutra 2.46*

Definitions and Cuing Possibilities for Effort and Ease

The balancing action of stability with comfort and of relaxation with determination supports integration and wholism. In the end (i.e., over time), *sthira* and *sukha* become one; they become integrated and opposites dissolve (cf., Yoga Sutras 2.47 and 2.48). This integration contains stillness in movement and movement in stillness; effortless effort and contented ease. Integration incorporates a relaxing into things as they are, a "growing openness to the unpredictable unfolding of the world as it is, a freedom from the constant effort to bend things to our liking, to make them conform to our conditioned notions of good and bad (p. 39)" (Hartranft, 2003).

The coalescence of effort and ease signifies wholism and leads to us to the middle way (Boccio, 1993). It brings with it the dissolution of grasping and wanting, of aversion and hatred, of ego attachments, of fear and worry, and of confusion and delusion. *Integration of sthira and sukha helps us transform avidya into vidya, relinquish the kleshas, and to bring about lucid mind states free from kleshas- and gunas-flavored (i.e., biased) vrittis.* In other words, when balance of sthira and sukha is achieved in and across all koshas, the body becomes resilient and stable, energy flows freely and without impediments, the mind finds concentration and lucidity, emotions are clear and even-keeled, actions are based in positive intention and serve the greater good, and relationships become compassionate and loving.

Integration and balance of effort and ease can happen across koshas and/or across time. For example, in a challenging shape, we can invite an easeful breath to have an overall sense of balance. If the body is working hard, we can invite the mind to stay open and resilient, not adding even more effort or tension to the effort in the body. A vigorous *asana* sequence can be balanced by gentle, calming, and cooling shapes or movements that bring balance back over time.

Sthira – Balanced Effort and Steadiness	*Sukha* – Balanced Delight and Sweetness
• Working toward purpose • Practicing with meaning and intention • Being committed to certain values • Letting action be guided by ethics • Practicing and living with fire or passion • Entering the practice and living life with endurance • Finding heart in all you do • Investing energy in your actions • Finding a way to persevere • Trying again in a new way • Sticking with the practice even when it gets tough • Engaging sufficient muscle action • Energizing the breath or energy • Finding mental fortitude • Bringing emotional commitment • Working with clarity	• Working with compassion • Practicing with playfulness and a sense of humor • Being calm and serene • Letting actions be gentle and sweet • Practicing with pliability and resilience • Entering the practice with flexibility and plasticity • Finding lovingkindness in all you do • Inviting heart into your actions • Finding ways that are loving and sweet • Exploring ways to release tension • Knowing when to let go of trying too hard • Releasing unnecessary muscle tension and gripping • Calming breath and energy • Releasing mental strain and wanting • Releasing aversion and fear
Too Much Sthira	*Too Much Sukha*
• Hostile or aggressive • Controlling or controlled • Bossy or domineering • Dictatorial or overbearing • Always having a *right* way • Harsh or strict • Unforgiving or demanding • Uncaring or hard-hearted • Rigid or inflexible • Stiff or unbending • Uncompromising or adamant • Forced or obligatory • Harmful or injurious • Hurtful or unkind	• Meek or docile • Submissive or passive • Directionless or drifting (adrift) • Uncaring or indifferent • Heartless or halfhearted • Careless or unthinking • Monotonous or repetitive • Uninteresting or disengaged • Lifeless or lethargic • Sluggish or inert • Weary or tired • Purposeless or pointless • Dull or lackluster • Muted or unexciting

Finding balance (and ultimately integration) of effort and ease can be cued by inviting exploration and union of opposites (or dichotomies) and/or the exploration of students' habitual extremes (i.e., a student who habitually sinks into *sukha* can be invited into *sthira* and vice versa). A few juxtaposed concepts that can be explored and balanced include the examples in the following list. This list is by no means meant to be all-inclusive. It serves as a way to show just in how many aspects of life the balance of opposites, the integration of effort and ease, of challenge and support can be applied. *As teachers we can invite student to explore and balance their various tendencies* **in all koshas** *and all aspects of life and practice.*

Balance, and ultimately integration (i.e., seeing the wholeness of what appear to be opposites), can be invited in some of the following tendencies or concepts and, of course, in many more:
- Deepening and softening
- Flexibility and firmness
- Strengthening and mobilizing
- Heating and cooling
- Vitalizing and calming
- Upregulating and downregulating
- Challenging and supporting
- Lovingkindness and discipline
- Exertion and rest
- Energizing and calming
- Activating and releasing
- Inner focus and outer focus
- Zoning or blissing out and attending and concentrating
- Embracing challenge and inviting surrender
- Over-efforting versus and-efforting
- Striving and falling into laxity
- Stimulating and soothing
- Compensating and healing
- Expansion and grounding
- Open-mindedness and the ability to take a stand
- Independent thought and adopting our tribe's opinions

Abhyasa (Practice) and Vairagyam (Non-Attachment)

The integration of effort and ease in all koshas is the requisite for the essence of our yoga practice, namely, the stilling of the fluctuations of the mind (YS 1.2: *yogas chitta vritti nirodha*). When we couple effort or movement with awareness, we are meditating. When we couple ease or stillness with awareness, we are meditating. In other words, ease and effort are integral to all practices of yoga and move us toward connection and collectedness. Their importance cannot be overstated and their cuing and integration in all we teach is tremendously auspicious and helpful – regardless of whether we are cuing asana, pranayama, pratyahara, dharana, or dhyana.

Effort and ease thus understood are closely related to the yogic concepts of *abhyasa* (practice) and *vairagya* (non-attachment). These practice concepts reflect both effort and tranquility and non-attachment to results or outcomes and are foundational to the work in all limbs of yoga. They are the very basis of moving yoga toward the stilling of the mind – toward lucidity, tranquility, equanimity, and vidya. We relinquish obsessions with desired outcomes or results, we enjoy the travel without seeing the destination; we live for the process, not the goal.

***tatra sthitau yatnah abhyasa* (Yoga Sutra 1.13)**
"Practice (**abhyasa**) means choosing, *applying the effort*, and doing those actions
that bring a *stable and tranquil state* (sthitau)."
(retrieved from https://www.swamij.com/yoga-sutras-11216.htm)

drista anushravika vishaya vitrishnasya vashikara sanjna vairagyam
(Yoga Sutra 1.15)
"When the mind *loses desire even for objects seen or described in a tradition or in scriptures,* it acquires a state of utter (vashikara) desirelessness that is called non-attachment (**vairagya**)."
(retrieved from https://www.swamij.com/yoga-sutras-11216.htm)

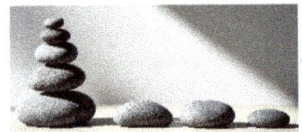

Obsession with results produces tension, which generates headaches, backaches, worries, and restlessness. Expectations lead to disappointments. When we have only the results in mind, obviously we can cannot pay attention to the task at hand. But if we let go of whatever we are trying to achieve and apply our whole mindfulness and attention to the effort we are making, we have a chance to succeed without creating tension.
Ayya Khema, Be An Island, 1999, p. 75

Cultivating Grounding, Expansion, and Stability

Finding balance and integration of effort and ease, of commitment and serenity, of movement and stillness, of abhyasa and vairagya, in our yoga practice and daily life is integrated into *invitations to access grounding, expansion, and stability* during yoga practice (Boccio, 1993; Farhi, 2005, 2011; Mitchell, 2019; Schiffmann, 2013). These concepts, while often most notable in asana practices, apply equally to breathing and inner practices. Grounding, expansion, and stability combine to cultivate physical, energetic, mental, and emotional wholism. Each one of these concepts is most auspiciously applied when integrated and balanced with *ease and effort* (i.e., we invest ease and effort in grounding, in expansion, and in creating stability) and honor, integrate, and balance the commitment of abhyasa and the non-attachment to a particular outcome of vairagya. With this integration, these concepts become balanced and create resilience. What, then, is meant by balanced and resilient grounding, expansion, and stability?

Rootedness of Grounding

Grounding – in the context of a yoga practice – is the practice of settling ourselves, with auspiciously balanced ease and effort, into the present moment and the current space to feel rooted and connected. Perhaps we ground into a set of values, a deeper motivation and purpose, the earth, our community, or a practice. When we are grounded and rooted, we have access to greater peace and equanimity. Grounding can settle an anxious mood or an agitated nervous system. It can invite the body to relax and the breath to ease. Grounding can facilitate a sense of safety and support and is a conscious technique that can be used with anxious, stressed, unsettled, panicked, distracted, even traumatized students or clients. Grounding is a lovely way to helping participants find less intensity in their affect, less distraction in their mind state, more softening in the body, and more access to a longer exhalation.

- Grounding can be invited physically through rooting into the earth and feeling the rebound of ground reaction forces. It can happen through the senses by finding a visual focus, or drishti; a sound on which to concentrate; a smell that is pleasant; a taste that is pleasurable; or even a tactile contact that feels safe, supportive, and calming.
- Grounding can emerge energetically or affectively through soft and gentle breathing with emphasis on the exhalation or tactile contact with the belly to feel the rising and falling of the abdomen, or the air flowing in and out of the nostrils. It can happen naturally through cuing a steady breath that is functional, gentle, soft, and inaudible. It may be achieved by connecting to the breath vayu called apana, a downward and outward moving energy.
- Grounding can be honed mentally by offering a point of focus for the mind, settling distraction or dysregulation. The point of focus could be an object in the room, a mantra, sensing into a particular alignment from the inside out, or engaging the mind in another deliberate, intentional, or purposeful way.
- Grounding can support us emotionally and relationally through co-regulation with the teacher and other students or clients, through tone of voice, pacing of speech, and environmental cues of safety. Grounding into community or sangha can be facilitated through cuing as well as through the deep connection of relationships that develop between teacher and students and among participants – often completely nonverbally.

Often participants find the easiest access to a sense of grounding by creating a strong physical foundation. This physical grounding arises auspiciously from downward and strengthening lines of energy wherever the body meets the floor. Sample cues for finding a physical foundation may be as follows (more sample cues are shown in the table below):
- Firmly ground through the body parts that meet the floor
- Imagine growing roots into the earth to ground deeply
- Use the exhalation to support physical and affective settledness, a grounding energy
- Invite a clear experience of grounding your life energy into the earth
- Feel the support of the earth beneath you
- Find a bounce-back or uplifting energy through pressing into the ground
- Ground the limbs in line with gravity
- Invite the body to become pleasantly heavy, releasing its weight into the earth
- Entrust your physical being to the support of the earth
- Connect into inner awareness of sensation (interoception)
- Surrender to the earth through the parts of the body that are making contact with it

A couple of cautions related to grounding:
- Be mindful not to let grounding become heavy or weighty in a way that pulls us down
- Do not mistake grounding for lassitude, rigidity, heaviness, immobility, or immovability
- Maintain a sense of freedom and space in the downward and inward energy to avoid feeling limited or trapped
- Be careful not to indulge any physical propensity for lethargy or inaction, not to feed habitual tamas or dorsal vagal autonomic nervous system patterns
- Continuously monitor the balance of strength or engagement with flexibility and expansiveness (with expansion)

Sample Cues to Create Grounding		
In Annamaya Kosha • Root down through the feet • Plug the feet into the ground • Ground through the three/four corners of your feet • Plant your … • Anchor your … • Deepen your connection to … • Press your … into … • Settle your … into… • Grow from the ground up • Sense your … being held by … • Feel the natural support available from the earth … • Sense the ground rising up to meet you … • Feel the bones in your body • Feel the sturdy base of your … • Feel the earth meeting your … • Align your bones to meet gravity with • Receive the support from the earth • Invite a drishti to anchor the pose • Align in collaboration with gravity • Ground through being mindfully present • Sense into your connection to the earth	**In Pranamaya Kosha** • Breathe out to create grounding • Steady the breath • Release into the breath … • Find grounding in the breath • Anchor the breath • Release into the support of the outbreath • Awaken to how the breath sustains you in this movement • Find a downward energy (apana) that grounds and settles you **In Manomaya Kosha** • Bring attention to where body meets the floor • Settle your mind into … • Anchor your mind to … • Bring the mind gently and firmly to … • Steady the mind on a point of focus • Find a sense of mindful attention • Find a steady focus for the mind • Invite your emotions to settle • Ground into the pleasantness of the moment • Connect to your intention	**In Vijnanamaya Kosha** • Notice the intuitive desire to be supported • How can you intuitively create a sense of being more rooted/grounded … • Invite intuitive movements that help you feel grounded/rooted/supported • Sense into your inner emotional rootedness • Yield to your urge to anchor • Sense into the ground meeting and supporting you freely **In Anandamaya Kosha** • Notice the relationship of your … to … • Notice how the how … connects you to … • Is there a sense of joy/bliss/gratitude … • Invite a smile/gratitude/connection … • Ground into your community … • Ground into a sense of joy … • Sense your connection to … • Revel joyfully in your connection to … • Find peace in a smile of connection

Openness of Expansion

Expansion – in the context of a yoga practice – is the auspiciously effortful and easeful practice of opening ourselves to something greater, to find a joyful path or a compassionate purpose. Perhaps we create more space and freedom for movement, spacious and freeing breath patterns, an expansive and open mind, joyful and engaged emotionality, open-hearted relationships, or buoyant actions. When we are opening up to spaciousness or expansiveness, we invite flexibility and joy into our lives. We open ourselves to more possibilities and interact with the world in a spacious, open-hearted, and open-minded way. We open our bodies, expand our breath, let go of rigidity in attitudes and beliefs, free our emotions, and open our hearts to others and ourselves as we truly are. Expansiveness invites interaction and light-heartedness; it honors interdependence and co-arising. It embraces new possibilities and embodies a greater purpose expressed with a wide-open body, heart, and mind.

- Expansion can be invited physically through letting the body's edges find space, lift, and flexibility. It can happen through freeing ourselves to wiggle, shake, dance, and move intuitively, grandly, and joyfully. It can happen through letting the body rise up or open wide.
- Expansion can emerge energetically or affectively through a breath that is spacious, light, and open. It can happen very naturally by breathing in a way that fully recognizes the exchange of the inner and outer in each breath; by breathing in the nurturance that is freely offered to us; by freely releasing the breath out to give something back to the world. It may be achieved by connecting to the breath vayu called vyana, an expansive and clarifying energy, as well as through the vayu called udana that is a light energy of exultation with a strong ascending movement.
- Expansion can be honed mentally by opening the mind to new possibilities, new ways, new ideas, new and attitudes. It is invited when we open to a continuous process of learning, unlearning, and relearning. The expansive mind has purpose, clarity, and direction – not in a way that seeks a particular outcome, but in a way that is open to new discoveries, surprises, and a life of meaning.
- Expansion can support and lift us emotionally and relationally through the development of an open and welcoming heart that invites connection and community. Communal expansion serves to gain and give support, nurturance, kindness, and other ways to create connection.

Often participants find the easiest access to a sense of expansion by creating a sense of expansiveness, opening, and open-heartedness through body and breath. These tangible forms of expansion arise auspiciously from upward/uplifting and open lines of energy marked by the crown of the head and edges of the body (e.g., fingertips) reaching for the sky or the breath becoming spacious, open, and light. Sample cues for finding uplifting and expansive energy may be as follows (more sample cues are in the table that follows):

- Find spaciousness, expansion, and openness wherever possible – the crown or the extremities
- Once grounded and stable, invite joyful extension at the edges
- Invite joy and lightness into the practice/the body/the breath/the mind
- Invite the crown of the head to rise or lift upward toward the sly
- Invite a lightness into your hands as you reach for the sky
- Invite a sense of energy flowing from the core to the edges, allowing that energy to guide the edge of the pose (sometimes finding flow means backing away, sometimes it means dancing or playing at the edge, and sometimes it means exploring reaching farther)
- Maintain a light-hearted focus and soft attention, using drishti (not laser-like gaze), especially in balancing poses
- Invite the heart to be lifted with joy

A couple of cautions related to expansiveness:
- Be mindful not to hyperextend, overmobilize, or overstretch
- Do not mistake expansiveness for striving or reaching a particular outcome
- Maintain a sense of anchoring and rootedness amidst the outward and upward energy
- Be careful not to abuse your own physical, emotional, or relational propensity for flexibility or hypermobility
- Continuously monitor the balance of strength or engagement (groundedness) with flexibility, expansiveness, and expansion

Sample Cues to Create Expansion		
In Annamaya Kosha • Draw the crown of your head up toward … • Imagine someone is pulling your … gently/with love/with compassion • Create space between the vertebrae • Release … • Reach through the crown of the head • Create space in … • Make space between … • Extend… • Grow… • Lift… (upper body/crown of the head) • Shine outward • Radiate with … • Fill the space … • Wake up your … (body part) • Move freely upward	*In Pranamaya Kosha* • Breathe yourself longer • Shine your inner light • Open your heart • Wake up the breath • Release the breath … toxins .. • Bring life to … • Energize your fingers/toes/ extremities/crown of head… • Invite a new way of aligning *In Manomaya Kosha* • Open your mind… • Imagine … • Transcend the habit to … • Set your emotions free • Invite mindfulness of … • Invite a new way of thinking about … • Free your thoughts … • Unfold your emotional possibilities …	*In Vijnanamaya Kosha* • Let your awareness become spacious/open/wide • Notice intuitively how you can grow and expand here… • Find yourself opening to something greater … • Notice where can you create a sense of spaciousness, openness, or expansiveness *In Anandamaya Kosha* • Notice your open-hearted nature … • Invite a smile that connects you to … • Open your mind • Open your heart • Revel in your vast net of relationships/networks • Feel the open-hearted support of your community …

Courage of Stability

Stability is the naturally balanced (effort and ease; abhyasa and vairagya) practice of connecting to inner balance, fortitude, resilience, and clarity. We can stabilize physically, energetically, mentally, emotionally, behaviorally, or relationally. When we are stable and balanced, our life and way of being reflects steadiness, steadfastness, resilience, resoluteness, commitment, persistence, and continuity. We feel dynamic, capable, and empowered; we sense our own agency and make our own path – never forgetting our embeddedness in a greater context and web of life. In stability, we rest in the opposite of our lives – we combine and integrate the extremes; we find the middle way; we find the most auspicious path into and through our lives.

Stability reflects our capacity to:
- Live life with endurance, steadiness, firmness, and sturdiness
- Engage in constant adjustment and readjustment to load factors like compression, tension, torsion, and shear
- The ability to reregulate in all koshas after disturbance
- Find resilience and dynamic resistance to sudden force, load, or disturbance
- To adapt and regain postural equilibrium with mobility and ongoing micro-adjustments
- To support joints during movement
- Let our movements, energetic presence, mental presence, emotions, and relationships be defined by ease, not by tension

When we are stable, we are able to withstand the challenges of life with resilience and a sense of resoluteness and dynamic persistence that invites equilibrium and equanimity. Stability allows us to meet life from a base of dynamic solidity – a place of being able to roll with the punches and flexibly from a platform of clearly sensed capability, agency, and self-efficacy. With stability we and our clients connect to inner strength and fortitude, able to meet what life brings our way with an open heart, flexible mindset, and sense of courage.

- Stability can be invited physically through dynamic adjustments that are responsive to the physical demands of a given situation. It can happen through engagement of the core; bringing dynamic and easeful effort to the core (rather than the periphery) of the body; stabilizing joints involved in movements; planting our scapulae on our back; and similar ways of balancing and aligning our anatomy responsively and in line with gravity. Stability in body and energy is allostatic – the very flexible process of adaptability that ultimately allows us to reach homeostasis after challenge.
- Stability can emerge energetically or affectively through balancing the breath or adapting the breath dynamically to situational demand. It can happen very naturally by vitalizing the breath when we feel tired, exhausted, or lethargic or by calming our breathing rhythm when we are upregulated, anxiety, or overly activated. A stable breath moves us into our ventral vagal space and serves as an anchor that holds us steady without weighing us down.
- Stability can be honed mentally by finding clarity and concentration of mind, settling distraction or dysregulation (a process that overlaps with grounding). A stable mind is able to transform disorganized, dull or distracted mind states into concentration, attention, lucidity, and spacious awareness. Mental stability allows us to problem-solve flexibly, to roll with the punches, and to lean into challenge with curiosity and a mental set of discovery.
- Stability can support us emotionally and relationally through adapting to specific demands of a relationship or situation, leaning into our capacity to meet ourselves and others where they/we are. Emotional stability comes from a resilient coping style that allows us to rest in balanced equanimity and compassion regardless of the emotional demands that arise.

Often participants find the easiest access to a sense of stability by creating a sense of balance, steadiness, adaptability, and continuity through body and breath. These tangible forms of stabilization arise almost naturally (especially once noticed and reinforced consciously) from dynamic, yet calming lines of energy that emanate from the inside of the body and a collected, quiet breath. Much of physical and energetic stability in a yoga practice is autonomic – in fact, sometimes rigid alignment cues can actually get in the way of the inherent wisdom (emanating from vijnanamaya koshas). Our prefrontal cortex may override stable movement that is inherent within because of goals, samskaras, even culturally and contextually (BPSC-based) imposed ideas of what yoga is, or teacher-offered instructions. Sample cues for stable and balanced inner energy that helps us withstand challenge and stress and invites us into our agency and power may be as follows (more sample cues are contained in the table below):

- Engage the core and other muscles needed to achieve and maintain the form or movement
- Identify the deep core muscles and ways/tricks/hints to engage them (e.g., laughter or coughing to find the deepest layers that are often 'asleep')
- Work from core to edges, encouraging strength at the center and flexibility at the edges
- Engage muscles around the major moving joints before lengthening, moving, or opening
- Use the breath as a stable anchor, deepening core strength through allowing the breath (exhalation is easiest) to support engagement of the deep abdominal muscles

- Find a steady and supportive breath
- Adapt the breath to specific demands – vitalizing collapse or calming excessive arousal
- Invite a stable mind anchored in a soft focus

<table>
<tr><td colspan="3" align="center">*Sample Cues to Create Stability*</td></tr>
<tr><td>

In Annamaya Kosha
- Draw the navel/belly button toward the spine
- Imagine you could draw the hip bones toward each other
- Create a stabilizing corset action with your deep inner core muscles
- Bring the low ribs toward the hips
- Draw the … inward with steadfastness …
- Hug/draw the knee caps toward the hips
- Lift the pelvic floor
- Isometrically engage …
- Courageously move from your core …
- Imagine you are zipping up pants
- Feel the strength in your core
- Notice the stability at your center
- Trust your inner experience of steadiness …
- Release into stable alignment …
- Draw into your own strength and courage

</td><td>

In Pranamaya Kosha
- Direct the breath into your core
- Feel a sense of strength as you exhale/inhale/hold the breath …
- Stabilize or steady the breath …
- Calm the breath to find your focus/strength/stability
- Stabilize the breath to sense into your own power …
- Invite a steady rhythm of breath
- Stabilize your energy to invite resilience
- Notice your emotional state and invite a sense of courage …
- Come into a ventral vagal space
- Connect to your inner fortitude and vitality

In Manomaya Kosha
- Empower your mind …
- Anchor thoughts back into …
- Notice if the mind wanders and invite it back into steady focus …
- With agency, anchor your attention to …
- Settle into thoughts with care …
- Tune into your inner emotional courage
- Venture into a balanced mind state

</td><td>

In Vijnanamaya Kosha
- Invite a sense of deep presence and awareness …
- Notice intuitively what may create more stability/courage/fortitude in …
- Notice if the default mode network is kicking in and return to a stable point of focus
- Trust in your inner wisdom and strength
- Rely on the wisdom of your inner teacher

In Anandamaya Kosha
- Find faith in your strength/courage …
- Invite a stable smile …
- Recognize your strength from connection to community
- Sense into the support and love from your community

</td></tr>
</table>

No cautions are needed with regard cuing stability (unlike for expansion and grounding as indicated above) because stability is by definition the calibration of all koshas into a state of balance. Stability is equanimity embodied. We do not trade flexibility for strength – we integrate them. we do not trade range of motion for healthful alignment – we honor both in the most auspicious way. We do not trade excess movement for safety and wellbeing – we recognize what is most helpful and wholesome in any given moment. Stability is the dynamic (not static) basis for allostasis and homeostasis in our physiology and energy. It is the basis for an open, yet inquisitive and discerning mind that honors difference without losing sight of a basic adherence to compassionate humanity, ethics and values, and purposeful living. Stability is about the journey and the process, not about a specific outcome or goal.

Anatomical Notes about Stability

Auspicious posture or embodiment of a shape is defined by ease; inauspicious postures or embodiment of shapes are defined by tension, pain, even fear. Interoceptive awareness is a key aspect to finding auspicious alignment. To bear load, muscles need to contract around the joints that move, which in turn limits range of motion in these areas of the body and makes a healthy trade off – in other words, it is important not to trade range of motion for risk of joint injury. "When under stress, stiffen; when enhancing movement, unload (p. 9)." (Clark, 2016). Unfortunately, modern postural yoga is often about flexibility and large range of motion, instead of stability and auspicious, healthful alignment and posture. Healthful therapeutic, holistic, integrated yoga is about stability and healthful, conscious range of motion, adapted to the reality of all the factors of influence at hand.

A neutral spine is central to overall stability. A neutral spine is stable and at ease in the sense that there is the least amount of tension as well as good bilateral balance on the joints, fascia, other connective tissues, and muscles. This type of stability is dynamic, not static; it is a constant adjustment to load factors like compression, tension, torsion, and shear. We are always in motion, readjusting to factors that affect posture, shapes or movements.

We are constantly rebalancing and readjusting (i.e., creating stability) to accommodate and dynamically adapt to all of the flowing influences and more:
- Environmental influences, such as soft or uneven surfaces, temperature, humidity
- Muscular involvement, including muscles that are relaxed versus engaged, active versus passive movement, bracing versus collapsing, habit versus novel movement, and more
- Joint alignment, both healthful alignment as well as extant injuries or pathologies
- Other connective tissue issues, including form (that followed habitual function) that resulted in pattern locks in the fascia, ligaments, and tendons, even bones
- Exteroceptive sensory inputs, such as visual distractions, nociception, noises, smells, inner ear balance, etc.
- Inner sensory inputs, such as proprioceptive and interoceptive inputs, even neuroception
- Nervous system inputs, such as neuroception, polyvagal states, fears, reactivity

It helps to notice this often-autonomic dynamic aspect of stability and to allow it with consciousness. *This* is what defines healthy postural alignment, not the outer shape. Movement creates various types of stresses; namely, tension, compression, torsion, and shear. As we move further away from neutral spine alignment, load increases – all types of loads, especially shear. It is auspicious to reduce load in spinal flexion and extension, for example via the use of props (e.g., place blocks under the hands and arms in camel to reduce load on the spine by co-carrying load in the arms; place blocks under the hands in a wide-legged forward fold, for the same reason. It is also auspicious to contract the muscles around the joints that are moving, even if this reduces range of motion.

Also, larger bodies have to bear a greater load when the spine departs from neutral. It is important to load properly and not to be tempted into excessive range of motion. Skinny people can have greater range of motion because their body weight give them less load and their compression edges are wider. However, less body weight comes at a cost – heavier bodies are less likely to develop osteoporosis. Always practice in harmony with your spinal structure.

Working with Lines of Energy

The work with lines of energy interacts profoundly with grounding, stabilization, and expansion. Energetic work can happen in all koshas, though it is most notable in the tangible koshas, of body, vitality, and mind, including emotions.

Physical Lines of Energy

The work with physical lines of energies cultivates embodied or somatic awareness, imbued by our vitality. We cue students or clients to:
- Notice upward (uplifting, lightening) physical lines of energy – remember the concept of expansion
- Notice downward (grounding, strengthening, rooting) physical lines of energy – remember the concept of grounding
- Find energetic arcs of movement that may reach beyond the physical expression of a pose
- Allow for a withdrawing of energy when and where appropriate to facilitate rest, relaxation, or deeper stretch – remember *sukha*
- Allowing for a deepening of energy when and where appropriate to facilitate firmness, commitment, and empowerment – remember *sthira*
- Recognize the physical impact of the gunas and/or polyvagal state – the autonomic nervous system states of *tamas* (or dorsal vagal complex activation), *rajas* (or sympathetic activation), and *sattva* (or ventral vagal activation) related to giving up, under-efforting, and collapsing; to hypermobilization, overefforting, and gripping; and to integrating, being physically responsive, and exhibiting resilient
- Recognize the physical effects of the kleshas in bodily sensations and physical movement – the affective and arousal states (or kleshas) that can be observed related to physical forcing or ambition out of *attachment (raga)*; disliking, spitting venom, or hating out of *aversion (dvesa)*; wanting and pushing for a particular outcome out of *ego (asmita)*; worrying, avoiding, or shying away out of *fear (abhinivesa)* of the unknown or fear of changing; and not understanding, feeling confused, getting jumbled or disorganized out of *lack of clarity (avidya)* and understanding
- Both gunas and kleshas in the physical sense might relate to bracing, buckling, and yielding (see below)

Life Energy or Pranic Lines of Energy

Working with affect and arousal-related lines of energy cultivates vitality and energetic awareness. We cue students or clients to:
- Sense onto the direction and nature of the breath, attuning to observable and subtle dimensions of breathing
- Have a sense of the *prana vayus* and how they affect energy, including affective tone, arousal level, and energy budget in all layers of human experience :
  - inward and upward energy (*prana*): vitality and sensitivity – smoothly flowing energy that provides the ability to direct energy for growth and development
  - outward energy emanating from center to the periphery (*vyana*): expansion, expansiveness – pulsating energy that creates resonance or integration at all koshas

- o stabilizing energy moving from the edges to the core (*samana*): peacefulness – stabilizing energy that instills the ability to contract and hold steady
  - o downward and outward energy (*apana*): groundedness, drawing inward – descending, releasing, and grounding energy that connects us to the earth
  - o upwardly ascending energy (*udana*): lightness, expansion, exultation – uplifting, inspiring energy that helps us take a broader perspective that is deeply informed and wise
- Recognize the energetic impact of the gunas and/or polyvagal states, noticing arousal and energy, perhaps as activation or tiredness, hyperarousal or lethargy, vibrancy or settledness
- Recognize energetic effects of vedana (or feeling tone: pleasant, unpleasant, neutral) in breath and energy – we might see this especially well in texture, rate, location, and volume of the breath
- Notice the interconnection of breath and movement as reflections of vedana or affective and arousal tones, even the kleshas
- Notice the interconnection of breath and mind as reflections of vedana, kleshas, mind states, and vrittis
- Notice the interconnection of vedana with community and relationships

Energetic body budget regulation works with depletion versus overconsumption or excess and with contraction versus expansion. It cultivates energetic sensitivity, the awareness of when we are depleting versus replenishing our energy. We cue students or clients to notice and find several possible expressions, including the coolness of *langhana*, the heat of *brahmana*, and the balance of *samana*.

The following descriptors offer a bit more detail:
- *Langhana*: coolness, release, letting go, inward focus
  - o an energy of reduction, release, quietude, support, restoration, relaxation
  - o this energy is said to be purifying and calming
  - o this energy is accessed via the exhalation, a horizontal physical position, focus on apana, and release of the bandhas
  - o it is associated with forward folds, inversions, letting go, relinquishing over-efforting, and introspection
  - o perhaps similar to a socially engaged parasympathetic state with focus on ease and grounding (ventral and dorsal vagal states)
  - o langhana is intentionally applied when there is excess or a sense of overabundance in the body, breath, or mind
- *Brahmana*: heat, expansion, power, strength, outward focus
  - o this is an energy of nourishing, expansion, power, strength, and vigor
  - o this energy is said to help with stress resilience and healthful activation
  - o this energy is accessed via the inhalation, power positions, a focus on prana, and activation of the bandhas
  - o it is associated with backbends, powerful standing and arm standing postures, and invigoration of sluggish energy
  - o perhaps similar to a sympathetic state of resilience with a functional vagal brake (ventral vagal and sympathetic arousal states)
  - o brahmana is intentionally applied when there is deficiency or a sense of depletion in the body

- *Samana*: bringing homeostasis, this is an energy of integration and equalization; this energy supports balance and essentially synonymous with the samana as one of the vayus; it is associated with *asana*, *pranayama*, and interior practices that are stabilizing and balancing (e.g., twists [which combine *langhana* and *brahmana*], *nadi shodana*); perhaps most similar to a ventral vagal socially engaged energetic state

Emotional and Mental Energies

Working with emotional and mental lines of energy invites recognition or mental and emotional states, guiding individuals toward acceptance. It is important to note that this is not acceptance in the sense of resignation, but in the sense of acknowledging the reality of a situation so as to develop the resilience, equanimity, and concentration to work with that reality (as opposed to living in denial, repression, or interiorization).

To draw attention to mental and emotional energies, we might cue students or clients to:
- Notice the impact of positive mental energy (e.g., smriti as a way of finding ease and familiarity) in form, movement, and breath
- Notice the impact of negative mental energy (e.g., smriti as a way of forcing a remembered but not currently available way of being in a posture) on form, movement, and breath
- Transform negative energy into positive through mental or physical techniques, such as generating resilience, grounding into your intention, transforming habit energy, or caring about something greater

Cuing Mindfulness, Attention/Attunement, and Awareness

Another set of practice principles that applies across all koshas and limbs is the cultivation of presence. It is the collection of ourselves into the present moment and present space that invites the emergence of samadhi, which in fact can be defined as exactly that collection and presence through which we unite with ourselves and all there is, fully present and fully aware. To understand the many ways in which we can cue students or clients to arrive in the present moment, whether in body, vitality, mind and emotion, or wisdom, whether during asana, pranayama, or the interior practice, it is helpful to define the difference between attention and awareness.

Attention and Awareness: Presence with Focus or Spaciousness

Attention is focused on a particular set of stimuli which then may lead to thought or action. Attention in daily life tends to shift to whatever seems most salient to the intention we bring to a situation. Awareness is the background of our experience – we are always aware of the sights, sounds, textures, tastes, smell, and other sensations of our inner and outer world. Attention, or a focus one a specific set of inputs, arises out of awareness as something catches our attention and shifts our concentration to a salient inner or outer feature. Awareness can arise out of attention when we broaden our focus from being exclusive (a single stimulus or set of stimuli) to inclusive (spacious and open without a specific focus).

In that sense, and commensurate with Buddhist thinking about attention and awareness, awareness is primary and always diffusely present in the background of experience. It may be more or less conscious, depending on circumstances. In other words, sometime we are aware that we are aware; other times, we are not aware that we are aware – and yet awareness is always present. From awareness arises sensation (i.e., sensory experiences received via neuroception, interoception, proprioception, and exteroception), which interact with intention. The combined experience of sensation and intention helps direct attention. Where and how we focus attention contributes to our mental and emotional experience of what it is we are attending to. In essence, there is a chain of events that moves from spacious or broad awareness to an interaction with intention and sensation to create attentional focus and attentional shifts to thoughts and emotions.

Attention is the mental focus we hone through concentration practices in yoga. However, it is clear at this point that attention, awareness, intention, and sensation are intimately linked and likely interdependent. How awareness leads to attentional choices and shifts (based on what we notice of salience) is deeply affected by intentions and perceptions of sensations and experiences. There is a profound interaction with polyvagal states and neuroception. If we are aware with a predisposition toward the detection of danger or threat, we may shift our attention to the sources of threat, when neuroception conveys signals of possible peril. If we have a predisposition toward the detection of emotional safety and social engagement, our nervous system in the same outer circumstances may signal safety and create a different focus of attention. Creating awareness of how we interpret sensory signals and how they combine with intention may help us direct attention more consciously and may support engagement of the prefrontal cortex, avoiding amygdala hijacks. The latter has been identified as a positive outcome of meditation.

The more information comes our way, the greater the risk of distraction and attentional drain. When we lose the capacity to attend, almost every aspect of our life can suffer, including our relationships and social connection. Humans are terrible at multi-tasking (at dividing attention). In fact, we cannot really do it. Instead, we rapidly shift attention back and forth, which after a while wears us out, makes us distractable and unconcentrated, reduces efficiency, interferes with understanding (including no longer being discerning about what is or is not important – we lose the signal in the noise), and impairs empathy – probably because we are really not working with relevant information but with anything that comes our way and captures our attention.

It is the magic of the human mind that allows us to broaden and constrict our experience of attention and awareness as relevant to each moment of our lives. Like a zoom lens, we can hone in with keen attention when we need a more microscopic view; then we can zoom back out when we need a vaster perspective. Reality is unchanged – we simply change how we look at it: from up close or from farther away. As we develop more skillfulness, we can hone in on attention without losing the capacity to maintain a vast perspective. In small ways, we do this all the time: We can attend to cutting vegetables with a sharp knife while enjoying the beauty of Vivaldi's Four Seasons. However, the more we are in *doing* mode, the less we are in *being* mode – we trade degree of attention for degree of awareness. This is not a value judgment. We need both. We cannot successfully run a meeting being blissfully attuned and spaciously aware of all that is. We will do a better job if we carefully attend to the matters at hand – all the while maintaining awareness of the 'feeling tone' of the meeting, the responses or reactivities of all participants, shifting attention as needed and salient with wisdom and compassion.

As teachers, we take care to differentiate between *mindful attention* <u>versus</u> *mindful awareness* (also called natural meditation or Dzogchen) as we cue students or clients into presence. To cue attention, we refer to full (yet soft) concentration, the creation of a single point of focus; to cue awareness, we refer to spacious and open presence – more inclusive than a single point of focus and yet fully absorbed in the moment (sometimes leading to a sense of awe or amazement). Following are a few helpful hints for cuing first attention, and then awareness.

Cuing Attention

When we cue *attention*, we invite participants to be attentive to what is unfolding with curiosity and a beginner's mind. We invite a presence that is strong, stable, observant, at ease, and present-centered with focus on an identified inner or outer object (e.g., breath, an outer object [e.g., candle flame, a Buddha statue, a sound], or a state of mind [e.g., compassion, lovingkindness]).

Sample languaging includes:	*Invite students or clients to let go of:*
• Be softly/gently, lovingly present with what is	• Resistance
• Recognize what is present/coming and going	• Judgment
• Notice what arises/unfolds	• Comparison
• Open yourself to sensation	• Evaluation
• Stay present with what is	• Expectations
• Observe what is coming and going	• Interpretations
• Recognize the short-lived nature of sensation	• Planning
• Can you become curious about what is	• Control

Cuing Awareness

When we cue *awareness*, we focus on instructions that invite a sense of being spacious, open, inclusive, wide, and timeless. There is no single point of attention, focus, or even soft concentration. Instead, there is an open spacious exploration of all experiences in all koshas, as well as external stimuli and their reverberation in our consciousness. As such, we cue spacious awareness of the *natural state of the body*, the *natural state of the breath*, the *natural state of the mind, and the natural state of the heart*. We remind participants that awareness is always present, even when we are not aware that we are aware. We invite them into awareness of all layers of consciousness, asking them to notice their profound connection to themselves and everything around them – all beings, contexts, biopsychosociocultural realities. This is meta-awareness – being aware of being aware.

Befriending the Present Moment

Yongey Mingyur Rinpoche (2009) asserts that the *only true obstacle* to practice (full disclosure – for him "practice" means meditation; I think it applies to yoga practice as a whole…) is lack of awareness, the forgetting to watch and be present for each moment of our life. In fact, he teaches that awareness is the antidote to all barriers to practice and enlightenment. We can use awareness to befriend everything that is present in our lives.

Awareness means being fully present for the five aspects (*skandhas*) of our human physical, energetic/affective, and mental/emotional experience (the whole of which is greater than the sum of these parts), namely,
- Physical form (*rupa*) and all matter (things, beings, objects) we come in contact with (associated with annamaya koshas)
- Feeling tones of our experiences; i.e., pleasant, unpleasant, neutral (*vedana*) (associated with pranamaya koshas)
- Bodily perceptions, i.e., the interpretation and evaluation of as well as the labels we give to our sensory experiences (*samjna*) (associated with manomaya koshas, especially manas)
- Mental formations such as volition, habit, reactivity, conditioning, impulse, conditioned states (*samskaras*) (associated with manomaya kosha, especially ahamkara)
- Consciousness of all of these aspects (vijnana) (associated with vijnanamaya koshas)

These five aspects of our humanity are not the causes of suffering in and of themselves. We observe our experiences, our environment, our perceptions and feeling tones, our mental fluctuations and states to become aware of *our relationship to the them*. It is *that* relationship, flavored by the gunas and kleshas, that leads to suffering.

Thus, in teaching yoga, *we invite students or clients into an aware, conscious, and attentive relationship with themselves.* We encourage participants consistently to be aware of body, breath, and mind and to use the feedback from and relationship with their experiences to make choices about their personal practice in class and in life off the mat, at home, at work, and in all settings and relationships. We liberally invite students to experience the present moment, to be aware of experience, feeling tones, perceptions, and habits or conditioning in all koshas. We consistently invite awareness, exploration, and understanding of neuroception, proprioception, interoception, and exteroception.

We cue mindfulness, attention/attunement, and awareness as relevant and appropriate, with keen clarity about the differences between these concepts and when to encourage the experience of which most optimally. As such, we cue mindfulness as a practice of being in the moment, in the current space and circumstance, without judgment, with curiosity and an open heart and mind. We cue attunement as practice of safely noting sensory inputs from within and without allows to help clients make discerning choices about their body, breath, energy, mind, and actions based on accurate and up-to-date information and inputs.

As students become more accurately attuned to their own resources and needs, they begin to make choices in line with these realizations. We cue awareness as a way to stay consciously anchored to our higher self, our ability to step back and recognize reactivity, the causes of suffering (i.e., kleshas), and the capacity inherent in all of us to transform our relationship with our experiences, feeling tones, and mental formations (vrittis and samskaras) to make different choices, to respond with new discernment.

Mindfulness, attention, and awareness are also modeled by teachers who remain equally attuned to their personal experiences, sensory inputs and needs, and relationships to them to make commensurate personals choices. Awareness in this sense is practiced on the mat and then taken into daily life off the mat. Providers who are mindfully attuned, attentive, and aware can hold space in the classroom with clarity and safety on behalf of themselves and their clients. Such teachers or clinicians observe participants in their entirety – recognizing their presentation and needs in all five koshas. They observe how inner and outer relationships are unfolding and how they may be improved through mindfulness, attention, and awareness.

If we have this skill as teachers or clinicians we are capable of the following:
- We help clients become mindful of their inner physical states – sensations, feeling tones, and perceptions – via learning to pay attention to signals that come from the body.
- We help clients recognize how they interpret information from the body and if there is self-protective reactivity that may suggest that a particular body signal triggers a sense of danger or threat (gunas) or attachment, aversions, ego, fear, or confusion (kleshas).
- We help clients learn to differentiate sensation from the body that truly signals danger versus sensation that has a conditioned danger (trauma) response – student may begin to realize that their associations with particular body signals are conditioned by prior experiences and challenges and do not actually pose a threat in the present moment; this may help transform their relationship with particular body states from fear to acceptance to health.
- We cue and invite practices that help clients tune into their capacity to self-regulate, to self-soothe, and to self-calm – for example, after a particular activity that may result in nervous system arousal, we can invite attunement with the reality that heart rate, breathing, and arousal reregulate (and co-regulate) automatically.
- We titrate cuing for interoception and neuroception based on reactions, reactivities, and responses noted in our students, especially in healthcare settings that bring us students with trauma histories – we start small (and always in a context of having established environmental and relational safety) and carefully, alternating challenge with ease, arousal with calming, exploration with predictability.

A Caution: Remember that attunement, awareness, and mindfulness mean that clients stay safely connected to themselves. *Students may also need to stay safely connected to the teacher so that they can co-regulate through the teacher's stability, groundedness, and capacity to remain in a ventral vagal space.* This means that if the provider has a day of dysregulation and distress, less invitation for client interoception, neuroception, and vulnerability may need to be cued so that teacher and student do not dysregulate together. In other words, the provider needs to maintain a safe and boundaried container for the work of awareness and attention.

The Four '-Ceptions' – Our Portal into Experience and Being

Related to cuing attention, awareness, and mindfulness, as yoga professionals, we cue the four -ceptions in such a way that participants gain access to various sensory inputs from within and without at the most auspicious time during a practice or sequence (Brems, 2024b). As students or clients sense inputs from inside and outside of themselves (sensations arising from the body and outer world), they may begin to gain awareness of nervous system reactivity, energetic and affective reverberations (feeling tones or vedana), and mental or emotional perceptions and narratives that arise in response. Four primary sensory inputs can be explored in yogic practices, including (or perhaps especially) in asana and pranayama, namely, neuroception, interoception, proprioception, and exteroception (sights, sounds, smells, tastes, touch). Good timing and pacing of cues for the four -ceptions are helpful so students are ready to engage, have enough time to be with sensations, perhaps notice their ripple effects, and can be guided back to a regulated nervous system before the end of a session.

- *Neuroception* – cue recognition, awareness, or mindfulness of current level of safety; cue exploration of presence or absence of sensations that result in a felt sense of safety, danger, or life threat, followed by a commensurate nervous system response that activates either the ventral vagal complex (safety), sympathetic nervous system (danger), or dorsal vagal complex (life threat); be familiar with polyvagal theory XE "Polyvaga(Porges, 2022; Sullivan et al., 2018a)(Porges, 2022; Sullivan et al., 2018a) to use this type of sensory cuing

- *Interoception* – cue to help develop the capacity to attune to, receive, process, and integrate signals about the internal and affective state of the body; cue somatic mindfulness, attention, or awareness; cue a felt sense of the body and its energetic and affective state; this cuing may tap into the capacity to sense the physiological state of the body from within via sensations arising from various physiological systems of the body, including but not limited to the respiratory, cardiac, gastrointestinal, thermoregulatory, and nociceptive systems; it will carry with it a sensing into the feeling tones that arise from these sensations

- *Proprioception* – cue to help cultivate the ability to grasp the body's alignment and positioning in space; this is a helpful exploration of physical patterns in the body that are not conscious for the student; clients may discover that what they perceive from the inside does not align with the actual placement of the body; this too increases somatic awareness and mindfulness, along with interoception

- *Exteroception* – cue for the ability to attune to stimuli from outside the body, to perceive and take in stimulation from the outside world – conscious and mindful perception of these visual, auditory, olfactory, gustatory, and tactile stimuli can then be integrated with stimuli arising from inside the body (i.e., interoception) and help inform neuroception of safety, danger, or life threat; exteroception can also be used to recognize how much stimulation is present on the outside that we habitually tune out yet that still is likely to affect the nervous system; this may help prepare students for pratyahara as the first step of sense withdrawal is noticing that the senses are being stimulated from the outside (and of course from the inside)

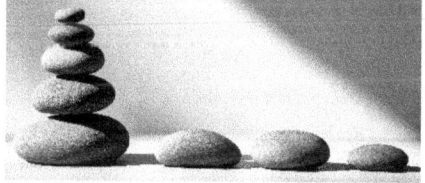

	Pathways of Sensory Processing Engaged in Integrated Yoga
Neuroception	Unconscious and spontaneous evaluation of current level of safety that results in a felt sense of safety, danger, or life threat, followed by a commensurate nervous system response that activates either the ventral vagal complex (safety), the sympathetic nervous system (danger), or the dorsal vagal complex (life threat); the ability to read internal physiological reactions, along with exteroceptive inputs, translate them into an assessment of our sense of safety, and react to them quickly and efficiently to mitigate possible dangers or threats to life or safety; all of this happens outside of conscious awareness or control, being based in the pre- or subconscious and *not* mediated by conscious cognition
Interoception	Capacity to attune to, receive, process, and integrate internal signals about the internal physical, affective, and energetic state of the body, including the capacity to sense the physiological state of the body from within via sensations arising from various physiological systems of the body, including but not limited to the respiratory (e.g., breathing rhythms), cardiac (e.g., pulse or heart rate), gastrointestinal (e.g., butterflies in the stomach), thermoregulatory (e.g., temperature) and nociceptive systems (e.g., pain and discomfort)
Proprioception	Capability to grasp the body's movement, force and speed (with which our body is moving), alignment, and positioning in space based on stimuli that arise from within the body itself, including stimuli that are received through the senses; proprioception is mediated by the cerebellum and brainstem resulting in ongoing (often unconscious) adjustments of the body in response to proprioceptive signals from receptors in muscles, tendons, and skin
Exteroception	Attunement and responsivity to stimuli originating outside the body, to perceive and take in stimulation from the outside world through the exteroceptors of the five senses of sight (i.e., photoreceptors), hearing (i.e., mechanoreceptors), touch, smell, and taste, as well as outer temperature, pressure, pain stimuli; conscious and mindful perception of these outer stimuli can then be integrated with stimuli arising from inside the body (i.e., interoception) and help inform neuroception of safety, danger, or life threat

Adapted/expanded from: Brems, C. (2020). Yoga as a mind-body practice. In J. Uribarri, & J. A. Vassalotti (Eds.), *Nutrition, fitness, and mindfulness: An evidence-based guide for clinicians.* (pp. 137–155). Springer Nature.

LET Be

LET Be is another way to help participants cultivate mindfulness, attention, or awareness. This process facilitates identification of and caring for sensations in all layers of human experience (*koshas*) through systematic exploration via four steps. This paradigm can be used to cultivate mindfulness, attention, or awareness. It can be used in the context of form and movement (*asana*), breathwork and functional breathing (*pranayama*), and any of the inner practices (including *pratyahara*, *dharana*, or *dhyana*), as well as in daily life as a brief check-in with experience and reactivity.

The process begins with simply locating of a point of interest, then invites open-minded and open-hearted experience of all that is present in this point of focus, followed by tending to experience that arises (e.g., via directing breath, compassion, or gratitude), and ends with open presence and being with what emerges. Following is a detailed description of the four steps. Two examples of guided *LET Be* experiences can be found on YouTube (https://youtu.be/wu-ksCtkaR8 [60 minutes with short didactic] or https://youtu.be/a_OUfTFeHEI (45 minutes]). Clients can be taught how to do this practice on their own.

- **L**ocate – begin by noticing (i.e., become mindful of, be attentive to, or find spacious awareness of) a particular part of the body or by noticing where a particular body part is located in space, where the breath is felt most directly, or where the fluctuations of the mind find embodiment; locating can be repeated in multiple steps (e.g., as might be done in a body scan [dharana] or in directing students to notice various alignment foci in a posture [asana] or in inviting students to feel various aspects of the breath [pranayama])

- **E**xperience – once a part of the self has been located, tune into the sensations (with mindfulness, attention, or spacious awareness) that emerge from that location in the body, breath, or mind; be particularly attuned to neuroception and interoception; explore and meet whatever arises with curiosity and an open heart and open mind; there is no need to change anything – simple meet what is present and invite yourself to experience it fully

- **T**end to – if desirable, direct attention, movement, breath, compassion, kindness or other ways of caring to that part of the self to support or increase a sense of ease or equanimity; for example, you might send breath to a tense or painful body part to be able to stay with a difficult sensation, perhaps inviting the transformation of suffering into pure sensation

- **Be** present – once you have attuned and tended to sensation, let go of all "strategies" and simply be present for what remains – no desire or need remains to change or alter anything – not even a desire to sense more deeply or to become more aware; there is no need to control, deny, repress, force, or tighten – there is acceptance without giving up; what remains in this moment is presence with what is; simply let be…

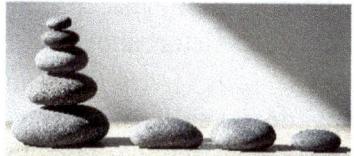

Embracing Trauma-Informed Yoga Principles

There are many forms of trauma and many roads to healing. The information in these pages is not sufficient to support a claim for being a trauma-informed, much less trauma-trained, yoga teacher or clinician. It simply serves to create awareness and openness about language and cuing that demonstrate basic sensitivity. Yoga professionals who want to specialize in trauma work have to take additional training to prepare for the specifics of the trauma-affected population with which they work (Badenoch, 2018; Justice et al., 2019; Schwartz, 2024).

Types of Traumata

A partial list of types of traumata is offered below. It is intended to raise awareness and increase thoughtfulness. Each listed type can vary further by whether it is acute (e.g., one-time traumatic event), chronic (e.g., repeated exposure to a particular type), or complex (e.g., repeated exposure to many types) Some individuals also can experience multiple sources of trauma – at once or across time.
- Trauma related to adverse childhood experiences
- Sexual trauma
- Domestic violence trauma
- Racial trauma
- Combat trauma
- War trauma (living in a war zone)
- Traumatic loss
- Trauma due to natural disaster
- Trauma due to victimization
- Medical trauma
- Historical trauma
- Ancestral trauma
- Secondary trauma

Trauma makes itself felt in all tangible koshas (Badenoch, 2018). Teachers may recognize signs of trauma in their students. They can also begin to teach with the potential for trauma in mind. In all likelihood, at least some students in the general population and a large portion of participants in healthcare settings will have had trauma experiences and may have integrated these experiences into their body, energy, mind, emotions, and relationships. It is important to note that not all students will benefit from trauma-informed teaching principles – this is a common misconception. Yoga professionals need to know their population and teach wisely with discernment and compassion at all times. Following are a few examples of how trauma may manifest and be observed:
- *Trauma in the body* (e.g., muscle and fascial tension and constriction, reduced range of motion, pain – acute or chronic, fatigue, numbness, disconnection from the body, GI disturbances, immune impairment, sleep disturbances)
- *Trauma in the breath, energy, and nervous system* (e.g., autonomic nervous system disruption – cf., polyvagal therapy, dorsal collapse or agitation of sympathetic arousal, hyper- or hypovigilance, disrupted breath, exhaustion, adrenal burnout)

- *Trauma in the mind* (e.g., distractibility, difficulty concentrating, mental preoccupations, rigid thought patterns, worries, catastrophizing, shame thinking)
- *Trauma in emotions* (e.g., anxiety, panic, depression, sense of loss, dissociation, shame, anger, disgust, loss of resilience)
- *Trauma in relationships* (e.g., loss of trust, inability to feel safe with others, effects on intimacy, emotional distancing, ingrained expectations of being hurt, dependence, inability to maintain boundaries)

As outlined elsewhere (Justice et al., 2018, 2019), there are several aspects of yoga services that can benefit from sensitivity to the reality that many individuals come to the mat with a range of traumatic experiences in their lives. Many trauma-informed yoga (TIY) principles are useful as general practice principles. However, they cannot be indiscriminately applied; for some population, especially those with persistent severe mental illness, TIY principles may be less than auspicious.

TIY principles guide yoga professionals toward open-hearted cuing that emphasizes self-agency, empowerment, and choice. TIY sessions are focused on creating safety via returning control to the client or student by giving choices, options, and freedom to find highly individualized practices based on client introspection, the four 'ceptions, and moment-to-moment need. Given this reality, cuing is non-directive and invitational. Such cuing may not be appropriate for individuals who are actively psychotic, have attention deficits, are dealing with cognitive challenges, or may otherwise be in need of clear, concise, and unequivocal cuing. In other words, while it may be tempting to default to TIY principles at all times, discernment is necessary about how to temper the open-ended nature of this cuing with come clienteles.

Beneficial TIY Principles and Practices to Cultivate

Beneficial practices useful to individuals with a trauma history or a need for self-reflection, self-compassion, and nervous system regulation (i.e., the majority of humans) focus on:
- Creating the opportunity for the experience of safety
    - provide a space that encourages personal boundaries for students (mat orientation, participant awareness of exits, minimal outside disruption)
    - invite student engagement in setting up and modifying practice space
    - engage in minimal instructor movement throughout the session – teach from the mat
    - provide stability and consistency
- Engaging the parasympathetic nervous system, supporting participants' access to their ventral vagal (or sattvic) state
    - breathing practices to reduce hyperarousal (e.g., prolonged exhales)
    - breathing practices to activate hypoarousal (e.g., emphasis on inhalation)
    - restorative poses
    - gentle and careful yin practices
    - soothing sequencing with lots of opportunity for recovery
- Cultivating interoception – all -ceptions, really …
    - invite access to inner experience and offer safety nets
    - use repetition and slower pacing to help clients find an inner experience
    - integrate observation and awareness of breath

- Invite mindfulness that draws attention inward
  - offer guided meditations that focus attention on the body, breath, or even mind from the inside out
- Offering variations and adaptations
  - offer a practice that is adapted and tailored to individual needs
  - promote safety through appropriate variations (e.g., modifications to sexually suggestive postures)
  - demonstrate variations that clearly communicate the emphasis on tailoring the practice to individual needs and resources
  - use props selectively and intentionally with sensitivity to individual reactivity or needs
- Using invitational language
  - empowering language that offers participants agency and self-determination
  - accessible language that emphasizes options, choices, adaptability, exploration, variation, and individual differences
  - make highly selective use of Sanskrit (with appropriate definitions, translations, and explanations)
  - make word choices that express egalitarianism, respect, and empowerment
  - offer sufficient guidance and clarity – neither being too forceful nor too vague
- Understanding power dynamics
  - recognize that clients may ascribe power and directiveness to you – whether you feel those characteristics or not
  - students see you as the expert – be sure to avoid letting that mean that power is transferred to you over their choices
  - empower clients into agency and self-determination while offering clarity about wholesome functional movement
  - continuously give power back to participants
  - invite students into agency and self-determination
  - respect participants' boundaries; in fact, encourage them
  - take responsibility for creating an environment of equality, inclusion, agency, and empowerment
  - relate and speak with humility and caring
  - avoid fragility language or intention
- Engaging in ongoing provider self-care
  - have a personal resilience practice
  - maintain self-protective personal boundaries, roles, and scopes of practice
  - be certain that you stay grounded and in a ventral vagal space – use your yoga practice to practice what you preach
  - check in with yourself regularly to make sure that you are neither burning out nor being caught up in secondary trauma
  - cultivate resilience and equanimity to be able to remain in your ventral vagal space in the face of dysregulation
  - consult, consult, consult – never assume you have seen and learned everything; debrief with peers, teachers, mentors, therapists
  - seek continued education – the field is constantly changing and emerging; stay at the forefront of trauma science – and maintain an attitude of lifelong learning

Contraindicated Practices in TIY To Avoid

Non-beneficial practices or contraindications that can get in the way of an auspicious yoga experience for individuals with a trauma history, with a need for self-reflection, self-compassion, and nervous system regulation (i.e., the majority of students). The following listing is food for thought; it is not necessarily all-inclusive.

Environmental triggers
- Excessively large classes
- Excessive proximity (lack of space) between students
- Triggering sounds (e.g., fan or HVAC sounds)
- Lighting consideration – too bright versus too dark

Surprises
- Changes in routine
- Lack of predictability
- Teaching off the mat
- Walking up behind students
- Walking around the room in unpredictable patterns

Sustained engagement of the sympathetic nervous system
- Breath retention
- Rapid or activating breathing
- Complicated breathing practices
- Overly activating vinyasa, kriya, or even form practice (e.g., deep backbends; rapid movement from form to form)

Excessive engagement of the dorsal vagus for students with that predisposition
- Excessive slowing of the breath
- Excessive calming down of energy
- Overly interior practices
  - excessive self-reflection or inward focus
  - excessive reliance on forward folds

Indiscriminate touch and common studio practices
- Touching without prompting and/or therapeutic relevance
- Touching without ongoing, repeated explicit consent
- Non-intentional physical adjustment or touch (even if consent was given)
- Sequences that include many postures positioning the hips in vulnerable ways, overly complicated breathing practices, or prolonged silences
- Large classes in which participants are positioned very close to one another

Unskillful cuing – content and process
- Excessive directiveness
- Force or aggressiveness
- Overly vague directions
- Too much silence or stillness

Conducive and Non-Conducive Interventions for Trauma Informed Yoga

Conducive Interventions to Use	Non-Conducive Interventions to Avoid
<ul><li>Create the opportunity for safety</li><li>Provide stability and consistency</li><li>Engage the ventral vagal system</li><li>Cultivate interoception and neuroception</li><li>Offer variations + adaptations</li><li>Use invitational language</li><li>Understand power dynamics</li><li>Engage in self-care</li><li>Seek ongoing education</li></ul>	<ul><li>Avoid large classes and excessive proximity with others</li><li>Do not surprise students</li><li>Avoid excessive engagement of the SNS or dorsal vagal system</li><li>Be sensible about touch</li><li>Do not offer physical adjustments without a plan</li><li>Do not direct or force</li><li>Do not be too vague either</li></ul>

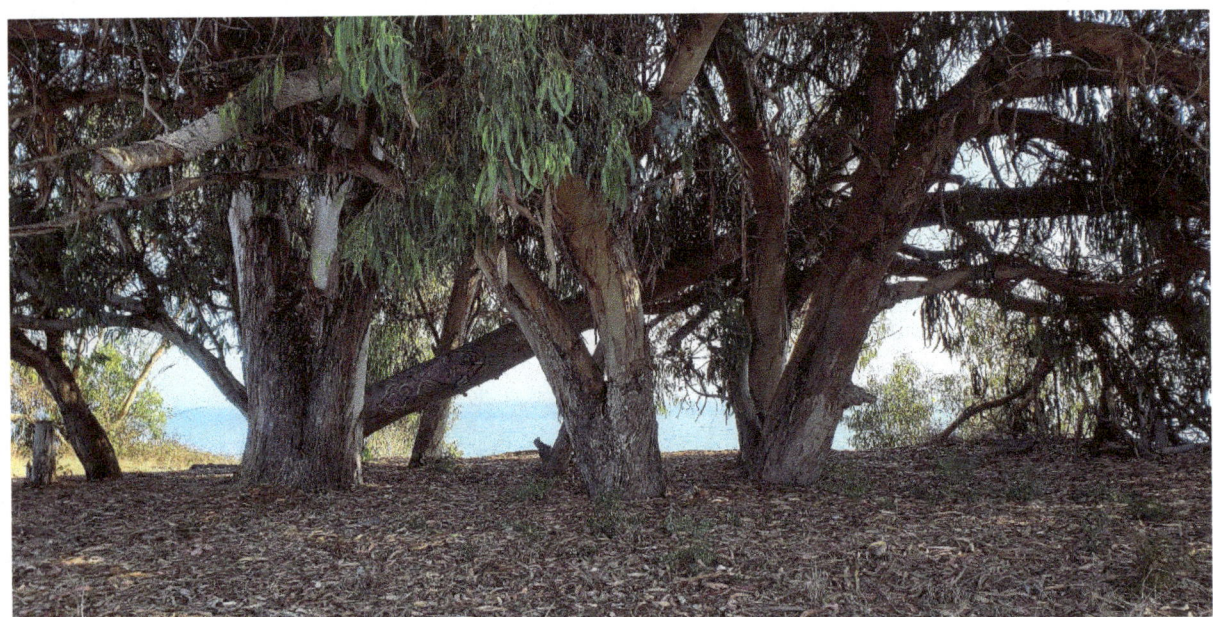

Chapter 9: Cuing, Demonstration, and Observation

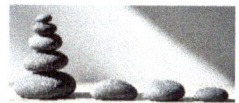

A well-sequenced session is rounded out by appropriate language choices in cuing, as well as well-chosen demonstrations by the yoga professional and mutual observation by provider of client and by client of provider. Careful observation of students will help guide teachers into appropriate language and demonstration choices that are adapted and attuned to students' needs, cultural contexts, experiences, and backgrounds. Language and demonstrations help create a psychological space that invites clients to find peace, balance, resilience, and discernment (including, clear decision-making and problem-solving ability).

Language choices in cuing have to do with inclusivity, accessibility, cultural appropriateness, safety, nervous system regulation, trauma sensitivity, and clarity. Some of these aspects of language (e.g., for accessibility and trauma or cultural sensitivity) have already been alluded to. Focus here is on word choices related to specific cuing of various yoga practices (from movement to breathing to meditation) and optimizing the student-teacher relationship.

Demonstration considerations have to do with decisions about which version of a shape to demonstrate, purpose of the demonstration (with care not to let ego of the teacher guide the choice), and needs and skills of students in the room. The latter is, of course, guided by in-the-moment observation of participants, their skill level, striving, and capacity for self-regulation and self-guided adaptation and modification.

Observation in the context of cuing and demonstration means that the yoga professional is aware of the impact of chosen cuing and demonstration on clients in the classroom or clinical practice. This is different from observation that informs the teacher about needs of the client that are inherent in the client's presentation and needs (which is covered elsewhere). Observation of participant reactions to cuing and demonstration is multifaceted and nearly endless in its complexities and layers. Observation takes in nonverbal communication about clients' relationships to their bodies, sensations, feeling tones associated with sensations arising from the body or environment, perceptions and interpretations of energy and feeling tones, mental formations and fluctuations, habitual reactivities in all koshas, and relationships to all human ways of processing the world. Clinicians can observe students in all koshas; from that, we can glean endless information about client's ways of being in the world and in relationship – with themselves and with others.

Choices for Successful Cuing, Speech, Action and Class Leadership

While the content that follows raises important considerations, offered ponderings and ideas are not to be applied *ad absurdum*. We can find something wrong with everything we say or do and could throttle ourselves by being too cautious or worried about language misuse. Yoga professionals simply hold offered cautions in their awareness to avoid the most egregious pitfalls. From there, they can have fun and be willing to explain and apologize as necessary. ☺

Thinking Before Speaking and Doing

In Buddhism, a series of queries is offered to doublecheck that, before we speak or act, what we are about to say or do is wholesome, appropriate for context, and auspicious for the recipient and the one taking the action. The four suggested questions invite discernment in speech and action and are as follows:
- Is it necessary or helpful?
- Is it true?
- Is it kind?
- Is my intention pure?

These questions offer yoga teachers a great way to ponder their cuing. Will we consciously ask them before *everything* we do and say? Probably not – things unfold rapidly in a class and we often have to be quick on our feet, so to speak. However, pondering later if what we said and met these guidelines can help shape auspicious habits in cuing. We become increasingly able to discern very quickly if what we are about to say or do will truly serve a purpose, is driven by the right intentions, will help the student, and is compassionate or kindhearted.

Is it necessary or helpful?

Over time, we begin to be more discerning about whether a particular cue, demonstration, or action was truly necessary given the students and circumstances or if it was based on some other need that arose from within us (rather than from the context). For example, we begin to notice if our action or speech was driven by habit, anxiety, the need to fill space, or another reason that really was neither germane to the present moment nor the client's need. Over time we gain experience whether a particular cue, demonstration, or offering actually helps students find wholesome alignment, states of mind, vitality, or other actions we are targeting. We become more discerning if what we say and demonstrate is truly helpful to moving students into a wholesome practice and experience or if it is potentially useless, harmful, or counterproductive.

Is it true?

Offering helpful cues and demonstrations is predicated on being truthful and accurate. Teachers review new science and engage in ongoing learning surrender speech and actions that may be based on outdated, inaccurate, or less than factual information. Teachers discern whether claims they make about alignment, benefits, risks, and other facts are based in truth as we learn it from ancient wisdom and modern science. Teachers, to the best of their knowledge, refrain from wrong or misleading statements and are open to feedback about new facts as they emerge.

Is it kind?

Even if a possible cue or demonstration is necessary, helpful, and factual, as teachers, we still need to discern whether our speech or action is kind. If we only show the most difficult version of a shape, are we being kind to all students in the class? Are being truthful if we do this? Cuing is most wholesome and auspicious if it is offered in an invitational manner, with compassion, lovingkindness, and non-attachment, especially to our own ego.

Is my intention pure?

It is helpful to stay anchored to the overall intention and theme for the class or session. Even more importantly, teachers remain aware of the intention that fuels their cuing, demonstration, assisting, and other actions. Are we doing what we are doing based on wholesome intention that serves our students? Or are we coming from a place of serving our own needs, perhaps showing off?

Considering the four questions helps teachers stay grounded in their own practice and is a great way to remain vigilant. They cultivate discernment and wisdom along with compassion and lovingkindness. In other words, the four questions keep us anchored to yoga ethics and the brahma viharas in our relationships with ourselves and our students.

Perspective-Taking in How Cuing, Speech, and Action May Land

In cuing and action, we, as teachers or clinicians, need to have clarity about how we affect your listeners – each individual student, the student body overall, and co-teachers or assistants in the room. Gaining such clarity requires taking the perspective of the listener – we imagine hearing and understanding what we say from our client's point of view and unique perspective. Phrasing, word choices, questions versus statements, specific ways of expressing something, even tone of voice and style of delivery can affect how students (as well as co-teacher and assistants) receive our communication.

Actions, as involved in demonstrating particular shapes and using props, speak very loudly. How we decide to model a shape and how we offer props (verbally and via demonstration) can make a large difference in how the practice lands with students. Our words and actions can lead to students feeling empowered or disempowered; invited and included or excluded and alienated. Following are some considerations about how our words and actions may land with students and others in the room (such as assistants or co-teachers). We ponder our intentions, thoughts, words, actions, and impacts (including possible unintended consequences).

The following questions can be helpful in making this self-assessment before, during, or after use. Specifically, we ask will, does, or did the chosen language, cuing, demonstration, and other action serve to:
- Empower or disempower
- Embody or disembody
- Embrace or reject
- Distance or bring closer
- Normalize or marginalize
- Include or exclude
- Shame or honor
- Embarrass or respect
- Support or undermine
- Respect or disrespect

Statements versus Questions

As teachers, we also ponder whether what we are trying to express or invite is best posed as a *statement* or a *question*. Plenty of opportunities exist in which we can invite clients into their own power and agency by asking them a question or inviting them to notice something rather than offering a directive, or even an invitation. When we ask questions, we invite interoception, exteroception, proprioception, neuroception; we support awareness and mindfulness. We encourage students to tap into inner resilience and resources to frame their own unique solutions to return to inner peace and balance in all their layers of experience.

Phrasing and Language

As we frame invitations, cues, and suggestions – verbally or behaviorally, we continuously and retrospectively consider the implications and applicability of each choice. Our intention may guide some of these choices, as will (perhaps more so) the needs and biopsychosociocultural contexts and experiences of our students. What may be appropriate in one context, may be less auspicious in another. As yoga professionals we need to have clarity about what we are trying to accomplish and adapt our language accordingly. We do not sell our students short – they are smart; they can learn jargon and anatomically and psychologically appropriate language. We do shy away from teaching them new words or concepts; however, we do so humbly and matter-of-factly, not as a way to aggrandize ourselves or make ourselves better and smarter.

Possible Connotations and Meanings of Questions, Cues, and Statements

To have clarity about the implications of language choices, we need to understand and ponder the many connotations our choices might have. We stay curious about how cues, statements, or questions may be heard, perceived, and understood by students. To think about this point, it might help to ponder the following questions (though there are surely many other questions to ponder in this regard):

- Who – or which layer of self or level of consciousness – is invited into action and agency?
- When (under what circumstances) may an action, question, cue, or statement serve?
- Whom does this action, cue, question, or statement serve? A particular student? All students? The instructor? An assistant who is also present?
- When might a particular cue, question, statement, or action not serve? Who is left out, offended, excluded, advantaged, disadvantaged?
- What or who is engaging in versus inviting the action?
- Will the action, statement, cue, or question lead to a clear and desirable goal?
- Will the cue, statement, question, or action support student autonomy and agency?

Observation of the Impact of Cuing, Speech, and Actions on Students' Experience

To notice how cuing, speech, and demonstrations can affect the students' attitude toward their experience, we can ponder the following questions, possibilities, and impacts:

- Is the cuing, questioning, or demonstration an invitation for students to open up to experience?

- Does the cue or demonstration close students down to their own experience (e.g., by suggesting, however indirectly, how students "should" move, feel, or experience a particular practice)?
- Does the cue, question, or action invite students into being with what is – without suggesting that they must accept all experiences as a given and unalterable reality?
- Does the cue invite students into the experience or exploration of something new, unexpected, curious, or different?

Neither the goal to open up to something new, nor the goal to experience something habitual and perpetual is good and bad; however, both goals are best expressed with intention and planfulness. This requires being thoughtful about whether cuing or questioning is consistent with the intention of either being with what is already there versus inviting a new perspective or experience. For example, cuing can be framed to invite:

- Interoception, mindfulness, and other inner experiences that facilitates students' experience of the present moment
- Beginner's mind that opens students to new possibilities, perhaps to reshape experience and action, not from a place of judgement but from the wisdom of discernment and compassion

Being Open to Experience: Coming Into the Present Moment

Cuing for being open to experiencing what is present in this moment in time and space invites students into mindfulness and awareness of what is naturally unfolding. There is no desire to change – simply to notice. Sample cues that invite openness to being with what is may include the following:

- If this feels challenging, can you be with it, accepting that this may be natural right now?
- If you feel yourself pushing against …, is it because you expected something different?
- If you notice strain in your …, this may be typical or it may invite you to ….
- Can you notice if this is your usual way of responding to …?
- What seems to be your predictable approach to … ?
- Maybe … is something that feels instinctive for you?

Alternatives to the word "normal" are helpful linguistic offering that help students explore the present moment as it presents. These words can be used to highlight that there is no need to change anything; they are simply invited into an opportunity to note what is showing up naturally. It also helps students become curious about "normality", nit tuning something out, just because it is familiar.

Here are some suggested words to help students notice their "normal" or "natural" experience:

- Ordinary, familiar, commonplace, unremarkable
- Typical, predictable, characteristic, usual
- Natural, likely, accepted, effortless, inherent, learned, instinctive
- Conventional, predictable, standard, expected

Maintaining Beginner's Mind: Inviting Openness for Something New

Cuing for being open to experiencing something new invites students into beginner's mind, into an attitude of non-expectation and freedom from assumptions. There is an invitation to change typical perception – to open up to new experiences and ways of perceiving or interpreting. Sample cues that invite openness to exploring new ways of being include the following:
- Can you let yourself settle into this unexpected sensation?
- What emerges that is surprising?
- I invite you to find an expression of … that is new or unique to you
- How can you make this next breath fresh or novel?
- What might you notice that was unforeseen?
- Can you give yourself permission to create a shape that is deeply yours, uniquely yours in a new way?

> Helpful language for encouraging students to explore the "extraordinary" helps them transform experience, perception, and action that has become stagnant or conditioned. There is no need to invite huge changes; we simply offer an opportunity to invite new possibilities.
>
> *Here are some suggested words to help students notice the extraordinary and open up to novel experiences.*
> - Special, particular, unexpected, remarkable
> - Surprising, unpredicted, unexpected, unforeseen, unanticipated
> - New, original, fresh, innovative, novel
> - Different, atypical, unique, distinctive

Considered Use of Specific Language Constructions

Grammatical Constructions

Considered use of grammar refers to conscious choices about appropriate person (I, you, we) and tense for the specific context and intention. Several considerations can be explored:
- Ponder the impact of the use of present participles: *-ing* words (e.g., moving, sensing, being)
    - When used in a yoga or meditation context, *-ing* words are often present participles that reflect an incomplete verb phrase, such as *"moving the hands overhead"* (as opposed to *"move your hands overhead"* or *"we are moving our hands overhead"*. This construction creates more distance from the doer and invites less embodiment.
    - *-ing* constructions may be useful for instruction in meditation when a less personalized approach is desired to direct attention away from a *self* and toward an observer or observing ego – importance is placed on the movement, not the mover
    - *-ing* constructions in yoga may increase disembodiment and dissociation from being an active and empowered agent
    - Different situations will require different cuing – the main thing is to have a clear intention when using this particular grammatical construction

- Ponder the impact of the use of the 1st person plural: *we ...; our ...* (s opposed to I and mine, or you and your)
  - The use of *"our"* versus *"your"* may create a strange unification (even inappropriate blending of boundaries) of all individuals present – e.g., *let's breathe into our belly* versus *I invite you to breathe into your belly*
  - At times, this use of 1st person plural may be intentional to signal community, shared experience, or co-regulation
  - The use of this 1st person plural may serve to distance students from their own body, experience, and breath
  - It is important to decide discerningly when this grammatical choice is appropriate – a decision that very much depends on context and intention
- Ponder the impact of the use of 2nd person: *you...; your ...*
  - This construction is generally a good choice for yoga as it invites students into own their body and experience
  - It invites action and agency; it empowers and delineates boundaries
  - In some contexts, it could potentially distance (yours *versus* mine or yours *versus* ours)
  - Relatedly, "the" instead of "your" may distance or disembody as it disowns the body part being cued – e.g., *let the arm float up* versus *move your arm outward and upward*

To practice discernment about how *-ing*, 1st person, and 2nd person constructions may resonate, compare the following cues:
- Lifting the hands overhead and bending to the right side …
- We are lifting our hands overhead and are bending to the right side
- Lift your hands overhead and bend to the right side
- Let's lift our hands overhead and let's bend to the right side
- If we lose our breath, we can …
- Notice if we are feeling challenge anywhere …

Efficiency, Poignancy, and Student-Centeredness

As teachers, we want to make statements count: we communicate what we want to communicate and direct this communication to whom it needs to reach. We keep students' perspectives in mind – a goal that can be a balancing act of knowing how neither to under- or overcue and -do. At the same time, we can remain aware and okay with the fact that however we phrase things, our words will not land equally with all students – so be kind to yourself. That said, we can ponder the following considerations to reflect on the effectiveness and efficiency of our communications:
- Avoid fillers without being too unclear
  - use smart parsimony in cuing: don't cue so much that students get overwhelmed but enough to create clarity and prevent confusion
  - optimize repetitive phrases and habitual expressions
  - do not get too flowery
- Use synonyms or let actions speak, instead of words
  - e.g., instead of constantly "inviting" verbally, create an atmosphere in class that makes it clear that everything is an invitation

- Beware of getting lost in stories or tangents
    - make cuing about the students, not about you, the teacher
    - if you choose to tell a story or self-disclose, know why you are doing it; have a purpose
- Adapt language and vocabulary to student body with respect and consideration
    - do not "dumb down" your language
    - teach students new vocabulary that invites efficiency and clarity
    - develop short-hand language with students

To ponder this concept in a bit more detail, look at and consider the impacts of the following samples of possible "extra" versus poignant or respectful verbiage:

- *Next, we will ...* - *Now we are going to ...* - *From here we will move to ....* - *When I am doing this I feel ...* - *I invite you to ... [used over and over]*	- *roll the acetabulum – or your hip socket – over the head of your femur* - *...observe the action of your rib basket – why might this word be preferable to rib cage?*

Attention to Language Connotations

Note if there are connotations that may run counter to inclusivity, accessibility, cultural appropriateness, safety, nervous system regulation, and clarity (Lasater, 2021). Look at the following samples to identify potential issues, challenges, and/or problematic connotations (a few hints are offered in parentheses):

- *Take one last breath* (ponder existential implications…)
- *Take a deep, deep breath* … (ponder anatomical and physiological accuracy)
- *Take a big deep inhale* ...
- *Continue to think about...* (ponder being versus doing; thinking versus feeling)
- *If you can't access this, try* ... (ponder disempowerment or implied judgment)
- *You can try the regression of xyz pose by ....* (ponder judgment of better vs. worse)
- *If you need to modify, do ...* (see above)
- *Place the hands alongside the torso in line with the breasts ...* (ponder binary language)
- *Place the block under your back, along the bra line ...* (ponder gender neutrality)
- *Float your arms up ...* (ponder agency)
- *Drop to the ground ...* (ponder agency and polyvagal state)
- *Stomp your heel down ...* (ponder aggression)
- *Hold this shape as long as you can ...* (ponder competitiveness, working with edges)
- *Push into the pose ...* (ponder self-harm or physical tuning out)
- *Let me help you with ...* (ponder agency and power)
- *If you are able to ...* (ponder fragility language)
- *Allow your arms to ...* (ponder agency)
- *Letting the legs ...* (ponder disembodiment and passivity)

Types of Language

Language used in cuing can be invitational and explorative versus directive, prescriptive, or commanding. Language can be active and clear in purpose or passive and somewhat vague in intention. Not any single type of style of language and cuing is right or wrong. However, it will be helpful to match the type of language to the purpose of the communication and the circumstances in which cues are offered. It is not helpful to use a passive, explorative, or invitational cue when a student is in danger of imminent harm. Such a circumstance calls for a directive and active intervention.

Whenever appropriate to context and student group, yoga professionals are well serve to use invitational and explorative versus directive, prescriptive, or commandeering versus assertive and intentional language. We use language that guides or leads (versus language that might lack clarity or direction) when guidance or leadership is necessary and helpful. We carefully consider under which circumstances guidance may become more important than completely open cuing.

Look at the following samples to tease out what may be invitational versus directive:
- *I invite you to … versus I want you to …*
- *You might choose to … versus now do xyz*
- *Consider moving your back foot to … Versus always move your back foot to …*
- *Explore which position feels more auspicious for your neck … versus I want you to roll you neck back to the right and left*
- *Try out which hand position might be most compassionate for your wrist in this moment versus come on, place the hand directly under the shoulder joint*
- *Notice which positioning might be most useful for your ankle … versus now turn your ankle to forward to create a 45° angle*
- *Softly scan your body for xyzzy … versus find the place in your body that xyz*
- *What do you notice? … versus feel the tension/ease/stretch in ….*
- *Meet your body where it is … versus your body should be …*
- *What might happen if you try? Versus now try ….*
- *Can you tune into your experience? Versus feel the tension*

Look at the following samples to tease out what is active and clear versus vague or passive. Compare the pairs of directives to gain a sense of what this may look like. For each sample of two, ask if one option is preferable to the other? Under which circumstances? What are the subtle differences in what is communicated and how it is offered?
- *To protect the forward knee, try to center the knee directly above the ankle versus you might consider centering the knee above the ankle*
- *Keep the neck in line with the spine, especially if you regularly have neck pain versus see where the neck feels best for you in this moment*
- *Allow the breath to move naturally so as to keep the belly soft versus explore how the breath wants to move in and out of your body in this moment*
- *Move your arms up and overhead with intention and engagement versus float the arms up*
- *Let the shoulder blades release forward and up as you press the hips up into down dog versus invite auspicious placement of the scapulae*

Adjectives to Invite <u>Intentional</u> Alignment and Breathing Choices *(aka alternatives to "auspicious" – my favorite descriptor ….)*		
• Auspicious • Conducive to success • Skillful • Beneficial • Timely – right choice for this moment • Fitting – right choice for this space • Propitious for … • Valuable as related to … • Thoughtful • Supportive of … • Helpful to … • Useful	• Loving • Kind • Caring • Generous • Compassionate • Empathic • Gentle • Open-hearted • Soothing • Comforting • Peaceful • Calming • Patient • Compassionate	• Sweetly • Regulating for … • Non-habitual • Open-minded • Novel • Inspiring • Innovative • Inventive • Creative • Imaginative • Respectful • Considerate of … • Lovingly • Humble about …

Wisdom of Intentional Demonstration

Demonstration is most auspicious and helpful when done in in such way that the teacher's body is easeful, optimally aligned, gentle and compassionate, humble, joyful, exploratory, safe, and true to needs (i.e., not overstretched, over-efforting, strained, misaligned, or showing off). Awareness of the profound modeling that demonstration entails is key to making good choices about which variations to choose for demonstration. The offered approach emphasizes that there is no yoga practice for which there is a single peak or final expression of a shape. All forms, movements, breathing, and inward practices have a range of expressions (or variations) that are idiosyncratic and unique to each yogi who engages in them. It is important to remember that in any moment, there are as many variations of an offered yoga shape or movement as there are individuals in the room.

Given this reality, yoga professionals learn to make auspicious decisions about how to demonstrate certain practices and how to choose variations and adaptations. The default is to offer choices and options in every practice, teaching students from the very beginning that they are in charge of their chosen expression of any practice. All options, whether variations, adaptations, or alternatives rely on ample use of yoga props. It is notable that in integrated holistic yoga, the words *adaptation* and *variation* are used – as opposed to *modifications* or *regressions* (even progressions) – for their less judgmental connotations.

In demonstrations be clear about intentionality, emphasize skillful alignment, role-model humility and prioritize accessibility, equality, and beneficence. Following are a few suggestions and recommendations; no doubt more considerations could be named.

- Role model intention, skillful alignment, and humility
  - demonstrate with ease and appropriate effort, choosing variations that are appropriate for class level as well as the teacher's own body
  - demonstrate for non-ego purposes (i.e., do not show off the teacher's own skill) that serve the practice of the students who are present in the room
  - demonstrate not just shapes, but – perhaps more importantly – transitions between shapes
  - narrate demonstrations to draw student attention to key principles and to provide multimodal learning access
  - know when it is and is not necessary to demonstrate
  - be clear whether the demonstration is happening in the same time as the students move into the same shape or transition or whether you are showing something that you want students to watch with attention and try afterwards
- Making auspicious choices of form or breath version for demonstration
  - when in doubt, demonstrate a modified version accessible to the majority (at least 90%) of the students in the class
  - demonstrate forms with the use of props
  - demonstrate the movement into and out of the form along with the form to show the flow and continuity of each shape
  - demonstrate in a manner that shows inward attunement, interoception, and proprioception
  - narrate the demonstration to make it instructive, not like performance art
  - adapt demonstrations to the needs and skill levels presented by students in a particular class
- Have clarity of purpose for each and every demonstration
  - have clarity why a particular demonstration is offered – tied to a teaching principle, an intention, a potential health issue, or a healthful alignment practice
  - do not demonstrate to perform or show off personal skill or accomplishment
  - at times it is helpful to have students demonstrate to each other – this requires discernment; in therapeutic classes this can be empowering and create agency; peer versus expert modeling can make a huge difference in how a particular shape is perceived

Wisdom of Observation: Holistic Seeing and Integrated Understanding

Yoga teachers tend to rely heavily on observation to understand their students and offer the most auspicious cuing during an integrated holistic yoga practice. Thus, in addition to utilizing formal assessment tools or mechanisms, yoga teachers and clinicians become skillful in the use of observation to refine their teaching and therapeutic yoga services. Such observation is focused on all layers of the human experience.

Seeing and Understanding People as an Integrated Whole

Seeing and understanding clients' bodies (anatomy and physiology; gunas), energy (arousal and affect; vedana and kleshas), and mind (thoughts and emotions; vrittis and mind states) guides our cuing, demonstration, and intervention – whether verbal or tactile. Seeing and understanding students' inner bodies, energy, and mind has nothing to do with judgment or evaluation. It is not a searching for outer manifestations, especially in the body, but rather an observation of inner experience as notable from the physically, energetically, emotionally, and behaviorally. As teachers, we do not look for outer shapes; we look for the inner body, the inner energy, the mind stories, and emotions. We try to understand the reflected health and wellbeing, not the superficial alignment or outer "looks". Observation is not a process of criticizing or finding what is wrong with students. Instead, we are trying to understand the structure and movement of students' anatomy, energy, and mind to best facilitate a tailored and individualized practice that serves them auspiciously and optimally. We are assessing energy and emotions that students bring to their experiences, especially as related to typical level of arousal (gunas), habitual affect or feeling tone (vedana), and kleshas and samskaras across all koshas. *Regardless of what we observe in students' inner bodies, energies, and mind,* <u>the power</u> *about how to move, breath, act, relate, and self-express and whether to follow our guidance* <u>remains with each student</u>. They are in charge of their body, breath, mind, emotions, actions, and relationships. We can make offerings, but we do not force a direction; we do not demand compliance; we do not expect to direct or command specific actions. We invite exploration, openness, and curiosity.

As we observe participants, we are especially careful in how to approach body reading (or assessment) and subsequent feedback to *make sure that we do not reinforce body hatred or engage in body shaming,* however subtly. If or when we give feedback to students (or to each other as teachers or fellow students), *we take care to start and end with noting the beauty and resilience we observe.* We resist focusing on or highlighting anything we observe as 'negative' or 'abnormal'; we are simply recording open-hearted and open-minded observations of individual physical and energetic expressions of body and energy. We keep in mind that for many students or clients receiving body feedback can feel like a judgment or confrontation; thus, we make our comments with compassion, lovingkindness, curiosity, and in an investigative and supportive spirit.

Equally important as not creating shame, defensiveness, or a sense of being judged, *we make sure that we not instill worry or anxiety about students' anatomy, vitality, or psychology.* We observe not to create fear, but to support the body, its inherent energies, and its relationship to mind and emotion to help students access their natural resilience and the recognition that homeostasis and adaptability will develop naturally through the practice. Unless we witness an extreme risk or imminent danger, we take care not to overreact to what we observe. Each body and mind is resilient in its own way and creative in overcoming challenges via useful physical, energetic, and emotional adaptations that may seem out of the norm but are actually auspicious or useful in action. This reality also means that we are patient. We do not jump to conclusions because we observed something one time; we do not notice something and immediately jump to cuing, assisting, much less adjusting. We patiently watch and learn; when we believe we have truly detected something of importance that can lead to cuing that will create an auspicious and meaningful change in the student's experience, then we cue, assist, and maybe even adjust.

A *rule of three* can be helpful. The first time, we as teachers or clinicians notice something interesting, we make a mental note. If we witness the same thing again, we become increasingly curious and begin to hypothesize the meaning or importance of what we are witnessing. If we see the same thing a third time, we can allow ourselves some cuing to see if there is resonance and more auspiciousness in the student or students to whom we are directing the cues. Assisting and adjusting may (or may not) follow from there.

The rule of three can be applied in multiple ways:
- Seeing the same thing in the same individual three times (e.g., a particular alignment in one type of asana; a particular breath pattern in one type of situation)
- Seeing the same pattern in three different contexts in the same individual (e.g., seeing a particular alignment in standing shapes, forward folds, and twists; noticing a particular style of breathing during the opening centering, during asana, and in savasana)
- Seeing the same uniqueness in three more individuals in our classroom (e.g., participants all adjust themselves in the same way; all participants engage in a similar breathing pattern – this will say more about *our cuing* than about the students' anatomy or energy!)

In observing participants, it can be helpful to have additional context. It can be useful for us as teachers to know a few key things about the students whose bodies, energies, and mind we observe (Brems, 2024b; Lasater, 2021). If we engage in this level of tailored instruction – especially if we incorporate tactile guidance, it might be helpful to find out if the student has received a physician's or other clinician's (e.g., psychologist's) clearance to practice yoga without limitations or special considerations. If there are physical, energetic, mental, or emotional challenges, it might be helpful to have basic information from the student, *if they are willing to share*. A few questions, the answers to which may provide helpful context, include, but are not limited to:
- Are there medical or psychological restrictions or contraindications (or a statement from the person that they have none)?
- Is there any hardware in the body (e.g., rods, joint replacements, pace makers)?
- Are there any spinal fusions? Other spinal issues? Osteopenia or osteoporosis?
- Is there a history or recent experience of accidents, surgeries, or other physical trauma?
- Is there any emotional/psychological trauma may be a contributing challenge in the practice? (be very discerning about whether and how to ask about this – again, consider your context!)

Basic Principles of Seeing and Understanding Students

As we observe our students or clients, it is helpful to stay attuned to all their koshas. It is easy to be distracted by the obvious nature of the body. However, breath – along with arousal (think *gunas*) and affect (think *vedana*) – can speak volumes not just about pranamaya kosha, but also about the relationship between annamaya and manomaya kosha. Indirect observations of mind and emotions are useful in that mind and body are connected – body influences the experience and expression of mind and emotions, and mind influences the experience and expression in body and breath.

The more connected we can stay to our clients, the more accurate our reading of their koshas. The connection between teachers and students maintains an environment of safety, a psychological container of clear boundaries and security, and a relationship of co-regulation and mutuality. It is in the context of secure connection and skillful co-regulation, that we, the teachers, look for the following aspects of our clients' experiences and expressions in all koshas during their time on the mat with us. As we look at clients, we note patterns and habits, effort and ease, abhyasa and vairagyam, lines of energy, evidence of awareness and attention (or their absence) across all koshas and practices. Following is a general overview of characteristics to observe in participants to offer them the most tailored and appropriate cuing, demonstration, and practice. This overview does not offer detail about *assessment* in the various koshas; it is strictly an invitation for observation of students or clients. More specific guidance about each koshas is offered in Volumes 2 and 3 (in particular, in the *asana* section, which offers guidance about understanding what is observed in the spine, posture, and pelvis; the *pranayama* section, which offers detailed inquiry about what to look for in students' breath and breathing-related physical, vital, and emotional layers; Brems, 2024b).

Annamaya Kosha Observations

- *Physical traits reflecting the inner body* (i.e., not getting distracted by aspects of the outer body that are often the focus of western society, such as beauty, symmetry, outer alignment, or 'classic' shapes of particular asanas), including but not limited to:
  o hypermobility versus restricted mobility (tensile and compressive resistance
  o tension or excessive strain versus laxity, collapse, or disengagement
  o strength versus weakness and their distribution across different parts of the body
  o comfort versus discomfort of students in their own skin
  o stress or strain in the body
  o evidence of acute or chronic pain, injury, or physical guarding
  o and more …

Pranamaya Kosha Observations

- *Energetic traits,* including but not limited to:
  o hypervigilance versus spaciness or being tuned out
  o breath patterns, textures, and rhythms; sound of the breath
  o hyper- versus hypoventilation; dysregulation in the breath
  o nasal versus mouth breathing; belly versus chest versus clavicular breathing
  o comfort versus discomfort with the energetic and affective demands of the practice
  o stress or strain in energy
  o and more …
- *Hints about arousal level,* including but not limited to:
  o hyperarousal, hypoarousal, or stable movement through various levels of arousal
  o physical and energetic expressions of the gunas (*tamas, rajas, sattva*)
  o polyvagal states (dorsal collapse, sympathetic activation, or ventral vagal equanimity)
- *Hints about affect,* including but not limited to:
  o feeling tones (*vedanas* of pleasant, unpleasant, and neutral)
  o activation of kleshas subsequent to the experience of a vedana, i.e., looking for grasping, clinging; aversion, hatred; fear, worry, anxiety, hesitation; ego investment and role expectations; confusion or misunderstanding

Annamaya and Pranamaya Kosha Observations

- *Experiences and expressions of effort and ease in body and energy,* including but not limited to:
  o balance versus imbalance of the two concepts
  o overefforting versus underefforting
  o lack of ease versus excessive ease or lack of engagement

- *Experiences and expressions of abhyasa* (integrated practice reflecting relaxation and engagement) and *vairagyam* (non-attachment to results or particular outcomes), perhaps as juxtaposed to ego investment in particular shapes, abilities, or expressions of the practice – in all koshas and actions
- *Grounding* and/or rooting, *expansion* and/or lengthening, and *stability* and/or balance in all koshas, that is, not just in the body but also in energy, arousal, affect, mind, mind states, thoughts, and emotions

Manomaya Kosha Observations

- *Emotional states and traits*, including but not limited to:
  - stress or strain in emotions
  - emotional distress versus equanimity
  - evidence of the kleshas – emotional expressions of attachment (e.g., clinging, grasping), aversion (e.g., hatred, anger, annoyance, impatience), ego (e.g., striving, being self-identified with an outer shape, being upset when personal expectations cannot be met), fear (e.g., worry, reluctance, shrinking back from new experience, anticipatory anxiety), or confusion (e.g., feeling lost, being unsure, being upset by not knowing what to do)
  - impact of the kleshas on actions and relationships in the present moment as well as off the mat (if the latter can be gleaned indirectly)
- *Mental states and traits*, including but not limited to:
  - mind states of disorganization, dullness, distraction, concentration and focus, or lucidity and clarity
  - stress or strain in the mind in its narratives or stories
  - presence of attention versus spaciness and distraction
  - evidence of the vrittis – preoccupation with memory, misperception, or planning
  - mental impacts of the kleshas – mental stories or narratives of greed, wanting, and attachment; of aversion and opposition; of ego with narrow role definitions for self and others (e.g., the teacher, other students); mental shrinking back in worry and anticipation of difficulty or challenge; or mental confusion about instructions with inattention to the teacher

Vijnanamaya and Anandamaya Kosha Observations

- *Evidence of wisdom and discernment*, including but not limited to:
  - use of props, adaptation, and personal tailoring of the practice
  - willingness to assert personal needs and to be self-compassionate and self-loving while holding oneself accountable
  - understanding of personal impact on other clients in the class, including compassion and lovingkindness toward others
  - appreciative and altruistic joy
  - equanimity in the face of challenge
  - clarity in problem-solving
  - openness to new experiences and more …
- *Evidence of joy,* including but not limited to:
  - sense of humor, ability to have fun with the practice

- light-hearted exploration, open-heartedness and light-heartedness
- connection to sangha
- appreciative and altruistic joy

A Few Helpful Hints for Observation

- Cultivate understanding and curiosity, not judgment
- Use tailored cues and practices (including alignment, percent of effort, breath, mind, emotions) to what is observed reliably and consistently
- Make sure the student always retains autonomy and power – invite, offer; never force, never direct – cultivate exploration and interest
- Do not engage in body shaming or reinforce body hatred
- Do not instill fear, worry, or anxiety
- Do not create – however inadvertently – a vulnerability mind state
- Place the emphasis of observation-based feedback or cuing on resilience, agency, empowerment, and intentionality, health and wellbeing – not outer shapes or alignment
- Be supportive and exploratory, inviting students into new ways of being, experiencing, and exploring
- Cue to direct students toward health and resilience based on what we see in all koshas
- Offer an "Oreo" of beauty and resilience: start with a positive and supportive observation; then make the offering of exploring a change; reconnect with the students around an observation of resilience, wellbeing, clarity, or skill
- Exercise patience – do not jump to conclusions; wait to see something at least three times before making an invitation for change or exploration
- Put the student and their inner experience in charge

Basic Aspects of Nonverbal Communication

Understanding nonverbal communication can be as helpful for yoga teachers as for clinicians. The following nonverbal aspects of behavior and self-expression can be attended to and are dealt with in much more detail in the section entitled "Non-Verbal Communication and Listening" in Brems's (2001) *Basic Skills in Psychotherapy and Counseling*. These aspects of communication are helpful in augmenting observations of students (the current context); however, they are also extremely relevant to how teachers and clinicians communicate their own intention, experience, and message to students. It is equally important to attend to students' nonverbals as to teachers'. A few useful categories that can be observed and expressed are as follows.

- Interaction between verbal and nonverbal communication – how nonverbal communication reinforces, contradicts, or alters verbal communication:
  - *repetition*: when verbal and nonverbal cues align (e.g., a teacher says "lovely expression" with a genuine smile and nod), they strengthen the message and help others feel assured of its authenticity

- o *contradiction*: a verbal statement such as "I am fine" paired with a slouched posture or sad facial expression creates confusion, indicating the need to read between the lines
- o *substitution*: sometimes nonverbal cues replace words altogether, such as a thumbs-up instead of saying "go for it"
- o *complementation*: nonverbal expressions, such as using animated gestures when sharing exciting news, add emotional depth to the verbal message
- o *accenting*: emphasizing key points with vocal tone, volume, or hand movements can help highlight critical parts of a communication, ensuring better understanding
- o *regulation*: nonverbal cues, such as pausing, leaning in, or making eye contact, guide conversational flow by signaling when to speak, listen, or end a dialogue
- Physical appearance – what is conveyed by nonverbal expressions that influence perceptions and interactions:
  - o *physical attributes*: traits like height, body shape, or physical abilities can unintentionally affect how others interpret confidence or authority – beware not to draw inaccurate conclusions or to succumb to stereotypes
  - o *fitness and health*: someone with a fit, energized demeanor may nonverbally communicate vitality and discipline, while visible signs of illness or fatigue might signal vulnerability
  - o *grooming and dress*: clothing, hairstyle, and personal hygiene may reflect social attitudes, cultural norms, or professional intent; for example, someone dressed neatly might convey competence, whereas an unkempt appearance might imply stress or indifference
- Kinesics – expressions and movements that are central to decoding emotions, intentions, thoughts, and more:
  - o *facial expressions*: smiles, frowns, or raised eyebrows provide immediate emotional cues; for example, a warm smile may foster trust, whereas a furrowed brow may signal confusion, aversion, or discomfort
  - o *gestures*: hand movements, such as open palms, signal honesty or openness, while crossed arms might suggest defensiveness or disengagement
  - o *body movements*: nervous habits, like fidgeting or shifting weight, might reveal discomfort or impatience. purposeful movements, like standing tall, suggest confidence
  - o *posture*: a straight, upright posture conveys attentiveness and self-assurance, while slouching may indicate disinterest or low energy
- Paralinguistics – the way words are spoken that conveys meaning beyond literal content:
  - o *speech fluency*: smooth, uninterrupted speech may suggest confidence and preparedness, whereas excessive hesitations or fillers like "um" or "uh" might indicate or be perceived as nervousness or uncertainty
  - o *rate of speech*: speaking quickly may signal excitement, or urgency; slow speech may suggest calmness, thoughtfulness, or deliberate emphasis or it may be due to uncertainty and hesitation
  - o *prosody*: variations in pitch, tone, and rhythm add emotional layers to communication; for example, a rising intonation may imply a question; monotone delivery might reflect disengagement or collapse
  - o *speech patterns*: repetition, pauses, or deliberate articulations can emphasize key points, helping others focus on the intended message
- Proxemics – use of space and what it reveals about comfort levels, relationship dynamics, and cultural preferences

- *proximity*: standing or sitting closer to someone may indicate familiarity or trust, while maintaining distance can signify formality or discomfort; for example, a yoga student who places their mat near the instructor might seek guidance, while choosing a far corner may indicate shyness or a desire for privacy
- *choice of positioning*: whether clients position themselves at the front, middle, or back of a yoga room or how they angle themselves (face forward versus to the side to avoid eye contact) can reveal level of confidence or intention to participate
- *orientation*: angling one's body toward another person tends to demonstrate engagement, whereas turning away may signal disinterest or withdrawal
- Timing – timing that reflects an individual's priorities, respect, and emotional state through behaviors and actions:
  - *chronic lateness*: repeated tardiness for sessions might suggest disorganization, lack of interest, or deeper issues such as anxiety or personal challenges
  - *missing classes or sessions*: absenteeism could indicate disengagement, overwhelm, or conflicting priorities
  - *specific actions at specific times*: timing of reactions (e.g., laughing at the wrong moment or responding to a question too slowly) may reveal miscommunication or discomfort; in a yoga context, someone who consistently aligns with the instructor's pace may feel unsure and desire additional support, whereas a student who times movement with their own breath rhythm may feel integrated and whole

Seeing and Understanding Collapsing, Contracting, and Yielding in All Koshas

Observations of collapse, contraction, and resilience are in a way a summary of all other observations and teaching principles discussed thus far. These ways of holding the body, expressing the breath, manifesting mind and emotions, and reflecting wise intuition integrate aspects of grounding, expansion, and stability (Brems, 2024b). They reflect lines of energy and speak of all koshas. They may reflect histories of trauma, polyvagal defaults, and current autonomic nervous system states and patterns, including arousal or energy. This way of looking at clients (or ourselves) – observing whether they are collapsed, gripped, or resilient – gives information about all koshas, reflects the gunas, gives evidence to vedana and kleshas, reveals the vrittis and samskaras – especially as flavored by the kleshas and gunas, and can provide profound hints about behavioral and relational patterns of our clients.

Noticing collapse, bracing, and yielding allows us to begin to notice, appreciate, even understand our clients' habits, conditioning, reactive styles, and unconscious responses to life in general and on the mat in particular. We can note if our students make conscious choices with discernment or react out of habit; we can see if they express and embrace a sense of agency, self-empowerment, and curiosity. We can appreciate whether students perceive possibilities or limits, openness or boundaries. Observation of these concepts is the culmination of our understanding and subsequently tailored and adaptive cuing for students. It is truly seeing students with an open heart and open mind to better teach and guide them in their practice on the mat and in their life. It is helpful to attend to how participants *embody a practice*. Are they collapsed and resigned, gripped and tense, or adaptable and resilient (Farhi, 2005; Mitchell, 2019; Porter, 2013; Schiffmann, 2013)?

Once the embodiment of asana is seen and understood, it is helpful to understand how collapse, contraction, or resilience manifest or fail to manifest in students' energy (arousal and affect) and mind (mental fluctuations as flavored by the kleshas, as well as emotions).

As teachers, we attend to collapse/resignation and contraction/tension versus resilience/yielding in students' expression across all koshas to notice how to issue invitations or cues for physical, energetic, mental, and emotional adjustments to create a practice that is honest, healthful, and reflective of students' current needs and resources. We can observe clients' physical, energetic, even mental or emotional presence to begin to get a sense of whether students have a tendency (or habitual way) to give up, resign, collapse, and buckle; grip, tense, over-effort, and grind; or respond, adapt, adjust flexibly, and yield to the demands of the practice (or life, for that matter). Patterns, habits, or ruts (samskaras in any kosha) can close down choice, shut down openness, and limit possibilities for practitioners. They tend to shut down agency, disempower, and short-circuit discernment and choice. Noticing tendencies and habits related to collapsing, gripping, or yielding invites us and our students back into beginner's mind, to a place of unlimited possibility, a place of exploration and options. It supports new self-awareness that can lead to greater agency, resilience, and self-efficacy.

As we observe students (or ourselves) in these ways and get to know them (and us) more intimately, we can begin to integrate cuing that is individualized and tailored, inviting students into a more intimate practice that is adapted to their needs. We invite clients into beginner's mind; we offer them opportunities to start over and reassemble a shape or breath in a new way, from a new foundation; we continuously encourage them to attend to grounding, stabilization, and expansion; we cue them into the experience of process, not the attachment to or seeking of particular outcomes, goals, or results. If we see their collapse, we can invite them into a rallying of resources, a deeper engagement, an experience of joy or pleasantness. If we see their bracing, we can offer them a pathway into ease, sweetness, softness, and gentleness; we can encourage them to release expectations, loosen their grip, free their straining. We help our students open up to new possibilities and new experiences. We invite them to surrender habit, stress, and expectations.

Teachers' observational skills of collapse, contraction, and resilience in students are honed over time. Once refined, the ability to observe these physical, energetic, mental, and emotional manifestations of students becomes an invaluable guide for cuing. When clients are observed to collapse, they may be invited to reengage, to rally resources to bring more energy into a form. On the other hand, when students are observed to brace, clench, or grip, they may be invited to find more ease, to access a softer approach and embodiment of the shape, to ease up on mental expectations about their performance, or to let go of excessive attachment to an outer form. Such invitations help students open up their bodies, hearts, and minds; they help students learn, unlearn, and relearn.

Of course, as yoga professionals we also note these tendencies in our own practice and life and remind ourselves to maintain vigilance about falling into physical, energetic, mental, or emotional habits, routines or ruts, or patterns that create reverberations in the practice on the mat, in our personal lives, and in our teaching.

Collapsing or Buckling

The practice of clients who are collapsing or giving up tends to be on the disengaged end of the spectrum, perhaps unintegrated and lethargic. It may be marked by sagging, slackness, lack of engagement, and under-efforting in body or energy and may be accompanied by limited mental presence and emotions of despair, helplessness, depression, or giving up. Buckling may show up as a collapsed resignation or crumpling into a shape, rather than a resilient and engaged yielding to it. There is neither much effort, nor true ease. The engagement and presence of abhyasa is minimal and lines of energy seem collapsed or non-existent.

Collapse can arise from *excessive grounding* or it may signal that the student is confusing relaxation with laxity or nonattachment with giving up. It may also signal a *lack of stability* and lack of engagement in key musculature leading to unprotected, loose joints and shapes or movements that lacks vigor and strength emanating from the center. Collapse may reflect a *lack of expansiveness*, purpose, or direction – showing up as a haphazard or half-hearted embodiment of a shape or movement.

Collapse may be a sign of lack of integration, disconnection from the body, apathy, or resignation. Anatomically and energetically, collapse is often accompanied by a deeply tucked pelvis (rolled posteriorly) with a rounded upper spine (arching forward) and head rolled up and back, with the throat hyperextended in front and the neck compressed in back. This may look like severe slouching, where all effort in the body has evaporated, and there is no joyful sense of ease. The back musculature is lengthened and the chest musculature is shortened pulling the chest and head forward while creating a rounded back. This anatomical embodiment of withdrawal or disheartenment can result in hyperkyphosis. This is alignment of the pelvis, rib basket, and head misaligns the spine and narrows the lower chest cavity, often interfering with a free and natural flow of breath. It typically results in shortened psoas and hamstring muscles (interfering with the natural relationship of the muscles with one another), often leading to hip and low back pain. Since shortened psoas muscles are a hallmark of a (reactive) self-protective stance, it is linked to chronic sympathetic arousal that can lead to burnout. Finally, shortened psoas muscles interfere with free diaphragmatic movement, impeding natural breathing.

Buckling or collapsing tends to be linked to a more tamasic nature and may – in extreme cases – signal dorsal collapse. It can also be related to burnt out chronic sympathetic arousal that has resulted in physical, energetic, and mental exhaustion. Collapse as a response to excessive challenge in one particular situation (e.g., type of pose) may simply be situational (a temporary *state* of being). Collapse as a general pattern (or *trait*) may reflect a more samskaric habit that may also manifest in life off the mat.

Possible manifestations of collapse across the koshas might be as follows (just a few examples):
- In annamaya kosha collapse may manifest as under-exerting, inadequate use of force or strength, lack of sufficient engagement or stretching in the muscles
- In pranamaya kosha collapse may manifest as shallow breathing, breathing weakly, collapse of the breath or energy, under-control of breath or energy; laxity in energy; absence of engaged emotion; lack of resilience and recovery in the breath; hypoarousal and unpleasant feeling tones

- In manomaya kosha collapse may manifest as sluggishness, depressive thoughts, not caring about what is happening, being hopeless, or giving up; the kleshas of fear and confusion may move into the foreground and may flavor thoughts and emotions and, in turn, physical and energetic expressions of the practice

Synonyms For Talking About Collapse			
Too Loose – Collapsed, Buckled			
• Buckling • Under-efforting • Tamasic • Dorsal vagal • Disengaged • Flaccid • Drooping • Sagging • Removed • Dispirited • Absent	• Limp • Nonresponsive • Uninvolved • Unintegrated • Indifferent • Fragmented • Hopeless • Withdrawn • Dissociated • Dissociative • Despairing	• Crumpled • Loose • Dull • Disconnected • Detached • Disheartened • Downhearted • Lax • Self-deprecating • Inattentive • Listless	• Having given up • Re- or unmoved • Disinterested • Indifferent • Apathetic • Slack • Careless • Haphazard • Resigned • Passive • Submissive

Contracting or Bracing

Contracting is marked by gripping, tension, and over-efforting, as well as a certain physical, emotional and/or mental rigidity or constriction. It can manifest as a fighting against or an active and stressful retreat from the present moment's demands, rather than a yielding to demands of the practice (or life in general). There may be an aspect of stubbornness and overcontrol in bracing that reflects a mindset of needing to be on alert, over-prepared, or simply over-ambitious about an inner state or outer form. Self-judgment and a chronic and pervasive sense of tension may emanate from the student who contracts into such tightness. There is an overabundance of effort, untampered by the sweetness of ease or delight. The joy has been sucked out of the practice. The engagement and presence of *abhyasa* errs on the side of effort and *vairagya* is often minimal to absent as attachment of outcomes overrides the joy and delight of the process. Lines of energy are forced and lack a sense of freedom or excitement. Everything looks like work; there is little to no play in the practice.

Contraction can arise from *excessive grounding* in the sense of trying too hard to find support and create a sense of connection. Bracing may signal that the student is confusing intensity with tension, commitment with obsession, persistence with perseveration. However, excessive grounding is not always part of this type of gripping. More often bracing signals an *excessive attempt at creating stability or safety* to the point of rigidity, forcing, clenching, or overcontrol. Contraction may include a *lack of expansiveness*, purpose, or direction – all force is directed inward or toward gaining a sense of control (often for self-protection of some sort). There is an inner tension and overcontrol that inhibits the path to joy and embrace of lightness that comes from expansiveness.

Bracing may be a sign of gripping and overcontrolling the body, forcing or muscling into shapes or movements in a way that creates tension, not joy or resilience. Anatomically and energetically, bracing is often accompanied by a slightly tucked pelvis (rolled a bit posteriorly, but close to neutral) with a lifted chest (rolled posteriorly), a head that is rolled up and back (with a hyperextended throat and compressed neck), and excessively depressed and retracted shoulder; at times, the belly is sucked in with an overreliance for stability on the rectus abdominus and an under-reliance on the more resilient and freeing transverse abdominis. This may look like good posture but on closer inspection, the body is held with excessive effort and tension; ease and joy are absent. The back musculature is shortened, compressing the spine in the low back and neck, muscles are tense around joints, and the chest musculature is lengthened, pulling the chest upward so the low ribs jut out. This anatomical embodiment of over-engagement and overcontrol can result in chronic muscle tension.

Further, as noted above, posterior alignment of the pelvis results in shortened psoas and hamstring muscles leading to hip and low back pain and interfering with free movement of the diaphragm, impeding natural breathing. It also leads to a braced core (rather than a resilient or strong core) that does not yield to load but is always overefforting and overengaged, contributing further to low back pain. This bracing is largely due to an over-engagement of rectus abdominis in pelvic tucking and a disabling of the transverse abdominis. All in all, the anatomic alignment that accompanies bracing interferes with spinal health, impedes natural breathing, and activates the sympathetic nervous system.

Contracting, bracing, or tensing is linked to a more rajasic nature and may – in extreme cases – signal sympathetic arousal. This SNS arousal can mean engagement at a level of fight, resulting in defensive or self-protective action that is overly engaged, aggressive, confrontational, or controlling in an attempt to gain control of a difficult situation. Alternatively, this SNS arousal can mean engagement at a level of flight, resulting in defensive or self-protective action that is in the service of extracting the students actively from a challenging situation via over-efforting in an attempt to avoid harm or escape a potential threat. Like, collapse, contraction can be situational (a temporary, even one-time *state*) or habitual (a lasting and deeply-patterned *trait*), the latter reflecting deeply ingrained samskaras or nervous system conditioning.

Possible manifestations of bracing across the koshas might be as follows (just a few examples):
- In annamaya kosha it may manifest as over-muscling, excessive use of force or strength, creation of traction (stickiness in the muscles), excessive tension (too much pulling or stretching) in the muscles; it may also show up as gripping in places irrelevant to the pose: e.g., gripping in the jaws or tongue; grimacing; or holding the breath
- In pranamaya kosha it may manifest as holding the breath, breathing too hard, freezing, over-control of breath or energy; stickiness in breath or energy; intensely unpleasant feeling tones; excessive arousal and possible hyperreactivity
- In manomaya kosha it may manifest as agitated thoughts, forcing a rigid story or expectation about the pose or the practice, being more attached to the outer expression of the pose than the inner experience, being driven toward achievement in the practice; the kleshas of clinging, grasping, aversion, or ego can show up forcefully

Synonyms for Talking about Contraction			
Too Tight – Contracted, Grasping			
• Bracing • Over-efforting • Rajasic • Sympathetic • Over-engaged • Tight • Reactive • Overinvolved • Inhibited • Overcontrolled • Grim	• Clenched • Too determined • Grasping • Obsessive • Forced • Strained • Hyper • Overactive • Overconfident • Self-judging • On alert	• Holding • Greedy • Gripped • Scrunched • Driven • Coerced • Constricted • Stressed • Overly ambitious • Squeezed • Strongminded	• Tense • Insistent • Resolute • Unbendable • Unyielding • Stubborn • Trapped • Restricted • Perseverative • Dogged • Tightly wound

Resilience or Yielding

Resilience or yielding means that the practice is well-balanced in all koshas. There is neither observable over- nor under-controlling; the student practices neither with reactivity nor resignation. There is neither laxity nor excess effort or tension. The student is clearly responsive to the necessary aspects of the practice – finding strength or engagement where it is needed and finding softness or gentleness where it is indicated. The balance of effort and ease is visible in all actions; there is engagement and interest without striving for a particular outcome – an abundance of abhyasa and vairagya. The client combines grounding, expansion, and stability in just the right proportions, truly finding the middle way in all koshas. There are clear lines of energy and clarity as well as pliability in mind and emotions. All koshas are present in the practice with (self-)compassion, (self-)care, joy, and equanimity. There is evidence of awareness, attention, and mindfulness; the student has access to all 'ceptions. Their window of tolerance in all koshas is optimal and wide, with an accompanying experience of agency and self-empowerment, embedded in compassion and lovingkindness.

Resilience arises from *stable and responsive grounding* that connects the student to an unwavering commitment to be present, engaged, and involved. It signals a *coherent sense of stability and integration* in key musculature, breath and energy, and mind and emotion. This stability is buoyant, resilient, steady, and adaptable. Resilience reflects a *purposeful expansiveness* – a joyful embrace of lightness, sense of humor, self-acceptance, and non-attachment to an outcome accompanied by clarity of purpose, direction, and meaning.

Resilience combines effort and ease; integrates all koshas; accesses grounding, expansion, and stability; combines all aspects of being human into holistic presence. Anatomically and energetically, resilience is often accompanied by a slightly tilted pelvis (rolled a bit anteriorly [~5°], but close to neutral) that allows for the natural resilient alignment of the spine along the vertical axis. The spine is elongated and open; it is flexibility and responsive; bones are aligned naturally in such a way as to minimize tension in muscle and connective tissue. The pelvis moves as a single unit and serves as the foundation for spinal movement and stability in all types of movements – whether sitting, bending, walking, standing, rotation. The rib basket is slightly anterior with the low ribs drawing toward the anterior superior iliac spine without shortening the front body. The head, too, is slightly anterior and rests well balanced on top of the spine at the atlas. This anatomical embodiment of resilience, of rolling with the punches, of adapting and responding, supports spine health, connective tissue cohesiveness, and muscular integrity and responsiveness. It frees the breath to move naturally and deeply into the body through resilient and dynamic movement of the diaphragm. The psoas and hamstring muscles are relaxed, elastic, and supportive of an upright position. They coordinate effectively (with each other, the core muscles, and the diaphragm) to create ideal balance. The core musculature is engaged but not tense, biased toward the use of the deep rather than superficial abdominal muscles. Resilience fully integrates and embodies *sthira* and *sukha*; it actively combines and expresses *abhyasa* and *vairagya*.

Resilience or yielding is linked to a more sattvic nature and tends to be associated with a ventral vagal nervous system response. The student rests in personal agency, expresses a sense of personal power, is available to (as recipient) and for (as provider) co-regulation, and can access adaptive responses to most if not all demands. Resilience shows up as an open-heartedness about the practice and about life that embraces and accepts with the ability to take action, confront challenge, access personal power, and be a free and compassionate agent.

Possible manifestations of resilience across the koshas are as follows (these are just examples):
- In annamaya kosha it may manifest as softness in strength and strength in softness; as stillness in movement and movement in stillness; as healthy muscle tone that supports the pose with easeful effort; as finding the physical middle way that integrates effort and ease and while expressing abhyasa and vairagyam
- In pranamaya kosha it may manifest as an easeful breath that is adaptive to respiratory needs; a smooth breath that is not dysregulated by increasing or decreasing demands; a balanced breath (or lengthened exhalation) that reflects a ventral vagal nervous system state; appropriate affective engagement with the practice and the community; balanced or easily rebalancing (i.e., adaptive and allostatic) levels of arousal; pleasant feeling tones or the capacity to easily reregulated in the presence of pleasant or unpleasant feeling tones
- In manomaya kosha it may manifest as clarity in thoughts, willingness to surrender habitual ways of viewing the practice; insight into the need for openness to using props and modifications; inspired ways of analyzing what is happening; clarity and presence; accurate appraisal of physical and emotional needs; willingness to explore something new

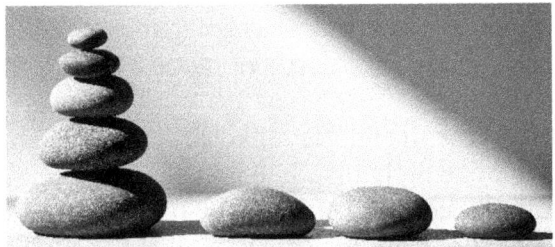

Synonyms for Talking about Resilience			
Just Right – Resilient, Yielding			
• Stable • Easeful effort • Sattvic • Ventral vagal • Engaged • Relaxed • Responsive • Peaceful • Balanced • Grounded • Self-compassionate	• Calm • Invigorated • Involved • Cohesive • Focused • Attentive • In the sweet spot • Integrated • Natural • Steady • With the middle way	• Unwavering • Committed • Established • Secure • Durable • Maintainable • Sustainable • Elastic • Resilient • Coherent • Nonattached to outcome	• Pliable • Uncomplicated • Safe • Hopeful • Fully present • Alert • Serene • Buoyant • Free • Lucid • Persistent not insistent

The tables with synonyms of these three concepts of bracing, collapsing, and yielding can be applied across the koshas. These synonyms can guide observation – allowing yoga professionals to better frame what they observe in the context of these three categories of practice experience and expression. These synonyms can also be used in cuing to help clients transform the extremes of buckling or grasping toward resilience and yielding.

> **To do anything well you must have the humility to bumble around a bit,
> to follow your nose, to get lost, to goof.
> Have the courage to try an undertaking possibly doing it poorly.
> Unremarkable lives are marked by the fear
> of not looking capable when trying something new.**
> Epictetus

Next, we will explore how to offer practices that are tailored and person-centered. We will explore use of props, demonstrations, variations, and adaptations. The we will explore how to offer additional supports that invite a personally adapted and adjusted practice that meets students and clients were they are in all their koshas.

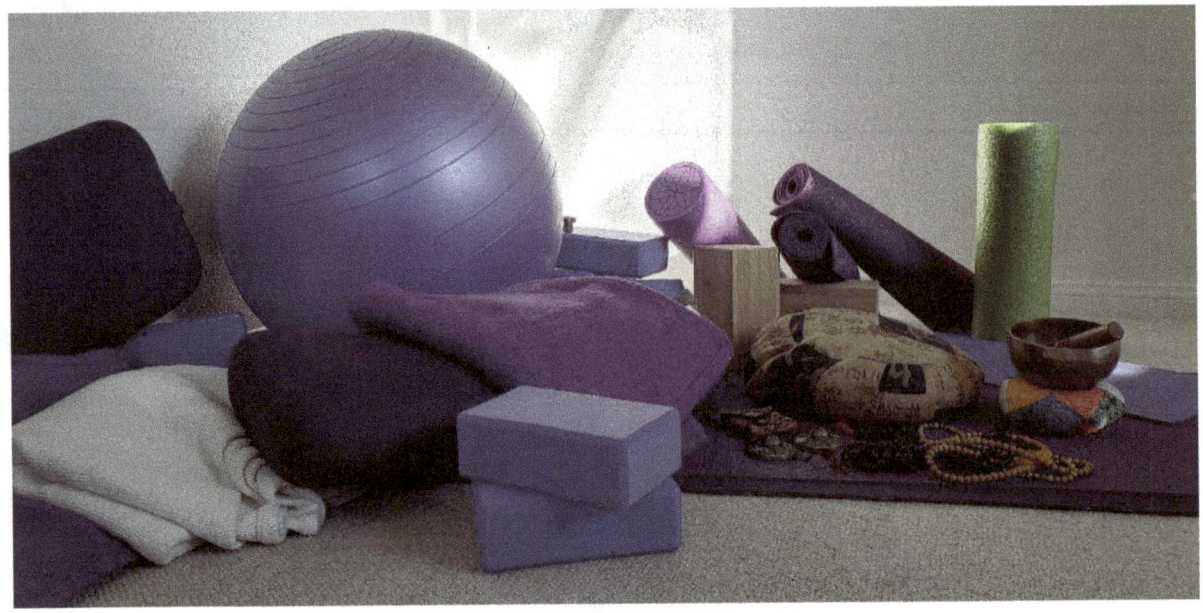
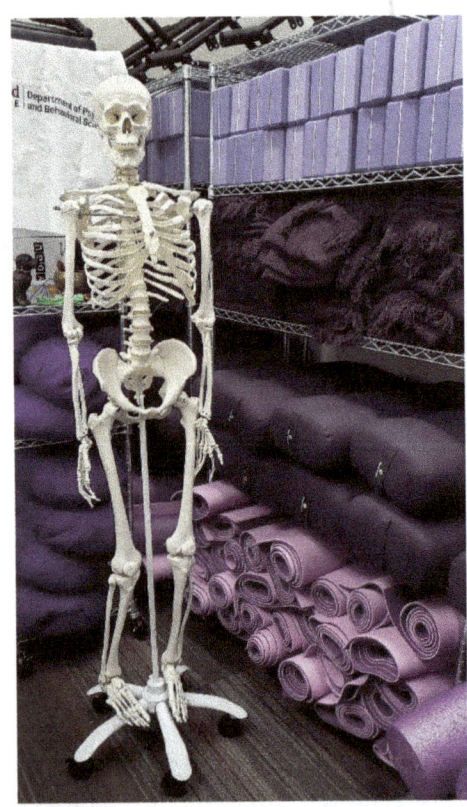
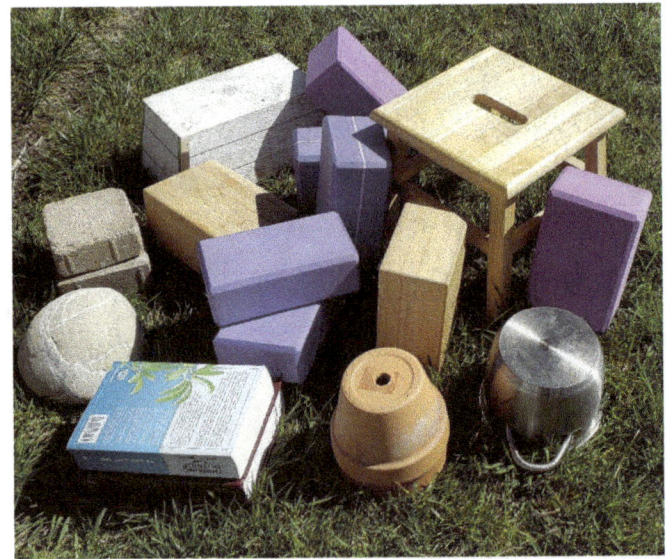

Chapter 10: Skillfulness in Providing Tailored Therapeutic Yoga

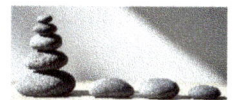

There is no yoga practice for which there is a single, peak, final, or complete expression. All forms, movements, breathing, and inward practices have a range of expressions (or variations) that are idiosyncratic and unique to each yogi who engages in them. Yoga practice reflects individuality, unique ways of moving, reacting or responding, individual nervous system adaptations, personal mind states, unique ways of thinking and believing, idiosyncratic emotions and hearts, as well as behavioral and relational tendencies.

Given the assumption of a unique expression of yoga for each practitioner, yoga professionals learn to make discerning choices about how to skillfully guide clients and students via cuing, demonstration, choices of variations and adaptations, and guidance that offers tailored assists and adjustments. The default is to offer choices and options in every practice, informing clients from the very beginning and all along that *they are in charge of the chosen expression of any practice*. All options, whether variations, adaptations, or alternatives rely on ample use of yoga props, introducing props as expressions of personal choices of *ahimsa, satya, asteya, brahmacharya,* and *aparigraha* toward oneself.

Offering props, variations, adaptations, and alternatives is the very essence of creating accessibility and doing no harm. Accessibility ensures that yoga professionals choose yoga practices and variations appropriate for students' state of health, nervous system, state of mind, and in-the-moment needs. All aspects of human experience, from anatomy and physiology, to breathing and arousal or affective tone, to emotional and mental presence, are subject to tremendous individual variations as well as to environmental or external factors. Anatomy (e.g., number of ribs, degree of thoracic kyphosis), physiology (e.g., hypersensitivity to carbon dioxide), psychology (e.g., polyvagal state), air quality, air temperature, type of movement, and many other variables affect experience and reactivity and, in turn, are affected by the yoga practice. These individual and environmental factors require that yoga practices of all types (whether movement, breathing, meditation, or relationships) be adapted to individual clients and their specific context and needs.

Wise Choices about Yoga Props

Accessibility includes the offering of appropriate props, such as blankets, bolsters, blocks, and more. However, it does not end there. Accessibility honors all layers of self and the biopsychosociocultural context of each person. Accessibility is reflected in the environment in which a session takes place (whether in a yoga or medical space) that may signal or fail to convey inclusivity and openness, equity and social justice, beneficence and compassion, professionalism and ethical commitment. Accessibility is reflected in language and cuing – via connotations of inclusivity versus exclusivity, authority versus autonomy, directiveness versus agency, compassion versus judgment, criticism versus open-minded exploration, and so much more. Clearly, whole books could be and, in fact, have been written about creating accessibility across a range of human dimensions. As yoga professionals, we must educate ourselves about how to make practices optimally beneficial and accessible by taking advantage of the wonderful resources that already exist (Bondy, 2020; Heyman, 2024; Johnson, 2021, 2023).

Creating or Impairing Accessibility Through the Use of Props

Props can create access to yoga practice in a variety of ways, including through providing support, limb extension, resistance, therapeutics, balance, introspection, joy, empowerment, extra load, decreased load, strength building, binding, warmth, comfort, ease, added effort, tethering, cushioning, lifting, safety, alignment enhancement, breath enhancement, meditative focus, sense withdrawal, concentration, calming, tension release, and more. Through all of these functions, yoga props often are used increasingly often as clients' practice advances.

Props are not affectations, 'crutches', items to make up for inability, or shameful implements that show up what we cannot do. They are items of personal choice, tools to express compassion for personal needs and preferences, avenues of access to different aspects of a pose or breath, expressions of personal agency and empowerment, and investments into personal wellbeing.

Props can also be presented and used in ways that inauspiciously or unconsciously hinder access to the yoga practice. Such use of props may be a reflection of cultural appropriation or otherwise hinders yoga practice from being embraced with an open heart, mind, and hand. For example:
- *Capitalism:* Western materialism and capitalism have created a usury yoga prop industry that suggests that yoga can only be available to those who can afford the expensive stuff that we see in conventional media, from $100 leggings to $70 folding chairs or $30 foam blocks. The appropriation of yoga and socioeconomic discrimination within western yoga due to capitalism must be named but does not have to rule our relationship with props. There are alternatives to expensive yoga props that are affordable; many fancy yoga props can be substituted with things most people already own; quite a few props can be made from scratch through creativity. Additionally, not everyone needs to have all props that exist in the yoga world. Yogis can decide for themselves which props will enhance their practice and feel important or even essential and put their resources into the acquisition or personal manufacture of those items (or their substitutes).
- *Cumbersomeness:* Use of yoga props can be cumbersome and hence yoga professionals need to use structure and discernment in how they demonstrate, introduce, and sequence with props.

Potentially Helpful Yoga Props

Yoga props come in many shapes, sizes, variations, and forms – just like people. They have a wide range of functions and students have diverse relationships with yoga props. Some students have a relationship of shame with props, having had the experience of being introduced to props as ways of making up for perceived deficits or lack of ability. Other students have a relationship of empowerment with props, having experienced props as supporting their practice compassionately, inviting creativity into the practice, and tailoring the practice to personal needs and resources.

It is helpful to invite clients or students to explore if they have a particular relationship with (or bias toward) yoga props in general or certain props in particular. Personal histories, especially trauma histories, may alter the relationship with certain items and may affect when and how props are offered. For example, items such as straps may create particular connotations for some students. Such reactivity may not imply that the item cannot be used; however, it does suggest care in how props are presented.

A good practice is for yoga professionals to inform new students or clients beforehand which types of yoga props will be used and to explore if any of these items may have special meaning for students that need to be addressed.

1. Mats
   - *Sample uses*: the obvious use ☺; also rolled up as a block or bolster substitute or as a support under the back when supine
   - *Notes*: select size to match student dimensions; choose ecofriendly material to prevent toxic or allergic reactions
   - *Alternatives*: large towel, blanket, carpet
2. Foam and Sturdy Blocks or Bricks
   - *Sample uses*: arm extenders in forward folds to reach the floor, lifts under feel, supports under various body part (e.g., under sacrum in bridge pose), supports during restoratives, implements for balance challenge (e.g., standing on a block in tree pose)
   - *Notes*: blocks come in various sizes; the most versatile is 4"x6"x9"; narrower blocks can be helpful for smaller people or certain body locations; egg shaped blocks are also offered; shoulder stand blocks are also useful; best to calculate at least 2 blocks per student; bamboo, wood, or cork blocks can be useful for some uses that involve significant weight-bearing or balancing
   - *Alternatives*: stack of phonebooks taped together; small foot stools; stack of blankets (e.g., for shoulder stand), chairs, upside-down cooking pots, bricks, logs (beware of splinters...)
3. Blankets
   - *Sample uses*: cushioning for select body parts or full body, lifts (e.g., under sitz bones), covers for warmth or privacy
   - *Notes*: they come in cotton or wool; wool is sturdier but more prone to trigger allergic reactions in some students; cotton is preferred – these come with or without tassels – we recommend the blankets without tassels; wash blankets regularly (cotton needs more washings than wool as wool sheds dirt better)
   - *Alternatives*: any regular blanket, large beach towel, rolled up mat (depending on use)
4. Straps
   - *Sample uses*: arm or leg extenders to reach other body parts, supports to hold body parts together in restoratives, tethering for safety, to create traction between or across body parts, to create isometric actions
   - *Notes*: straps may be contraindicated for some individuals with complex trauma history – explore carefully with each individual client before use; straps come in various sizes; it is best to have an assortment; the most versatile length is 8 feet
   - *Alternatives*: tie, scarf, towel, resistance band, blanket, soft belt from a robe

5. Bolsters
   - *Sample uses*: cushioning, supports, lifts, restorative supports
   - *Notes*: various shapes and sizes exist and need to be matched to function; e.g., pranayama bolsters are skinnier and longer; cheap bolsters tend to be less soft and don't not have handles
   - *Alternatives*: large pillows or small sofa cushions
6. Towels
   - *Sample uses*: hygiene (e.g., to cover bolsters, blankets, etc.), supports under ankles, sweat removal; can substitute for straps in TIY, eye covers, supports under various body parts
   - *Notes*: we recommend one large and one small towel per student; many studios do not provide these as they have to be washed after each use; if not provided, ask students to bring them
   - *Alternatives*: blankets, items of clothing
7. Walls and door jambs
   - *Sample uses*: leaning against, support, safety, alignment checks, balance, resistance
   - *Notes*: freely available in most studios (there should be no mirror or window) and yet very underused; completely available at home
   - *Alternatives*: teacher's body (obviously there is risk associated with this ...), chairs, doors, partners
8. Chair(s)
   - *Sample uses*: supports, assists for individuals who cannot access the floor, alternate seat for meditation, balance, resting place
   - *Notes*: the best chair is a metal folding chair, possible with no back panel in the frame for more space for body parts; chairs typically are best used on top of a sticky mat to prevent sliding, especially when used with inversions or half-inversions
   - *Alternatives*: headstander, stacked blocks, blankets, regular chairs, yoga ball, wall – all depending on purpose
9. Balls
   - *Sample uses*: seats, can substitute for chair, tension release method (e.g., foot rolls), strength-building, balancing, stretching, opening, dexterity (especially in the toes), therapeutics; can be used as a spacer that can be squeezed for muscular engagement
   - *Notes*: these come in different sizes (large enough to sit on; medium to squeeze between the knees; small enough to roll under the feet; tiny – like marbles to mobilize the toes); they come in various densities (from very hard to squishy); it is best to have multiple sizes and densities available to accommodate different purposes
   - *Alternatives*: chair; tennis or squash balls, anything round that won't burst, blocks, bolsters, cushions
10. Wedges
    - *Sample uses*: lift under wrists or heels, lift under sitz bones, support under other props whenever an angled support is needed, therapeutics
    - *Notes*: these are not often made available in yoga studios but have incredible utility; they come in various shapes and size and function dictates chosen form
    - *Alternatives*: blanket, towel, small foam block, books, small pieces of wood, shims

11. Foam rollers
    - *Sample uses*: lifts, supports, massage apparatus for tight muscles, therapeutics
    - Notes: these come in various lengths and it is useful to have short and long rollers; use of the soft foam rollers maybe preferable to hard (Pilates) rollers
    - *Alternatives*: rolled up mat, towel, or blanket; clothing; bolster, balls, and more depending on use
12. Resistance bands
    - *Sample* uses: can substitute for straps, strengthening methods, breath sensitivity, resistance, binding body parts, therapeutics
    - *Notes*: these come in different tensions (yellow – easiest; red – medium; blue – tough; black – toughest); best to have all tensions available to accommodate needs of students; best to calculate two per student; some come with handles or loops; some are bands and some are tubes – choose form based on function to be served
    - *Alternatives*: yoga strap, soft scarf, tie, soft belt from a robe (however, none of these substitutes provides the flex and variable tension of a resistance band …); small hand weights
13. Headstander
    - *Sample uses*: headless headstand, support for down dog or forward folds with tight hamstrings
    - *Notes*: these are the best investment for teachers who want to teach headstand – they reduce the highest risks from headstand (cervical spine injuries); this prop needs instruction for use by the teacher and is best used by a wall, not in the middle of the room, especially with students who are not yet advanced in their practice
    - *Alternatives*: two yoga chairs or two regular chairs padded with sticky mats and placed on a sticky mat
14. Eye pillows and weighted bags
    - *Sample uses*: calming the nervous system, aroma therapy, sensory withdrawal, grounding, support, guarding the senses
    - *Notes*: for eye pillows, choose the lightest weight as these can cause problems with regular use if heavy and placed directly on the eyes; place bulk of weight on forehead and let the fabric cover the eyes; for weighted bags try filling your own bags with sand, rice, beans, or other items, including scented materials (e.g., lavender blossoms); be mindful of scent allergies and always ask permission to use scented materials with students
    - *Alternatives*: wash cloth, sock, small towel, homemade bags of any shape and size with a variety of fillings (for eye pillows, flaxseed is ideal); 5-lb bags of rice or beans

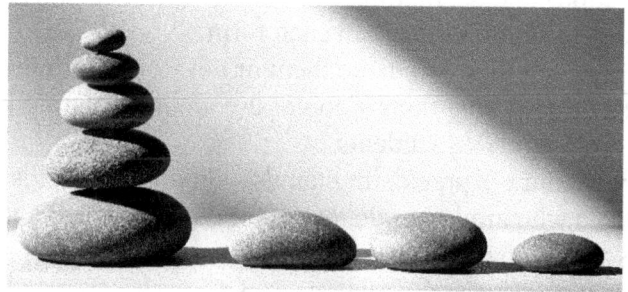

Planning for Variations, Adaptations, and Alternatives

Offering Variations to Meet People Where They Are

Auspicious teaching includes the offering of variations and adaptations to students' extant observable traits in all koshas, including any known physical (e.g., illnesses, injuries, and conditions), energetic, mental, or emotional challenges, illnesses, or conditions. Skilled teachers embrace the notion that for all asana and pranayama practices out of the basic (average) shape or action of a particular asana or pranayama an infinite number of variations can arise. There is no single expression of a form or a breath and there certainly is no "full expression" of a form or breath that is noted externally. The phrase 'full expression' – if that term is ever desirable –best refers to the *internal experience* of having found a variation of a form or breath in one's experience that feels integrated, whole, and healthful.

The following guidelines may be helpful as yoga professionals prepare for serving in a person-centered manner that honors participants' individual needs, resources, and strengths.
- Preplan variations and adaptations from the beginning
- Re-plan variations on the spot based on the people who arrive in your classroom – be creative in inviting personalized expressions of all shapes
- Keenly observe participants to glean needs from non-verbal communication – some individuals may not realize their own need for variations, may not be able to disclose needs or potential areas of injury, or may not realize that they have an injury or vulnerability – find ways of inviting them into variation without targeting them or stigmatizing them
- Verbally address – to the class as a whole – potential risks of particular forms or alignments (perhaps as you observe alignment issues in the room) and provide suggestions and invitations for their mitigation via adaptations, responsiveness, variations, and props

Recognizing and Drawing on Students Resources and Strengths

Be knowledgeable about participants' resources, strengths, needs, and presentations with attention that goes beyond the physical self, integrating as many koshas as possible. Ponder all of the following:
- Physical needs and resources (*annamaya kosha*)
    - use props and clarify that poses can actually be harder with props (demo example – e.g., Warrior 2 with chair)
    - demonstrate accessible pose variations – do not show off
    - be clear that variations and adaptations are not "less" but actually often "more" – encourage students to find their truth in each form
    - work with the gunas whether you name them or not; for example:
        - do not increase preexisting rajas – do not use an upregulating practice with already hyperactive or upregulated students
        - do not overly encourage preexisting tamas – do not use exclusively restorative poses with individuals who are lethargic, hypomobile, depressed, and so on
        - balance rajas with tamas and/or sattva
        - balance tamas with rajas and/or sattva

- if not sure about the student's presentation or if you have a very mixed class, teach a sattvic practice and empower students to self-regulate
- Emotional and energetic needs and resources (*pranamaya kosha*)
  - continue work with the gunas – with energetic/emotional (rather than physical) focus now
  - pay attention to the kleshas whether you name them or not; for example:
    - recognize attachment to outer manifestations of a pose – raga (attachment to pleasure and outcome, greed, desire, expectation to have things a certain way)
    - recognize misalignment due to lack of knowledge or misunderstanding of instruction – avidya (lack of wisdom, limited understanding, misinterpretation)
    - recognize aversion in the form of not wanting to engage in certain practice – dvesa (aversion to pain, hatred, enmity)
    - recognize ego in persisting with unhealthful expressions of poses or competitiveness with others or self – asmita (ego-absorbed individualism, identification with roles)
    - recognize fear or anxiety – abhinivesha (holding on to life, fear of change, anxiety about the new or unknown)
- Mental and cognitive needs and resources (*manomaya kosha*)
  - continue to recognize the gunas but now on a cognitive or mental level
  - continue to see the impact of the kleshas in the context of how they flavor cognition and mental fluctuations
  - work with the vrittis whether you name them or not; for example:
    - reinforce expressions of accurate perception, such as successful self-correction in a pose – pramana (right perception, verifiable knowledge)
    - invite exploration of misperceptions, such as helping students see misalignment or recognize loss of breath – viparyaya (misperception, faulty or illogical thinking; cognitive distortion)
    - invite the exploration of positive uses of imagery, such as guided meditations or imagining a version of a pose that is currently not accessible – vikalpa (fantasy, imagination, creative thinking, day dreaming)
    - support development of sleep hygiene, such as guiding sleep-supporting asana or meditation practices and talking about sleep hygiene (e.g., food, stimulation, lighting, circadian rhythms) – nidra (sleep, absence of thought, absence of the other vrittis)
    - explore use of memory and recollection as a positive guide for practice (e.g., remembering how to move into a posture mindfully) versus as a negative habit (e.g., having become habituated to a particular alignment that is less than healthful) – smriti (memory, recollection, remembrance)
    - discuss in all vrittis, as related to samskaras or habitual ways of responding, distorted cognitions, and harmful habits; discuss what fires together, wires together

Preplanning and Revising on the Fly

Yoga professionals may want to strive to have a clear plan for their chosen methods along with plans for making more refined, tailored, and discerning choices and revisions *once class has started*. Life often gets in the way of best-laid plans; it is helpful to remain flexible, alert, and open to changing course depending on observations and experiences in the classroom or office. Nevertheless, careful preplanning is helpful and can include the following – along with the flexibility to change all plans:

- Demonstrate responsive and beginning postures rather than advanced postures based on wat you see in the moment in the majority of your students
- Make ample use of props, with narrated reasons for use, in all forms and movements, basing selections on what you notice in your classroom as universal needs; if you address an individual need, ask participants to use discernment about whether they might want or need a particular prop
- Add or eliminate preplanned poses depending on needs presented by the people who are present – always have an outline that allows for flexibility to revise your plan based on what you see in class
- Always allow sufficient time for resting/recovery postures and closing meditations at the end of class

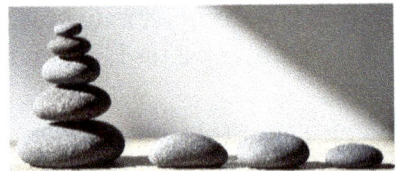

A Few Additional Considerations

Importance of Variations

Most shapes have excellent variations that make the practice available to most individuals. Decisions have to be made about which variation is shown by the yoga professionals in class and choices are most auspiciously calibrated to class level. Variations are terribly underused by teachers who tend to demonstrate the version of a particular form that is shown in yoga magazines or books. It is helpful for yoga professionals to think outside the box and to model more accessible versions of many forms. Here are some ideas:
- Wall versions
- Chair versions
- Multi-propped versions
- Simple-propped versions
- Accessible versions for people who are new to yoga
- Accessible and adapted versions for clients with particular needs

Importance of Adaptations and Propping

It is helpful to adapt practices, whether form, movement, breath, or meditation, to the specific needs of the people in front of us (Heyman, 2019). This may occur, for example, for individuals with an injury, a physical challenge, a missing limb, or similar circumstances. A few sample ideas follow (and can be gleaned above from the use of props). The possibilities for adaptation are truly unlimited and can create a wonderful sense of accessibility, empowerment, and agency in clients if offered freely and with the understanding that this is a compassionate and wise way to individualize and tailor a practice through a commitment to Limb 1 of yoga, to *ahimsa*, *satya*, *aparigraha*, *brahmacharya*, and *asteya*.

- A strap as arm extender in supine poses for individuals with tight hamstrings
- Blocks under hands in forward fold in case of low back problems or tight hamstrings
- Blanket or wedge under the seat if knees are too high (due to tight hips) in seated postures
- Blocks under hands in lunge posture to maintain open heart
- Chair under hands in down dog for tight muscles in back of legs or low back pain
- Sloped platform (made out of blocks, bolsters and blankets) for supine poses with individuals with low back problems or during pregnancy
- Chair under forward leg in warrior for individuals with balance issues or weakness
- Balancing postures with back at the wall for individuals with balancing issues
- Plank on forearms for individuals with carpal tunnel
- Blocks under an elbow or shoulder in case of a missing limb

Knowledgeability about Alternatives

Some shapes or movements may not be appropriate or accessible for some individuals or sometimes (e.g., full inversion for clients with glaucoma, deep backbend during pregnancy). When such practices are included in a general class environment, alternatives can easily be offered. A few samples follow, but only the teacher's creativity limits the options here. Clearly, the possibilities are truly unlimited.
- Child or puppy instead of down dog
- Legs-up-the-wall instead of headstand
- Handless small cobra instead of up dog
- Side-lying posture instead of supine posture
- Half lift instead of forward fold
- Windshield wiper instead of supine full twist
- Wide-legged forward fold instead of tripod headstand
- Bridge instead of shoulderstand (if shoulderstand is taught at all…)
- Half frog instead of bow
- Sweet seat instead of hero pose

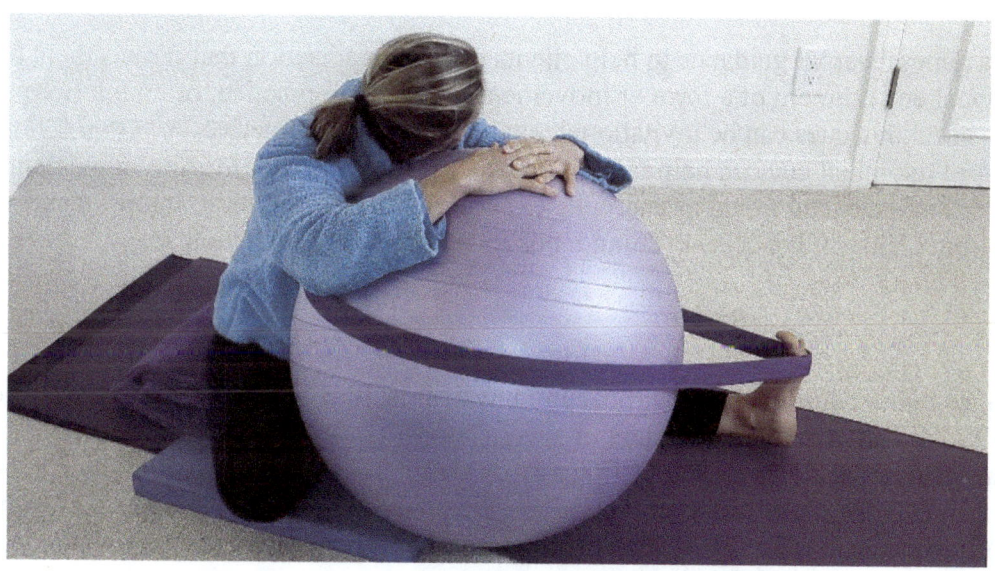

Guiding via Cuing, Assisting, Adjusting, and Adapting

Safety in yoga services arises not only from keen observation skills, proper demonstration, and the offering of variations, adaptations, and props. It also arises from the appropriate choice of client supports or guidance, including cuing, adjusting, assisting, and modifying. Such supports may be verbal or physical/tactile, with the safest default being verbal supports offered to the entire group of students based on in-the-moment observation.

Supports – instructions beyond initial cuing – are not offered routinely or randomly, but rather address a specific need in the moment either by an individual or several students. Thus, supports are predicated on the teacher's observational skills, student needs, and informed choices about least intrusive or directive levels of intervention to support and guide students toward increasingly healthful alignment, balanced breath, less dysregulated presentation, and emotional balance.

Supports have a clear purpose and are used with intention. Some are appropriate for the entire group of students; some need to be individualized by voicing to whom they may apply (e.g., special cuing about contraindications or risks, e.g., "if you have glaucoma, stay in a half lift rather than releasing into a forward fold"). Students may need to discern if a particular support is relevant to them and thus it needs to be clear from offered supports to whom and when they apply. All supports offer safe biomechanics, clear intentions, enhanced healthfulness of the embodied practice, and increased stability in body, breath, and mind.

Supports are offered in the spirit of increasing participants' sense of agency and autonomy, giving power of choice to students, and inviting clients to exercise their right to adapt the practice of yoga to their unique circumstances and needs. An occasion when this 'rule' might be broken is if an individual is in imminent danger of harm unless the teacher intervenes. Cuing, assisting, adjusting, and adapting (or varying) can intermingle and typically co-occur. It nevertheless helps to understand how each is defined and operationalized.

Cuing

Cuing is a general verbal guidance to help clients engage in an action that moves them toward their personal embodiment of a form or movement, a breathing practice, or an interior practice. Generally speaking, cues can be invitational, explanatory, or re-directive. A verbal follow-up or deepening of the initial cue can help facilitate further refinement of a form or movement, breath, mental focus or state, emotional or energetic experience, or attunement to intuition and interoception. Cuing and follow-up cuing tends to be directed to the whole class.

Adjusting

Adjusting provides additional verbal (possibly physical/tactile) support or guidance (beyond initial cuing) to help a particular student or several students achieve a small movement, subtle shift in any layer of self (physical body, energy or breath, mind or emotion, intuitive sense), minor positional change, or different type of muscle engagement (more relaxed versus more engaged). Adjusting is typically offered in response to observations of clients to help deepen their experience, find interoceptive awareness, or empower and invite personal choice. Adjustments are typically directed to the whole class though perhaps more relevant to some of the participants than others. If this is the case, the teacher verbalizes the conditions to which the cue is most relevant to invite participants to make their own empowered choice.

Assisting

Assisting integrates verbal or physical supports or guidance that help practitioners achieve a different depth of experience based on an intervention that is more significant than an adjustment. Assists are more likely to be physical than verbal and less commonly used than adjustments. They are used to enhance ease, decrease risk, or invite personal choice for a change in alignment or breath because of an observation by the teacher. Assists are offered when a teacher discerns that a participant could benefit very specifically from a particular change. Assists tend to be directed to specific individuals without necessarily calling them out by name, but by clarifying to what conditions or presentations the assist applies most directly.

Intervening

Directive interventions serve to create a necessary change in light of a potentially dangerous or risky expression of form, movement, or breath. They are typically used because of a student's known contraindication or potential risk that emerges from a participant's embodiment of an instruction or demonstration (e.g., asking a pregnant woman very directly no longer to lie in her back in *savasana* [though even this caution may be based on dated information – stay tuned]). Interventions can be verbal or physical. They are most likely directed to a specific individual or for a specific condition that is present in more than one person in the room.

Applications of Cuing, Assisting, Adjusting, and Adapting

Following are sample operationalizations of types of demonstration, cuing, adjustments, assisting, and adaptations – sequenced from least to most intrusive or directive. In each instance of using this succession, teachers proceed with caution and discernment tailored to the particular moment in time. In using these strategies, it helps to choose language that is supportive, invites agency, and empowers – as opposed to using language that suggests vulnerability or lack of resilience; much less lack of choice. Even when using these types of strategies, it is useful to offer choices and options when available so that accessibility of the practice is always at the forefront. All offerings are made in the spirit of imitating curiosity and exploration, yielding agency and power to the student as much as possible and reasonable.

It is also helpful to explain anatomically or energetically why certain safety cues or physical assists are offered and how they are helpful, especially in particular cases. In other words, the yoga professional's intention in offering one of these cues or assists is shared with the students. Such explanations are educational for participants and are more likely to help them generalize the learning to their personal practice at home. Additionally, explanation invites autonomy and empowers people in the moment. Risk of harm is directly addressed when it drives the intention behind a particular cue, assist, or adjustment.

Types of Demonstration, Cuing, Adjustment, Assisting, and Intervening

- *Demonstration* (see prior section) – yoga professionals (whether teachers or clinicians) demonstrate most relevant variations and prop uses for the particular students representing in a given class; always remember that demonstrations are for the benefit of the students who are present and need to seem relevant and accessible to them; demonstrations are not there for teachers to show off their practice or skill
- *Explanatory alignment or safety cues* are offered to entire class based on form, movement, or breathing practice being taught; in giving explanatory cues, it is helpful to favor the cuing of actions rather than outer shapes; this preference underscores that the practice is engaged in from the inside out, not the outside in – that shapes are brought and adapted to the student, not the other way around (i.e., we never force students to assume a particular outer shape or alignment, always remembering and prioritizing the bioindividuality of students' anatomy, energy and nervous system, and mental and emotional needs)
- *Corrective cues* to the entire class based on in-the-moment observations of common challenges, misunderstandings, or struggles; over time, teachers learn what to look for in a classroom and begin to note which types of corrections seem to be most commonly needed and useful; corrective cues are generally offered to the whole class, without singling out an individual student or subgroup of students; corrective cues based on a teacher's experience of common challenges in particular shapes or breathing exercises can be particularly helpful in online class settings when it is hard or even impossible to see individual students
- *Verbal adjustments* can be offered to specific students or particular groups of students in light of in-the-moment observation; these adjustments are just that: verbal; they are not tactile or touch-based; nevertheless, they are more specific than corrective cues in that they are most relevant to one or a few of the students and not as generically expected as corrective cues
- *Physical cues* that are less invasive potentially tactile contacts with students; rather than the teacher touching the student, these cues invite the student to bring a body part to or toward the teacher; the teacher uses her or his body as a prop in a way that invites the students to find an adjustment or alignment with a physical assist over which the student has complete control – in fact, the student can simply move toward the offered body part of the teacher without ever actually reaching or touching it; the student is in charge of the potential physical contact every step of the way; examples of such physical cues are as follows, with many, many more possibilities:
    - "what would happen if you brought your hand toward mine?" (e.g., teacher standing in front of a student in Warrior 2 to invite movement of the shoulder girdle forward to align above the pelvis)
    - "would you like to try what happens if you met my hand with your knee?" (e.g., teacher hovering a hand to the outside of a knee when the student is in a lunge with the knee collapsed toward the midline)
    - "notice how it might feel if you were to bring the back of your head toward my hand" (e.g., teacher's hand behind the student's head in downward facing dog)
    - "might there be more ease if you allow the weight of your arms to rest on my hands?" (e.g., teacher standing behind a student in Warrior 2 inviting the shoulder blades to release downward to ease excess effort or tension)
- *Physical assists* involve the teacher putting hands on the student. This is done gently, never forcefully or directive; preferably teachers do not move a student's body part but trace a

location on the body where a change to alignment may auspicious (e.g., tracing a V on the student's back to suggest retraction and depression of the scapulae); they guide the student toward a more healthful experience of the practice – see cautions and guidelines below for touch
- *RARE USE: Physical adjustment* tend to be longer physical contacts that encourage safe deepening or are offered as a support in a restorative or therapeutic form; they are gentle physical interventions that are never forceful or overpowering – see cautions and guidelines below for touch
- *SUPER RARE USE: Physical corrective actions* in light of imminent risk or danger is approached gently, with the least invasive and non-forceful touch; it is typically used after a verbal corrective cue was not successful in remedying a risk or contraindicated expression of a practice – see cautions and guidelines below for touch

Developmental and Respectful Approaches to Guiding Clients

- Understand the students' skill levels in offering supports – never push students beyond their safe developmental skill level or form expression, either verbally or physically
- Encourage participants to make clear choices about supports (e.g., offer flip cards that indicate whether a student is okay with physical touch; even if yes, always ask permission for informed, explicit, enthusiastic, and ongoing informed consent)
- Support client autonomy balanced with safety; empower students' decision-making and agency; educate, do not placate
- Assume participants are smart and capable – provide information and education; then invite people to self-adjust from there

Safety Considerations in Choices for Supporting or Guiding Clients

- Address or support safety issues (e.g., potentially harmful misalignments) before offering refinements
- Use verbal adjustments first; graduate to physical cues (inviting the student to bring a body part toward the teacher's hand) and then to light touch adjustment offered only with permission, with clear consent that is freely given and revokable
- Be precise in language when offering verbal supports
- If verbal redirects are not effective and it seems therapeutic or necessary to redirect the student for a very specific reason and in a very purposeful way, then a physical assist may be indicated; physical assists may also be offered in some settings in which students desire such intervention and are well-known to the teacher; the following section explores physical assists in some detail

Supportive Guidelines Related to Physical or Tactile Assists and Use of Touch

Touch reverberates into and best serves a purpose for all koshas. Touch may be tactile and physical in nature (directed most obviously to annamaya koshas), but it deeply affects and reverberates into all koshas, including energy, arousal, and affect in pranamaya koshas, thoughts and emotions in manomaya koshas, and relationship factors in vijnanamaya koshas.

Touch – however purposeful, consensual, and intentional – can be triggering. As teachers, we always are prepared to discontinue touch when we get the sense that the student is becoming reactive, uncomfortable, unsure, or otherwise uneasy in any kosha. We may be very well-intentioned, the client may have consented, and yet something feels off. We listen to our intuition and co-regulation. If we become uncomfortable, this may be a signal that the client is uncomfortable. If this happens, we gently discontinue the tactile contact while staying energetically and emotionally supportive and connected to the student.

The following guidelines are offered in the spirit of creating the greatest opportunity and likelihood for continued safety and wellbeing for participant and provider. They are not guarantees that everything will go smoothly. Learn to apologize if something goes wrong; learn to shift gears if something feels inappropriate. Always listen to the student; always observe and stay connected to all of their (and your own) koshas.

Explicit and Ongoing Informed Consent

Yoga professionals who are committed to integrated holistic yoga principles ask for and receive explicit verbal or otherwise clearly communicated permission that is freely, even enthusiastically, given and never coerced (however implicitly) for *each episode* of physical touch. Such a policy of ongoing informed consent optimizes the opportunity for safety as perceived by the participants – the individual who is receiving the cue directly and other students or clients who may be present if the intervention is offered in a group context.

The fooling suggestions or ponderings may be helpful:
- Become skillful in asking for consent to touch; it may not be as simple as saying "may I touch …" or "is it okay to place my hand …". Students may answer such a yes/no question with *yes* simply because they do not want to offend the teacher by declining the offer of support; instead consider asking permission in a way that offers choices; for example, you might state several options:
  - "I might be able to help you find greater ease in this shape. Would you like me to explain how you may adjust your stance, or would you like me to demonstrate how you could adjust by demonstrating it in my own body, or would you like me to use my hands on … to help you move …" With this invitation the student can choose a verbal adjust, a demonstration, or a tactile contact
- Become skilled at reading non-verbal communication when you ask for consent – there are individuals who may give verbal consent because they tend to yield to authority figures; however, they may give non-verbal indications that they are actually uncomfortable with being touched
- If you are doubtful about a client's authenticity and deeply felt sense of giving permission, choose not to touch and find an alternate means of working with the individual to find a more auspicious embodiment of the offered practice
- If the client has given verbal consent and tactile contact has been initiated and results in the individual's shrinking back or retracting from the touch, discontinue the touch and find a gentle and compassionate way to extract yourself from the tactile episode – not giving the participant a startle and definitely not embarrassing the person for having become reactive

- If you sense a <u>physical or emotional</u> pulling back or tensing in the individual *while* they give <u>verbal</u> consent, refrain from touch – give verbal adjustment another chance or cue the individual out and back into the practice in a new way
- If you are unsure about how the verbal and nonverbal communication align, ask again; then, if you move ahead with touch, monitor the student's reactions and be prepared to stop or even ask again while touching to give them opportunity to retract permission
- If in serious doubt, err on the side of caution and do not touch – just say that you changed your mind and offer more verbal assists

It is best to be clear that consent is given only for a specific episode of touch and that even within this episode, consent can be retracted at any time if students change their minds. As soon as there is evidence that an individual has changed their mind about touch (either explicitly or implicitly; verbally or nonverbally), touch is withdrawn as quickly and safely as possible (without either destabilizing the teacher or the student).

- Explicitly check in with the participant during the touch episode to offer opportunity to the student to retract consent
- End the touch immediately but respectfully, compassionately, and cautiously if the student shrinks back from it or seems clearly uncomfortable – consider this a nonverbal retraction of permission

Clear Intention with Explicit Verbalization of Purpose and Planned Action

Verbalize a Clear Intention

Have a clear purpose or intention for any request to provide physical adjustments or assists (Heyman, 2024; Lasater, 2021; Stephens, 2011) and name the purpose explicitly (time permitting in high-risk situations) when asking for permission/consent to touch a student. Do not touch randomly; have a clear intention and purpose for all offered physical contact. Not all purposes have to be specifically about alignment in a particular asana. The intention or purpose may also be connected to energy, breathing, or mental and emotional comfort or engagement.

Sample purposes or intentions may be as follows:
- Deal with an imminent risk, threat to safety, or specific danger
- Support greater healthfulness of alignment for a specific body part/region or for the movement of breath
- Clarify a verbal adjustment that was not understood but is necessary for the safety of the shape or breath
- Emphasize or direct attention to a particular region of the body where more ease or effort could be helpful to the shape, energy, breath, or level of comfort (including emotionally)
- Support the grounding or releasing of a body part/region, energy, breath, or emotional tension
- Invite greater comfort or ease into the experience of a shape, movement, energetic expression, or breath
- Support expansion or expansiveness in body, breath, or energy
- Stabilize or steady a body part/region, shape, or breath, emotion, or mental fluctuation

- Invite co-regulation of breath, energy, or arousal
- Help clarify directions, movements, or other actions that appear so confusing to a student that they cannot figure out what to do

Provide Specifics

Be specific about what you are offering in terms of physical contact with the participant. In other words, provide the what, where, why, when, and how of the touch or physical assist that is being offered (Lasater, 2021). Physical or tactile assists offered for energetic, mental, or emotional reasons need to be detailed in this manner as well, explaining both the type of tactile contact and its purpose.

Several issues are attended to, including, but not limited to the following:
- Give detail about the kind of touch you will use (defined in more detail with explicit examples below), with the following likely options:
  - *student-initiated touch* whereby the student is moving toward a body part (often the hand) of the teacher
  - *guiding touch* of the student by the teacher of the student to identify a particular body region or to suggest activation of a particular muscle or set of muscles
  - *directional touch* that guides a student's body region, limb, or the body overall in a particular direction without the teacher exerting any active force or effort
  - *supportive touch* in which the student gains an insight about or greater comfort in a body region, energetic movement, or emotional response to an asana or breathing practice
  - *stabilizing touch* in which the student may be supported by the teacher's body (typically via hands or arms) to gain greater ease in balancing a particular body region
  - *auspicious touch* of the student that invites a settling of a particular body region or the body overall
- Be explicit about the exact body part/region you are asking to touch, using appropriate anatomical (and clearly understandable) language:
  - students need to be clear exactly which part of *their body* will be touched and how
  - students need to be clear which body part of the teacher will be involved in the touch (e.g., hand, arm, leg)
  - do not touch sensitive or private body parts – even if the students implies that it is okay; never be invasive (not even potentially invasive)
- Give a timeframe for the touch:
  - clarify if the touch will be fleeting or lasting a few second
  - do not linger in a touch beyond what the student consented to or what seems appropriate
  - let the student know when you are about to initiate the touch
  - let students know when the touch is about to end to avoid destabilizing or surprising the students when the touch episode ends

Be Patient and Take Enough Time

It is very supportive and respectful to be specific about the details of what physical contact the teacher has to make and the necessary amount of time necessary for the interaction with the

student. Such specifics can be offered before, during, and after the touch episode. Following are a few considerations related to this specificity.
- Make sure there is enough time for the following steps:
    - to get permission – i.e., to gather and reaffirm consent
    - to inform – i.e., to make sure the student understands the purpose and specifics of the tactical contact
    - to attune – i.e., to stay relationally and emotionally connected to the student during the contact, and
    - to debrief – i.e., to answer questions during or after the contact
- If you do not have time to be deliberate and compassionate in collecting consent (e.g., in a very large or fast-paced class), do not touch unless there is an imminent threat or risk that must be addressed in a tactile manner
- If insufficient time is available to engage in consent and deliberate empowerment of the student, if a student is in a potentially harmful position, cue the entire class group to come out of the position rather than trying to offer a modification or intervention to a specific students (if at all possible)
- If there is insufficient time to complete the tactile contact in a manner that makes it truly helpful, do not engage in it
- If there is a clear emergency, intervene for the sake of safety (e.g., if a student is about to come to harm because of a fall or another participant's actions, step in and then be sure to debrief)

Continuous Yielding of Power and Agency to the Student

Ensuring Privacy

When you talk to a student about the offer of a physical assist, realize that other participants will be aware and may hear what you say. It is virtually impossible to guarantee privacy, much less confidentiality, in a group class and as the teacher, you need to stay aware of this reality. Consider the following issues related to privacy and transparency:
- The advantage of other students bearing witness to the episode of touch is that you can role-model for all in the class how you handle touch, which may add to a sense of safety for everyone.
- The challenge inherent in this situation is that you have to remain mindful of how you handle anything that may feel private or even confidential to the student to whom you offer the physical assist.

Choosing Least Restrictive and Least Intrusive Interventions

Do always yield the power during a physical assist or touch to the student to the greatest degree possible. Attempt to follow these guidelines of *least restrictive and least intrusive intervention*:
- Encourage student to move toward the teacher rather than teacher moving toward the student (e.g., "bring your head to my hand"; "reach your fingertips toward my palm")
- Encourage backing away more so than deepening

- Use the least amount of physical contact that is needed to achieve the stated intention – the smallest possible area, shortest possible duration, and the goldilocks amount of pressure (not too soft, not to hard – enough to be effective)
- Check-in with the student to invite the option to retract consent
- Check in with the student to see if the touch is "landing" appropriately
- Check in with the student to see how they perceive the touch and continue or discontinue commensurately

Do not deliberately or intentionally use physical touch that is intrusive or disempowering in any way. Try to make sure that you avoid touch that is or may be perceived as:
- Forceful, pushy, harsh, punitive, or aggressive
- Creepy, frightening, or suggestive
- Destabilizing or ungrounding *physically*
- Destabilizing or potentially perceived as threatening or intimidating *emotionally*
- Inappropriate (e.g., sexual, intrusive, interfering with student autonomy and self-determination)
- Random or not clearly intentioned/purposeful
- Unconscious or inadvertent – again without clear purpose
- Surprising, sudden, or unexpected

Do not touch or invade the following body parts (cf., Hansen-Lasater, 2021) as they are very sensitive, private, and potentially triggering – resist touching these areas of the body even if the student gives permission to do so!
- Face
- Chest, especially breasts
- Belly
- Buttocks
- Genital regions
- Inner thighs

Recognizing the Personal Impact

Notice and assess the potential physical, energetic, and emotional impact of your intervention and stance on the student, especially as related to how the participant's body or energy may move unexpectedly and how your own body is positioned vis-à-vis the individual during the touch episode. Beware of unexpected interactions and ponder the following issues:
- *Empower, do not disempower*:
  - notice the power impact of standing over student who is in a position lower to the ground – lower yourself to an appropriate level
  - do not straddle a student, especially when the student is lying down
  - do not inadvertently touch the student with one of your body parts that was not named in the touch for which you received permission
  - do not put your body weight on a student
  - do not push or exert inappropriate levels of pressure
  - touch where you said you would and do no not let your hands wander off from there

- *Use proximal, not distal, touch for physical safety*:
  - do not encourage movement from the edges of the students' body by touching too far away from the joints and muscles that you are inviting to activate
  - touch as closely to where the actual movement or adjustment needs to happen to prevent torquing
  - beware of maintaining appropriate *energetic and emotional boundaries* in touching at the proximal body parts
  - if the proximal body part happens to be a very private body part, do not touch – use verbal intervention or demonstration instead
- *Encourage active joint movement by students rather than passively moving students whenever possible*:
  - use touch to invite the student to initiate the movement from the inside out
  - do not move the student from the outside in with your own muscle power
  - never move a student forcefully – be gentle and minimal in the amount of effort
  - invite action from the inside out rather than the attainment of a particular outer shape
  - invite active decision-making by the students about how to actualize or operationalize the invited motion
  - beware of maintaining respect of energetic and emotional boundaries by yielding to student discomfort, resistance, or hesitation
- *Stabilize, rather than fostering reliance on the teacher*:
  - offer physical stability without taking on the student's body weight
  - do not destabilize students physically with quick movements or sudden movements
  - give notice of how touch will evolve as it does in the moment so the student is not startled, destabilized, or surprised
  - be aware of stabilizing the student's energy via co-regulation and coordination of breath rhythms (following the student's lead OR retraining a student's dysregulated breath)

Protections for the Yoga Professional While Using Tactile Assists

Just as it is important to attend to clients' physical, energetic, and emotional wellbeing during an episode of physical touch or tactile contact, it is important for yoga professionals to maintain awareness of their own personal body mechanics and safety when offering a physical assist. The type of physical assists that are endorsed here do not generally represent a threat to the physical integrity of the teacher's body as all touch is light and stabilizing. In other words, in most if not all situations when physical touch is offered, the teacher does not bear the client's body weight in any way. Nevertheless, it is important to stay mindful of personal posture and alignment as assists are provided to participants. If there is any weight-bearing on the part of the teacher, it is auspicious to make sure that we do not overly challenge or stress our lower back and that we use the strength of our legs to support any lifting or bracing.

It is helpful for teacher and student, to make sure that neither has loose pieces of jewelry or clothing that can get caught or get in the way. It is helpful to remain mindful of direct skin contact with students, as opposed to clothing on clothing. Direct skin contact may be more triggering to students or misunderstood. As yoga professionals, we can protect ourselves from being misunderstood if we can maintain a physical boundary (even as thin as a piece of fabric) between us and our student (other than our hands) when we make physical contact. This is not a hard and fast rule as this may not always be realistic given room temperatures. Yet, it is helpful to keep in mind that there is extra challenge the greater the area of skin-to-skin contact between provider and client.

Types of Tactile Contact Defined With Examples

A few types of touch are outlined below to demonstrate the vast range of possibilities for making tactile contact with students. The order is roughly in the order of least intrusive or directive to most profound with regard to the size of touched area and degree of strength exerted by the teacher during physical contact. In all these options, the teacher fully honors all rules of engagement outlined above, from gathering continuous consent, to a full description of what is involved in the tactile episode, to having clarity of intention, while always yielding the power and agency to the student. The yoga professional remains fully attentive to the participant during the episode, remaining responsive to verbal and nonverbal signals. The teacher's actions are guided by the student's response to the physical contact. The teacher also needs to continue to monitor the reactions and reactivities of other students or clients who are present and responds to their needs as well to the degree possible.

Student-Initiated Touch

Student-initiated touch is defined as touch whereby the student is moving toward a body part (often the hand) of the teacher. The student is completely in charge of the degree of touch, the strength of the contact, and length of the touch episode. If desired, the student does not even need to touch the teacher's proffered body part but can simply move in its direction without ever making full tactile contact. This may well be the least intrusive and most student-empowering form of physical (or almost physical) touch. This form of touch is the essence of the physical cuing that was presented above in the context of listing interventions with students from least to most intrusive or directive.

Examples:
- *Shoulder girdle alignment from past to present in Warrior 2* – the teacher stands forward of a student in Warrior 2 with her or his arm stretched toward the student – just ahead to the student's forwardly-stretched arm and hand – to invite movement of the student's shoulder girdle forward to align the shoulders above the pelvis; the teacher asks the student to move her or his fingertips to or toward the teacher's proffered hand or fingers
- *Shoulder girdle alignment from present to past in Warrior 2* – the teacher stands just back of a student in Warrior 2 with her or his arm stretched toward the student – just behind the student's backwardly-stretched arm and hand – to invite movement of the student's shoulder girdle backward to align the shoulders above the pelvis; the teachers asks the student to move her or his fingertips to or toward the teacher's proffered hand or fingers
- *Knee alignment in warriors or lunges* – the teacher kneels next to the student, holding her or his hand with the palm facing toward the outside of the student's knee while the student is in a lunge or warrior shape with the knee collapsed toward the midline; teacher asks the student to move the knee to or toward the teacher's hand; if the student chooses to touch the teacher's hand with the knee, some pressure between the two body parts can be added with the student's permission

- *Engagement of scapulae in downward facing dog* – the teacher hovers her or his hand behind the student's thoracic spine in downward facing dog; the teacher then asks the student to move her or his rib basket to or toward the teacher's hand to create core engagement and remove the collapse from the thoracic spine, engaging the core muscles while drawing the low ribs toward the hips
- *Engagement of head and neck into healthful posture in downward facing dog* – the teacher hovers her or his hand behind the student's head in downward facing dog; the teacher then asks the student to move her or his head to or toward the teacher's hand to create muscular engagement in the neck, emphasizing a chin tuck before the chin moves toward the back plan of the body to come into a more natural postural head alignment
- *Releasing effort in the shoulder girdle during Warrior 2* – the teacher stands behind a student in Warrior 2, with her or his arms out to side just under the student's arms; the teacher invites the student to release her or his shoulder blades downward to or toward the teacher's arms to create more ease and eliminate excess effort or tension in the shoulder girdle

Guiding Touch

Guiding touch of the participant by the yoga professional is a gentle and typically light, never forceful or heavy, tactile contact through which the teacher identifies a particular body region of the student with a discerning touch by the teacher's hand or hands (most typically). Guiding touch can be offered simply to help a student *become more aware* of where a targeted body region is (e.g., identifying a bicep muscle or a peroneal muscle). It also be offered to guide the student into *activation* in areas that are collapsed or into *release* of a particular muscle or set of muscles that are braced. The touch is guiding without exerting force; it is simply a placement of the teacher's hand on a body part that the student has trouble locating, releasing, or engaging on her or his own. It is accompanied by gentle verbal instruction about the intention: for example, noticing, releasing, or engaging.

Examples:
- *Encouraging hand engagement in downward facing dog* – very gently placing the teacher's hand on the index finger and thumb of a student who is in downward facing dog to encourage the engagement of pada bandha in the hand with internal rotation of the humeri to gain more lightness in the wrist
- *Encouraging release of a braced area* – gently and lightly placing the teacher's hand on a braced area (always avoiding the sacred areas named above) to encourage the student to find more ease in the muscles around this body region
- *Encouraging engagement of a collapsed areas* – gently and lightly touching a collapsed area to help the student identify a muscle that can support greater engagement and health in a particular muscle (e.g., touching the mid trapezius of a student who collapses while holding a plank even if activation of the shoulder blades has been verbally cued)

Directional Touch

Directional touch involves a *hands-on* or *fingers-on* touch by the teacher that guides a student's body region, limb(s), or the body overall in a particular direction without the teacher exerting any active force or effort. The touch guides the student in a direction that the student was not able to access through verbal cuing alone. Through this directional touch the student better understands the healthful alignment of the body region and muscles in question. The touch is very light and yet has a discrete directionality to it that guides the student toward a specific movement (as opposed to light touch which is not directional but simple invites attention to, release or, or engagement of the are being touched).

Examples:
- *Shoulder blade stabilization* – very gently, with two light fingers, tracing a V down the student's upper back to encourage the retraction and depression of the shoulder blades on the thoracic spine
- *External rotation of upper arm bones* – gently touch in a way that suggests external rotation of the humeri in extended mountain pose – the teacher's hands are gentle placed on the student's arms near the shoulder joint (above the elbow joint) to guide the student toward the type of external rotation that brings greater ease to shoulder (glenohumeral) flexion
- *Scapula retraction in plank* – gentle touch at the outside of a student's elbows, encouraging a movement toward the center of the body (i.e., medially) while the student is in plank pose to help guide the elbows toward each other to prevent the splaying out of the arms which – over time and with repetition – can be harmful for the shoulder joint
- *Deepening of spinal rotation* – gentle placement of the teacher's hands on the shoulders of a student who is moving into a seated twist; on the side same side of the twist (i.e., the right shoulder, if twisting to the right), the teacher places the hand on top of the shoulder with fingers wrapping to front of the shoulder; on the side away from the twist, the teacher places the hand on the shoulder blade; there is a directional hint into the direction of the twist but the teacher exerts no force at all; the student is in charge of the degree of additional rotation in the spine that feels auspicious

Supportive Touch

Through supportive touch, a teacher helps a student gain insight about or greater comfort in a body region, energetic movement, or emotional response to an asana or breathing practice. Supportive touch invites a deliberate action by the student to find either greater ease or greater engagement in a body part that is either over- or under-efforting, either braced or collapsed. Supportive touch is more substantial than light touch; however, its safety comes from the fact that the student remains in charge of the degree of engagement inherent in the touch and the length of the tactile contact with the teacher, being able to release from the tactile contact at any time without risk of destabilization.

Examples:
- *Human stretching rack with student gripping teacher's ankles* – the teacher stands above behind the supine student's head (permission for this is key as this stance can be triggering) and invites the student to grip the teacher's ankles; the teacher starts with knees in flexion and tension increases on the student's spine as the teacher straightens the knees
- *Side plank with hip support* – the teacher's hand is supportively placed under the student's lower hip in side plank to invite a lifting of the pelvic girdle toward the sky – eliminates collapse of the core muscles in side plank that often shows up as hips sagging toward the floor

- *Palm-on-palm lift-up for spinal extension in pigeon pose* – while teacher is kneeling or squatting directly in front of the student who is in pigeon preparation, teacher and student place their palms (teacher's right on student's left; and left in right) together providing support for the student as the student lifts up into spinal extension
- *Back and leg support in boat pose* – the teacher squats at the side of the student who is preparing to rise into boat pose; as the student lifts the legs off the ground, the teacher provides a supportive arm behind the student's back and possibly a supportive arm under the thighs, just above the backs of the knees; all along the teacher encourages the student to engage the core and to find the strength to hold her or his own legs
- *Lifting-up support in headstand* – the teacher stands to the side of the student; as the student reaches up from a tight downward dog to move toward headstand, the teacher supports the swing leg to help the student reach the inversion; from here the student is asked to self-stabilize and the teacher takes her or his hand away when the student is self-sufficient in the up-side-down shape; this assist can also be used for handstand

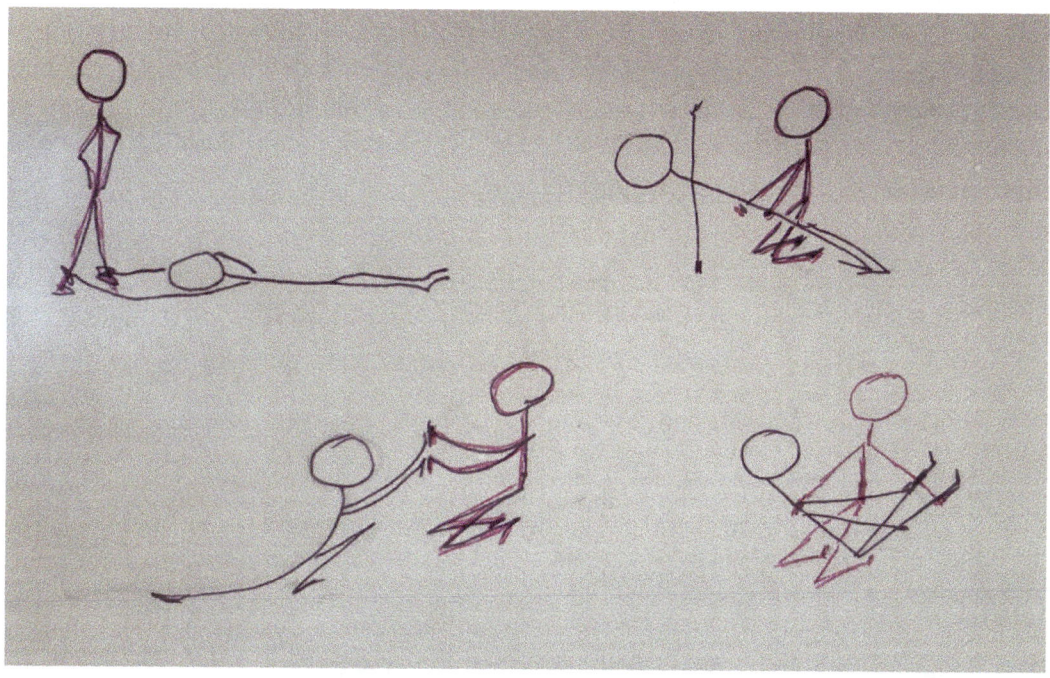

Stabilizing Touch

Stabilizing touch involves the teacher using a body part (most typically a hand or arm) to stabilize the student to gain greater ease in balancing or stabilizing a particular body region or the body overall. Stabilization is most commonly used in standing balances to help the student access the shape without the need to concentrate overly hard on staying upright. Once the student has accessed the shape with more ease and stability, the teacher can slowly and gently encourage the student to disengage contact from the teacher to move into a free balance, if desired. It is the student's choice to disengage from stabilizing touch; the teacher takes great care never to remove tactile contact with a student while the student's stability is still linked to the presence of the teacher's touch. The teacher makes sure not to destabilize the student.

Examples:
- *Stability in tree pose* – the teacher offers a hand or finger to the student (on the side of the student's lifted leg) to stabilize the pose; the student is in charge of grasping or touching the proffered hand or finger with her or his hand or finger
- *Stability in dancer pose* – the teacher offers a supportive hand or outstretched palm to the student's forward hand to stabilize, and possible deepen, the balancing backbend; the student is in charge of grasping or touching the proffered hand or palm with her or his hand or palm
- *Stability in half moon* – the teacher can stand behind the student so that the student may choose to lean into the teacher (in lieu of being stabilized by wall); the teacher does not carry the weight of the student but simply serves as a stabilizer to give the student more security in this open-hearted balance
- *Stability in Warrior 3* – standing in front of the student with the student's hands reaching toward the teacher as the student folds forward into the share, the teacher offers supportive hands with upwardly-faced palms onto which the student can choose (or not choose) to place her or his downwardly-faced palms for stabilizing support
- *Hands-under-shoulder support in crow pose* – while teacher is kneeling directly in front of the student, the teacher's hands are placed under the student's shoulders as the student moves forward into crow pose; this support helps the student feel less afraid of falling head-forward onto the mat as an attempt is made to lift the feet off the ground; the addition of a bolster in front of the student is also very helpful (no picture 😊)

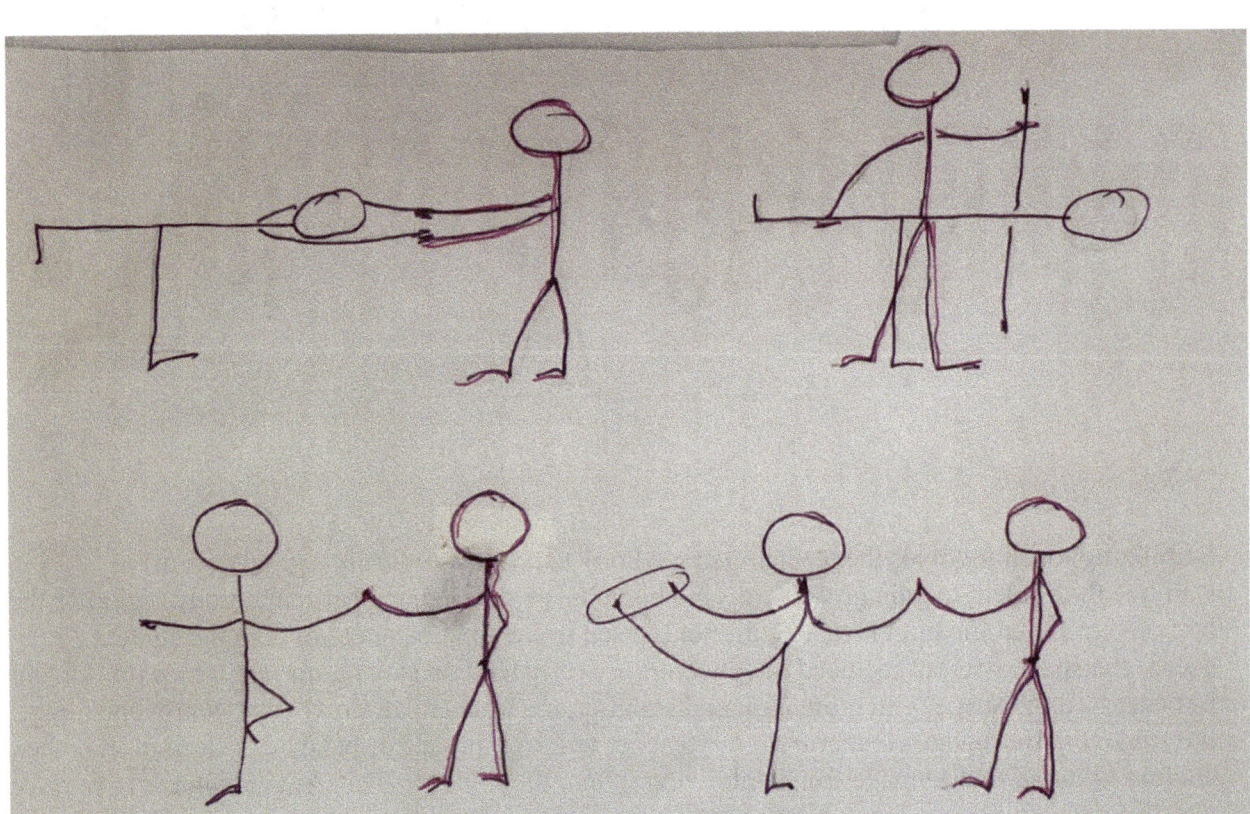

Auspicious Alignment Touch

Touch to support auspicious alignment involves the greatest amount of active physical engagement between teacher and students. Alignment touch offers the student access to changing placements in a particular body region or the body overall to gain more ease or healthful engagement in a particular shape. The teacher has a more active role and may actually move certain body parts of the students, always taking care to work closely to the joints that need to increase range of motion to access the alignment. Alignment generally brings more healthful assembly or stable engagement into a student's body, breath, or even her or his mind.

Examples:

- *Grounding through the back foot in warrior and related wide-legged standing shapes* – the teacher places her or his foot next the back-facing foot in the standing warrior or related shape; this allows the student to release weight into the foot in a grounded way; the contact between student and teacher is strong and relies on the power of the teacher to stabilize her or his own foot
- *Hip alignment in lunges and warriors* (asymmetrical standing shapes) – the teacher stands to the side of a student who is in a lunge or warrior, with a pelvis that is not properly aligned side-to-side; the teacher – with permission, of course – uses her or his hands to pivot the students pelvis into proper side-to-side alignment, supporting the moving backward of the hip connected to the forward leg and the moving forward of the hip connected to the back leg; the mobilization of the pelvic girdle is provided by the teacher and the student is then encouraged to maintain that hip alignment as the teacher withdraws her or his hands
- *Knee alignment with a resistance band* – there is no actual physical contact between student and teacher here; however, the teacher will exert significant force on the resistance band that connects from her or his hands to the leg of the student; the band is wrapped either directly above or below the student's knee to support proper alignment of the knee in the same line as the foot and the hip (i.e., side-to-side, NOT forward of or behind the ankle) (no picture 😊)
- *Anterior rotation of pelvic girdle in standing or seated forward folds* – the teacher stands to the side of a student who is in a forward fold (e.g., downward facing dog at the wall) and whose low back is rounded (i.e., the pelvis has posterior tuck); the teacher uses her or his hands – one at the outside of each of the student's hips – to rotate the pelvis into a more anterior tilt to bring the natural lordotic curve into the student's lumbar spine; the teacher attends to any strain by the student and cues bending the knees as needed
-

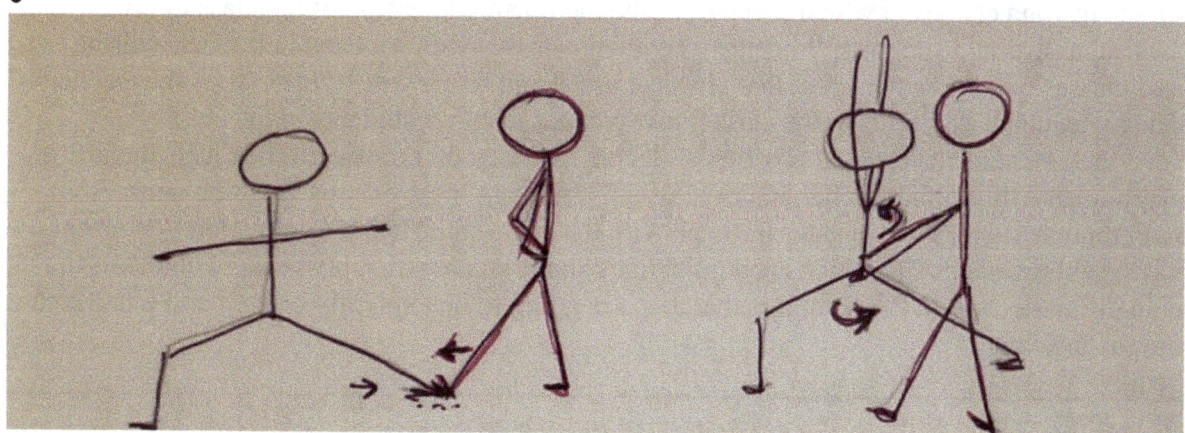

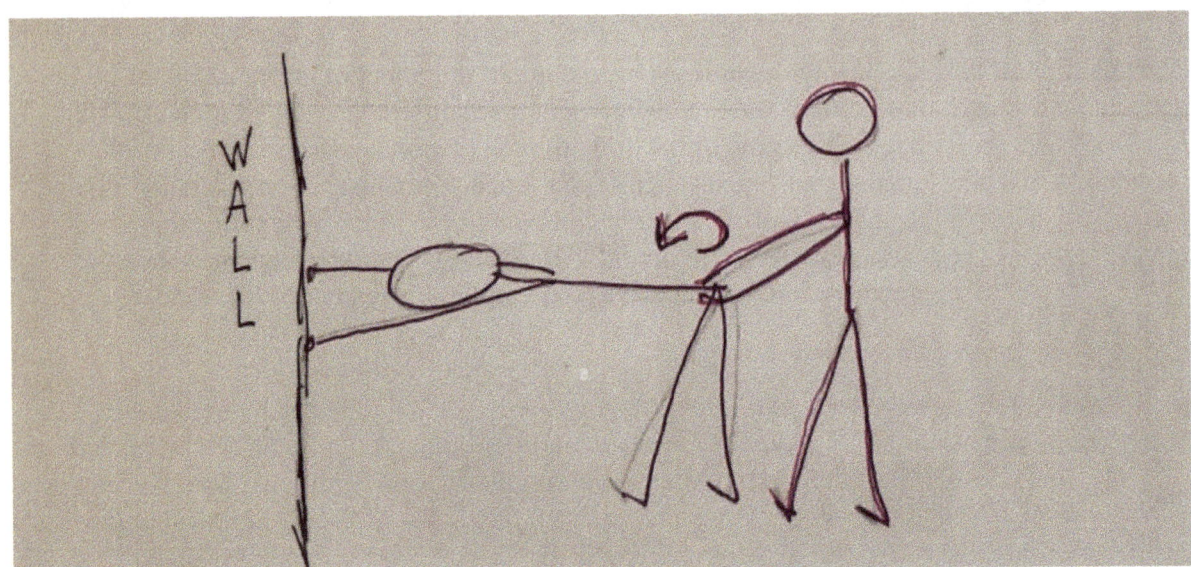

Another Perspective on Touch…

There are (at least) two situations in which touch may be integrated into the theme of the class and explicitly planned.

Partner Yoga –

In partnered yoga, by definition, students will touch each other and/or the teacher. Often partnered classes are taught to actual partners, but not always. Sometimes students pair up in class with a classmate they may or may not already know. Students who attend partnered classes give explicit consent to this form of touch and physical interaction; they know to expect it. If they have an unexpected reaction to the physicality of the class, they will need to decide what they want to do – they can choose to leave the class or they can get the essence of the shapes that are taught while doing them on their own.

Yoga Classes with Explicit Class Descriptions that Touch Will Be Offered

These are yoga classes in which it is part of the therapeutic intention of the class to give physical assists and supports. Students who attend classes with such explicit touch-will-be-used classes will know to expect that physical assist and touch will be offered by the teacher and any teaching assistants in the class (however, not by other students in the class). Nevertheless, students can – at any time – decide that they do not want to be touched and communicate this to the teacher and/or assistants. Even in these classes, ongoing consent is used, though after a few episodes of touch with the same student, such collection of consent may be abbreviated. All cautions and guidelines about touch still apply in these classes – the main difference is that the default is that touch is going to be explicitly offered and integrated into the teaching.

Chapter 11: Foundational Ethics and Commitments

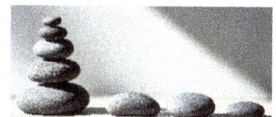

There are multiple foundations in yoga psychology to help guide ethical inquiry for yoga teachers. From the rich cultural traditions of yoga, we can draw upon the yamas and niyamas. Relatedly, guidance can come from the yoga-specific organizations that have struggled with defining ethical guidelines for yoga teachers and related yoga professionals (namely, the Yoga Alliance and International Association of Yoga Therapists). From a larger cultural perspective, ethical inquiry considers local laws and values to guide the work of yoga teachers, incorporating professional association guidance where available and relevant (e.g., looking at ethical codes for psychology, medicine, physical therapy, and similarly health and allied health professions). Finally, yoga professionals are encouraged to engage in their personal values clarification process to allow their inner system of morals and ethics to become relevant to professional ethical decision-making and debriefing.

Sources of guidance include, and are not limited to the following:
- Guidance from the yamas and niyamas
- Guidance from the brahma viharas
- Guidance from the ethical codes of conduct from Yoga Alliance and International Association of Yoga Therapists
- Guidance from relevant professional ethical codes of conduct
- Personal values clarification in the greater cultural context

Ethics Aspects of Being a Yoga Professional

Ethics in Relationship

Relational ethics in yoga are far-reaching, complex, and easily violated if clear goals and boundaries are not made a routine part of teaching yoga (Farhi, 2006). Many issues have to be considered and negotiated to assure that proper boundaries are honored for everyone – not just individual participants, but also the group of clients as a whole and the yoga professionals who are present (including assistants). Rights to privacy may conflict with being fully and optimally prepared about special needs of individual participants; individual desires can come in conflict with group rights and needs; teacher responsibilities for safety may be threatened by over-eager or inattentive clients.

These are but a few examples of the types of situations yoga professionals need to ponder, recognize, navigate, and consult about. It is impossible to be prepared for every eventuality and some challenges may arise that are beyond teacher preparation. None of this has to be a problem or ethical violation as long as teachers recognize their misstep and take appropriate action to repair, debrief, and regroup.

The ethics of proper relational and pragmatic boundaries:
- Avoid multiple relationship when possible
- Process and debrief multiple relationships if they arise (e.g., rural teachers may have multiple relationships due to the context of their environment)
- Do not self-disclose inappropriately (or at all if uncertain about proper limits)
- Do not engage in sexual relationships with current or former students
- Have clarity about class rules and expectations
- Begin and end class on time to honor your own time needs and those of the students

The ethics of respecting students' rights to privacy, self-determination, and autonomy
- Do not force self-disclosure or ask intrusive questions that are irrelevant
- Respect student choices in the class as long as they are within limits of safety
- Do not gossip, don't make inappropriate disclosures about others, and don't talk about students or other teachers in front of students
- Collect appropriate informed consent prior to class and within class in the context of giving students agency and opportunity to refuse or request physical assists
  - make sure consent about touch/no-touch is informed (student knows what you are asking or suggesting)
  - make sure consent is ongoing (re-collected each time a new situation arises that requires that the student give consent again)
  - make sure consent is enthusiastic or overt (student gives a direct affirmative answer as opposed to a vague or uninterpretable response)
- Consider the use of touch/no-touch cards on mats
- Use invitational, rather than directive, language when options are safe and indicated
- Whenever possible, offer choices to engage students in introspection and to grant them their own agency over their decisions and choices

The ethics of negotiating individual student rights and needs versus group rights and needs
- Manage/limits the amount of time dedicated to questions from students during class – find a middle ground of letting students process and engage in inquiry versus usurping everyone's time for their personal curiosity
- Manage/limit before and after-class availability to students lest you burn yourself out
- Have expectations about appropriate dress and use of language

The ethics of interacting with other care providers and teachers involved with your students
- Do not disparage other teachers
- Do not contradict recommendations students have received from healthcare providers
- Have a referral network of trusted teachers for students you cannot work with for any reason (including time, mismatch of need versus capacity, scope of practice, etc.)
- Have a referral network of healthcare providers for students who need help linking to supportive providers – be cautious, however; it is preferable to provide multiple names so the student has choices
- Offer to collaborate with, perhaps even meet, your student's care providers who interface with your scope of practice
- Develop relationships with community teachers and care providers

Ethics in the Yoga Room – Preparation, Teaching, Debriefing, and More

The complexity of ethical challenges, conundrums, and decision-making cannot be overstated. The more people a yoga professional instructs, the more opportunities exist for ethical faux-pas. Being prepared to navigate ethical dilemmas is key to success. Having clear policies and procedures protects providers and participants when questions arise about pragmatics (such as payment expectations, scope of practice, unkept perceived promises and more).

Honoring the ethical and lifestyle foundations of yoga Limbs 1 and 2 can prevent many potentially challenging ethical issues. Coming to yoga service delivery with the *yamas* at heart, honoring non-harming, truthfulness, non-stealing, moderation and non-greed, guides yoga professionals and their clients toward proper boundaries and respectful interchanges. Honoring the *niyamas* by integrating lifestyle choices of cleanliness, discipline, commitment, introspection, and devotion to a greater cause increases the likelihood of clear business practices, straight-forward and insightful interpersonal exchanges, and ongoing professionalism.

The ethics of being prepared include, but are not limited to taking responsibility for all of the following matters:
- Securing proper credentialing and training
- Working within the scope of practice
- Maintaining and continually enhancing skills
- Understanding liability issues
- Obtaining all necessary insurance, permits, or licenses
- Integrating the yamas and niyamas in day-to-day life
- Having clarity about payment and financial terms (e.g., pre-payment for courses; late fees for late payment; clear refund policies), making room for access to individuals with limited resources while also looking out for personal financial needs and commitments
- Developing appropriate paperwork for signing individuals into classes, including a proper informed consent form

The ethics of being prepared for classes or session ensure that yoga professionals:
- Make honest claims about what is being offered in a yoga class (truthfulness)
  - level of class (beginner, intermediate, advanced…)
  - size of class (know what you can manage safely and competently)
  - drop-in versus cohort classes
  - style of class
  - intentions of class
- Provide appropriate teacher-student ratios (non-stealing, non-greed)
- Select properly trained assistants and substitute teachers
- Collect informed consents from students (differences between legal and ethical issues in studio- versus clinic or hospital settings) (non-harming)
- Know and observe your students, including noting their progress, to be able to adapt and challenge properly
- Prepare session or class outlines and have clear plans for each class that is taught (discipline)
- Have the capacity to veer from the plan is needed given student presentation

The ethics of being, teaching, and engaging in the yoga room to make yoga accessible and inclusive translate into:
- Providing necessary materials (props) or require students to bring them (non-harm)
- Maintaining a healthy and sanitary environment (cleanliness)
- Maintaining a safe environment (scents, privacy, etc.)
- Keeping students, self, and others safe
    o being fully and mindfully present
    o monitoring and observing what is happening in the room
    o intervening in risky situation with calm and equanimity
    o being able to manage a crisis
- Answering inquiries honestly and be able and willing to say "I don't know"
- Offering necessary adaptations, modifications, adjustments, alternatives, and props
- Touching only respectfully and with explicit permission on each occasion
- Treating all students with respect and honoring student autonomy (see above)
    o being humble
    o being culturally sensitive, aware, skilled, knowledgeable, and humble
    o being inviting and grant access to all (while maintaining safety and boundaries)
    o being mindful and thought about your language
    o being mindful and thought about dress, jewelry, modesty, and other aspects of possible materialism or professionalism

The ethics of debriefing and consulting outside the yoga room are engaged in on behalf of personal and students safety by being sure to:
- Maintain student confidentiality when consulting with others about how better to help or support a student (of challenge)
- Maintain confidentiality about the identity of students in your class
- Have class rules about self-disclosure in class and student-about-student disclosure outside of class
- Seek supervision or consultation when a challenge has arisen that you do not know how to manage

The ethics of scope of practice ensure that yoga professionals:
- Use referral sources when a student health or mental health issue is outside the teacher's scope of practice
- Engage in ongoing continuing education and aspire to become a better teacher
- Teach only those students whom you are qualified to teach (e.g., take care with children, pregnant women, individuals with complex trauma, etc.)
- Teach only what you know and have experienced
- Be honest about what you know and don't know – admit when you run up against your own limits of knowledge and experience

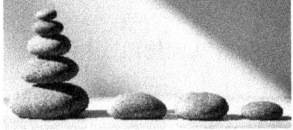

Relevant Ethical and Professional Resources

It is key to review extant codes of ethics developed by Yoga Alliance and the International Association of Yoga Therapists. These yoga profession-based codes of conduct are best supplemented by codes of conduct for the healthcare context in which yoga is provided (as relevant) and for which the yoga teacher may have a coexisting license or certification. It is the responsibility of each yoga professional to review and achieve facility with all of these ethical and professional resources. Following are a few items to attend to.

Yoga Alliance Ethics Code Topic Summary

- Adherence to law and ethical financial practices
- Adherence to scope of practice, including
  - appropriate conduct
  - teaching qualifications
  - informed consent
  - sources of information
  - advising and teaching within the scope of practice and training
  - credentialing
- Adherence to anti-harassment policies
- Adherence to sexual misconduct policies
- Adherence to "do no harm"
- Yoga equity and inclusion (more about this below)
- Respect in the student-teacher relationship (covered above)
- Integrity and honesty in communications and actions

Yoga Alliance Equity Position Statement

The Yoga Alliance position statement and the YogaX YTT commitment to equity (see policies and procedures), trainees are invited to recognize that:
- Inequities permeate systems in which yoga is taught and through which yoga is practiced;
- Yoga systems have perpetuated harm and exclusion of certain communities, populations, and groups and that all yoga community members are responsible for creating change that leads to equity, inclusion, and accessibility;
- Resources, supports, and opportunities must be distributed more equitable across diverse groups, populations, and communities; and
- Diversity, accessibility, and inclusiveness are essential commitments of a yoga school in line with yogic commitments to the ethical practices outlined in the yamas

Sample Yoga School Equity Commitment

YogaX at Stanford Psychiatry is an excellent example of a yoga school-based code of conduct and commitment to equity. The full document is available upon request from the author. Following is an excerpt:

Understanding the history of inequity and harm within yoga communities, YogaX is firmly committed never to discriminate against or refuse to provide teaching or training to any student, participant, or employee based on any protected class such as age, gender (including pregnancy), race, ethnicity, culture, national origin, religion, sexual orientation, disability, socioeconomic status, or genetic information.

YogaX teachers welcome, accept, and support all students regardless of religion, gender, sexual orientation, language, nationality, political, or cultural background. They embrace yoga equity and inclusion, doing their utmost to make yoga equitable, inclusive, accessible, and diverse. YogaX's emphasis on teaching, and practicing yoga honestly, respectfully, and with integrity requires that YogaX teachers actively promote equity, reduce harm, honor and leverage differences, and foster diversity and inclusion in all areas of yoga – while honoring the integrity and diversity of yoga's cultural and historical roots.

YogaX teachers are well educated in how to make yoga equitable, inclusive, accessible, and diverse. They apply principles of accessibility, equity, and inclusion to all training and teaching events at all times. All YogaX events integrate accessible yoga teachings so that all participants, regardless of background or ability, practice together and feel fully included, respected, honored, and valued. Accessibility includes yoga practices that are varied to suit students with disabilities, physical challenges, chronic illness, seniors, and anyone who may not feel comfortable in a typical studio class. Accessibility also includes making classes welcoming to everyone and teaching in a trauma-sensitive and trauma-informed manner.

Ethical Commitments and Professionalism in the Context of Yoga Services

Focus in this context is on assuring that teachers remain clearly aware of the ethical codes of conducts of their profession, practice within their proper scope of practice, and commit to practices that reflect utmost professionalism. Additionally, teachers commit to actions and teaching strategies that foster equality, social justice, inclusion, and accessibility.

- Secure proper credentialing, training, and maintenance of skills
- Collect informed consents from students (differences between legal and ethical issues in studio- versus clinic or hospital settings)
- Maintain professional, compassionate, and safe personal and physical boundaries
- Use referral sources when a student health or mental health issue is outside the teacher's scope of practice
- Integrate the yamas and niyamas in all teaching-related work and day-to-day life
- Create a teaching space where students may offer feedback
- Remain committed to the YA Code of Conduct, Scope of Practice, and commitment to equity, inclusion, and accessibility
- Remain committed to relevant professional Code of Conduct, Scope of Practice, and commitment to equity, inclusion, and accessibility
- Review the information above regarding timeliness, consistency, and cleanliness in the environment, interactions with students, and relationships with colleagues

Legal Commitments in the Context of Yoga Services

Legal aspects of the business of yoga are covered with focus on assuring that trainees/teachers remain clearly aware of local laws that apply to their yoga business, marketing and promotion, including proper scope of practice. Additionally, teachers commit to actions and business strategies that foster equality, social justice, inclusion, and accessibility.

- Understand liability issues and obtain all necessary insurance, permits, informed consents, and licenses
- Collect informed consents from students (differences between legal and ethical issues in studio- versus clinic or hospital settings)
- Collect liability waivers form students as appropriate to the local legal environment
- Use ethical and legal practices for invoicing
- Refer to the extant relevant Codes of Conduct for additional information about legal and ethical business practices as related to marketing, promotion, and other business and legal-related practices.

A Few Final Notes

- Be clear about personal scope of practice, given acquired registration, certifications, and other professional or healthcare licenses
- If scope of practice augmentation is desired, be sure to obtain all commensurate education and commit to securing relevant certifications, registrations, and licensure
- Develop a detailed yoga resume – tracking hours, describing experiences; developing spreadsheets to document work experience, educational attainments, teaching hours, types of clients served and more
- Understand how to build contextually appropriate relationships in your community
- Understand how to connect with other yoga schools, clinics, and hospitals
- Build a referral list with other physical, allied, and mental healthcare professionals who may facilitate networking opportunities within your community
- Develop a website to market services and display credentials
- Decide on the role of social media in your practice and marketing – the Yoga in America 2016 study found that the majority of yoga teachers actively promote themselves on social media (IPSOS Public Affairs, 2016)

Create boundaries, not barriers.

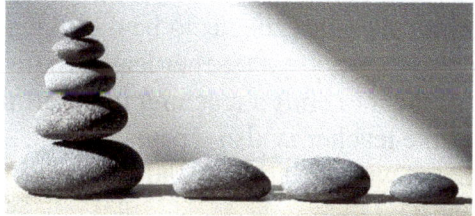

Professional Development Aspects of Being a Yoga Professional

Successful yoga service delivery is predicated on knowledge of and commitment to the legal, ethical, and professional practices of any profession, including the profession of yoga. Following are a few guidelines that help assure that a yoga services provider adheres to the ethical and lifestyle principles on which integrated holistic yoga practice and teaching are based.

Credentialing and Commitment to Ethics and Professionalism

It is important to understand the different scopes of practice within the realm of yoga service provision. Based on the desired scope of practice, different educational requirements need to be met and different types of credentials or licensed may be required. Yoga can be a singular activity for many (e.g., people who only engage in postural practice), a lifestyle for others (e.g., those who apply all eight limbs on and off the mat), and a profession for some (e.g., yoga teachers or yoga therapists). The heart of all applications – whether as a practice or a profession – is grounded in yoga psychology and yoga's deep roots in ancient wisdom traditions, evolved across the millennia and deeply affected by the biopsychosociocultural contexts in which yoga is practiced and applied. Below are some ideas about the range of yoga *services* and how this relates to yoga as a profession – a profession that can have many manifestations and applications. Yoga as a *practice* has been addressed elsewhere.

Services that can be provided by yoga professionals range widely, are often misunderstood, and may be confusing to the public and to healthcare providers whose patients may benefit from one type of yoga service but not another. It helps to look at this range of services from the perspective of scopes of practice and educational backgrounds of yoga professionals. The range can be roughly shown as a continuum from *yoga teaching* to *yoga therapy*, with *therapeutic yoga teaching* in the center – leaning toward the teaching end of the spectrum; and *therapeutic yoga applications in healthcare* – leaning toward the yoga therapy end of the spectrum.

Scope of Practice Definitions

As yoga teachers and yoga clinicians become more knowledgeable about health and mental health issues, it is crucial to continue to track and stay within an appropriate scope of practice. It helps to keep in mind differentiations within the yoga profession to adhere to the yoga services for which a teacher or clinician has been trained. It is equally important to clarify agreed-upon role(s) with any given client or student. For example, if the relationship was based on a pre-existing clinical contact, adding therapeutic yoga needs to be discussed and matched to the scope of practice of the healthcare provider. If the relationship was originally a yoga teacher-yoga student relationship, adding a clinical context needs to be discussed and within the provider's greater clinical scope of practice. When a yoga teacher learns more about mental health issues, for example, this will not be sufficient to shift a teaching relationship into a therapeutic or clinical interaction. However, if the teacher is also a psychologist, such a shift may become appropriate, if explicitly negotiated with the student and with appropriate shifts in relationship and focus.

From the integrated holistic yoga perspective, four broad categories of yoga services can be delineated. While I offer these simply as starting points for a conversation, I do believe they are fairly representative of the types of yoga services that are being actively offered in a variety of contexts. Yoga classes tend to be clustered in studio and other community settings (e.g., gyms) and are often fitness oriented. Yoga therapy is largely offered in private practice settings. The therapeutic yoga offerings between these two anchors might indeed cluster the way I suggest below; however, it is important to note that these clusters likely still miss or even obscure important nuances and variability that exist or are possible. It is the center of the spectrum that deserves careful attention in the future, as yoga evolves into a viable and clearly delineated therapeutic intervention in healthcare settings.

The center of the spectrum can perhaps be understood as driven from the bottom up, by community demand and patient need. Yoga therapeutics and therapeutic yoga can be tailored to specific collective and individual needs that emerge in a particular context and are provided by yoga professionals who are embedded in this same interpersonal matrix. In that sense, the center of the spectrum may be more culturally and emotionally responsive to communities than determined from the top down by professional organizations or business considerations. Their potential bottom-up, community-informed nature does not free the yoga services provided at the center from conscientiously and ethically adhering to professional needs and standards. It may simply invite a more flexible perspective on who is best situated and prepared to bring these services to the people who can most benefit from them. However, that idea is for another time.

The Spectrum of Yoga Services

Yoga Teaching
RYT200 & RYT500 Yoga Teaching credentials

Therapeutic Yoga
- In small-group settings with specific focus
- One possible pathway is a Yoga Alliance RYT500 with healthcare focus

Yoga Therapeutics
- Within a QHP's healthcare scope of practice
- One possible pathway is IAYT's IAYT-Q credentialling of QHPs

Yoga Therapy
C-IAYT Yoga Therapy Credentials

Yoga Classes

Yoga classes take place in studios, gyms, and even online and range widely from being strictly exercise-based to including accessible practices from all yoga limbs. Classes vary greatly in size and exposure to other students, and may be so large that they do not support an individual relationship between yoga teacher and student. Classes are not specifically tailored to individual needs, though they may promote self-agency through encouraging the use of props, adaptations, and variations. Yoga classes are not offered for specific therapeutic reasons; however, they may offer yoga practices that have benefits for physical and emotional wellness overall. It is highly recommended that yoga teachers minimally complete a 200-hour yoga teacher certification. Additionally, yoga teachers are best registered with Yoga Alliance to reassure the public that they have been trained to a minimum standard of teaching practice. Specialty teaching (such as for children or pregnancy) may require additional training focused on the relevant topic or population. Commensurate supplemental Yoga Alliance registration is recommended.

Therapeutic Yoga Classes

Therapeutic yoga classes tend to be offered for individuals with a particular characteristic, concern, or challenge. While some are offered in the same venues as yoga classes, they are well-situated in healthcare, allied healthcare, mental healthcare, and/or community health settings. Therapeutic yoga classes are provided and practiced in small groups, may have more than one teacher (and/or assistants), identify a health or mental health-related presenting concern (e.g., yoga for back pain; yoga for cancer survivors; yoga as stress reduction), and make explicit, deliberate, and demonstrated use of props, adaptations, and variations. An affiliative, direct relationship between student and teacher is encouraged. Teachers and assistants pay attention to individual students and offer specific directions and interventions that tailor the practice uniquely to each individual in the group. Therapeutic yoga classes, because of their shared and clearly-defined focus on a common physical or mental health concern, create more student-to-student relationships as well because of shared experiences, therapeutic interests, goals, or presenting concerns of participants.

It is recommended that yoga teachers who want to provide therapeutic yoga classes *minimally* complete a 200-hour yoga teacher certification *with specific focus on yoga in healthcare* (as opposed to fitness) settings. Training may focus on the populations the teacher wants to serve; it highlights how to bring yoga to individuals who can benefit from the practice, yet often do not have access to the practice for a variety of resource-, stereotype- or stigma-related reasons. To create more accountability to the populations they wish to serve, teachers who want to offer therapeutic yoga classes ideally seek certification at the 500-hour level of teacher training. This advanced credential holds them directly responsible for understanding the therapeutic yoga principles and practices that will most auspiciously support, honor, and address the needs of the potentially vulnerable individuals who access their therapeutic yoga class offerings.

Additionally, yoga teachers can choose to register at the appropriate level (i.e., 200-hour or 500-hour) with Yoga Alliance to assure their students that they have been trained to a minimum standard of teaching practice; and that they have the humility to recognize their responsibility to continue to learn more about the people they service and the services they provide. Additional specialty training may be indicated if therapeutic yoga classes are offered to specific clinical or age-related populations (e.g., therapeutic yoga for children or seniors; or yoga for specific healthcare topics, such as cancer, mental health, or pregnancy).

Yoga Therapeutics in Healthcare

Yoga therapeutics in healthcare are integrated and holistic interventions offered for individuals with particular characteristics, concerns, or diagnoses. They are offered in healthcare, allied healthcare, mental healthcare, and/or community health setting by a *qualified healthcare provider with training in therapeutic yoga principles and practices*. Yoga therapeutics are provided within the context of the healthcare professional's existing scope of practice, either individually or in small groups. In small groups, yoga therapeutics are offered similarly and require the same humility and responsibility as therapeutic yoga classes, except that groups are clearly marked as yoga-therapeutically led by a healthcare provider with an existing commensurate scope of practice. Yoga therapeutics in healthcare, because of their clearly-defined focus on particular patients or specified physical or mental health concerns, typically are grounded in a clear care plan or intervention plan. The provider has in-depth, assessment-based knowledge about the clients that guides the yoga therapeutics offered in group or individual sessions.

Healthcare providers who aspire to provide yoga therapeutics can become credentialed by the International Association for Yoga Therapists via a new pathway for qualified health professionals (QHP) who to want apply therapeutic yoga principles and practices to their extant healthcare practice. This new IAYT-Q designation documents that the QHP has specific preparation for using yoga therapeutics in the context of their defined healthcare setting. The expectation for the IAYT-Q designation is that yoga-therapeutically-trained QHPs honor their healthcare training and use therapeutic yoga principles and practices within an appropriate scope of clinical practice and therapeutic yoga specialization.

Yoga Therapy

Yoga therapy is offered one-on-one (perhaps one-on-two if a yoga professional has two clients with similar clinical presentations) and specifically tailored to the needs and presenting health or mental health diagnoses of the client. Client or patient and clinician create a clear understanding of the goals for the work together; explore needs and resources together; journey into a greater understanding of the client or patient over time; and have a clear set of ongoing assessment criteria that guide the healing journey. To honor identified needs and resources of each individual, tailored and individualized applications of props, variations, adaptations, and interventions are an assumed ingredient in the therapeutic work. Yoga therapy often occurs in collaboration with a referring healthcare provider (e.g., psychologist, physician, occupational therapist) and generally presumes a working relationship of the client with this medical or mental healthcare provider (depending on referral).

It is incumbent on yoga *teachers* who want to become yoga *therapists* to complete a formal yoga therapy training program. Ideally, such a program is accredited by the International Association for Yoga Therapists. Additional specialty training may be indicated if yoga therapy services are to be offered to defined clinical or age-related populations (e.g., yoga therapy for children or seniors; yoga therapy for specific health concerns or conditions, such as oncology, mental health, cardiology, neurology, and more).

Details about Yoga Teaching and Yoga Therapy Credentialing

Yoga Teaching – Certification Preparation and Credentials

The yoga profession at the teaching level of scope of practice is not well regulated. The term 'yoga teacher' is not protected; anyone can choose to call themselves a yoga teacher, regardless of training or qualification. What they cannot do is call themselves a 'certified' or 'registered' yoga teacher, unless they have the commensurate training (see below). Certification of yoga teachers (so that they may call themselves 'certified yoga teacher') can be accomplished via any yoga teacher training that offers a certificate program in yoga. Such programs are not regulated and competencies taught may range widely from program to program. Registration of a yoga teacher (so that they may call themselves 'registered yoga teacher') depends on the completion of a yoga teacher training program that is registered with Yoga Alliance.

Yoga Teaching – Registration Preparation and Credentials

Yoga Alliance (YA) is the organization that has taken charge worldwide of defining basic competencies and setting foundational standard for yoga teacher training to ensure the basic skills necessary for teachers to provide yoga classes to the public. Yoga Alliance embraces "a thoughtful, creative, and broadly community-centered approach" to yoga teaching that assures that everyone feels included, welcomed, and represented in a practice of yoga that reflects and honors a multitude of perspectives and voices (https://www.yogaalliance.org/Strategic_Plan). Teacher training programs that meet the YA requirements for their basic competencies and standards (including ethics and scope of practice commitments) can apply to become a Registered Yoga School. Once a yoga school is registered by Yoga Alliance, it can advertise itself as such (using a Yoga Alliance-provided logo), signaling to applicants and trainees that – upon graduation – they will be eligible to apply to Yoga Alliance to become a registered yoga teacher. Only graduates from *registered yoga schools* are eligible to apply to Yoga Alliance to become 'registered yoga teachers'. Registration as a Registered Yoga School by YA simply means that the school's program has met the minimum standards set for a particular level of yoga teacher training. Registration alone does not guarantee high-quality instruction or content as there are currently no checks and balances to investigate ongoing compliance by an RYS, once it is registered.

Registration for schools and teachers happens at two levels of education (200-hour and 500-hour). At the teacher level, there is also an experience-based designation defined by yoga teachers exceeding a certain minimum number of direct teaching hours. Specialty registrations are also defined. At different levels of registration, different requirements exist for ongoing continuing education. Ideally, CE is obtained from a Yoga Alliance Continuing Education Provider (YACEP), a teacher who meets minimum hours of experience with yoga teaching.

The following details summarize the current state of affairs related to registered yoga teaching credentialing:
- RYS200 – This designation identifies a Yoga Alliance-registered yoga school that provides 200-hour yoga teacher training that meets the basic standards set by Yoga Alliance.
- RYS300 – This designation identifies a Yoga Alliance-registered yoga school that provides 300-hour yoga teacher training (beyond the 200-hour teaching level) that meets the basic standards for a 300-hour training program by Yoga Alliance.
- RYT – This designation identifies a registered yoga teacher who successfully graduated from a teacher training program that is registered with Yoga Alliance. Such teachers must complete 30 hours of Continuing Education plus 45 hours of direct teaching every 3 years to maintain registration.
  - There are two levels of education:
    - RYT200 = These registered yoga teachers have completed a minimum of a 200-hour yoga teacher training program registered with YA.
    - RYT500 = These registered yoga teachers have completed a minimum of a 500-hour yoga teacher training program via programs registered with YA.
  - There are two levels of experience:
    - E-RYT200 = *Experienced* registered yoga teacher at the level of 200-hour yoga teacher training have completed a minimum of 1,000 hours of direct yoga teaching experience.
    - E-RYT500 = *Experienced* registered yoga teacher at the level of 500-hour yoga teacher training have completed a minimum of 2,000 hours of direct yoga teaching experience.
  - There are two specialty registrations:
    - RCYT = Successful graduates of a 200-hour teacher training plus at least 85 hours of additional child-specific training, both from an RYS, may call themselves registered children's yoga teachers.
    - RPCT = Successful graduates of a 200-hour teacher training plus at least 95 hours of additional pregnancy-specific training, both from an RYS, may call themselves registered prenatal/postnatal yoga teachers.

Therapeutic Yoga Preparation and Credentials

While yoga teaching is clearly under the purview of *Yoga Alliance* and yoga therapy is clearly under the purview of the *International Association of Yoga Therapists*, therapeutic yoga is largely undefined territory. There are 300-hour yoga teacher training programs that are therapeutic in nature (such as the YogaX YTT300; https://www.yogaxteam.com/300hr-ytt) and are clear about preparing yoga teachers for working in healthcare settings. However, Yoga Alliance neither has a clear educational pathway, nor educational standards for programs that train teachers to work in the breadth and complexity of healthcare settings. This leaves yoga teachers who have this professional interest to their own devices in locating and vetting possible YTT300s that can prepare them auspiciously for such work.

The *International Association of Yoga Therapists* has stepped into this undefined territory by creating a novel pathway (https://www.iayt.org/page/ACC-qhps-in-yoga-therapy) for healthcare providers who want to integrate therapeutic yoga principles and practices into their extant clinical work. This pathway for Qualified Health Professionals (QHP) became available in January 2024; the first program accredited under this novel initiative was the YogaX IAYT-Q program at Stanford Medicine/Psychiatry (https://www.yogaxteam.com/yogax-iayt-q-300-hour-program). Programs in the QHP pathway train healthcare professions in foundational therapeutic yoga principles and practices.

To become a healthcare provider with a QHP credential (designated as IAYT-Q) requires graduation from an IAYT-accredited *Foundation of Therapeutic Yoga Principles for QHPs Program*. The program must require a prerequisite of a healthcare profession or enrollment in the clinical phase of a healthcare preparation. QHP programs require 300 hours of training in foundations of therapeutic yoga principles and practices, and at least 30 hours of practicum. Maintenance of certification requires a minimum of 10 CEs every three years. There is a one-time registration fee and an annual membership cost (required for credentialing).

Yoga Therapy Preparation and Credentials

The *International Association of Yoga Therapists* (IAYT) is the regulating body for yoga therapy programs in the US and worldwide. IAYT certifies programs and teachers who want to provide yoga therapy, defined in IAYT's 2024 strategic plan as the "professional application of the principles and practices of yoga to promote health and well-being within a therapeutic relationship that includes personalized assessment, goal setting, lifestyle management, and yoga practices for individuals or small groups".

To become a yoga therapist, certified by IAYT (designated as a C-IAYT), requires successful graduation from an IAYT-accredited yoga therapy program. IAYT-approved yoga therapy programs must require a minimum of 800 hours of yoga therapy training (including at least 150 hours of practicum plus 30 hours of mentorship), in addition to a prerequisite of having already successfully completed a YTT200 (i.e., adding to a minimum total of 1,000 hours of yoga training). Maintenance of certification as a C-IAYT requires a minimum of 24 CEs every three years as well as successful completion of an ethics exam. A worldwide competency exam for C-IAYT applicants needs to be passed before certification is granted, even if the applicant graduated from an IAYT-accredited yoga therapy program. There is a one-time registration fee and an annual membership cost (required for credentialing).

IAYT has expressed a preference that CEs be obtained from IAYT-approved continuing education providers (APDs [which stands for Advanced Professional Development provider]) to assure that trainers (even of ongoing education) meet minimum therapy training requirements. IAYT provides many resources to its membership, including a quarterly newsletter, *The Yoga Therapist*, and a PubMed-indexed professional journal that is published annually, the *International Journal of Yoga Therapy*. IAYT sponsors two annual conferences, one geared to the entirety of its membership and one focused on research in yoga therapy.

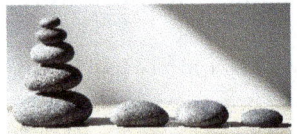

Summary and Definition of Relevant Acronyms Related to Yoga Services

Yoga Teaching - Certification

CYT = certified yoga teacher; any yoga program can offer certification of yoga teachers – regardless of whether the school is registered with Yoga Alliance or not and regardless of the number of hours required for graduation

CYT200 = certified yoga teacher at the level of 200-hour yoga teacher training (no experience level is recognized)

CYT500 = certified yoga teacher at the level of 500-hour yoga teacher training (no experience level is recognized)

Yoga Teaching - Registration

YA = Yoga Alliance – the only formal group that sets standards across the US and the rest of the world for the registration of yoga teachers

RYS200 – registered yoga school by Yoga Alliance with registration for providing 200-hour yoga teacher training

RYS300 – registered yoga school by Yoga Alliance with registration for providing advanced 300-hour yoga teacher training (beyond the 200-hour teaching level)

RYT = registered yoga teacher; only teachers who successfully graduated from a teacher training program that is registered with Yoga Alliance can become registered yoga teachers; 30 hours of Continuing Education plus 45 hours of direct teaching are required every 3 years to maintain registration

RYT200 = registered yoga teacher at the level of 200-hour yoga teacher training

E-RYT200 = experienced registered yoga teacher at the level of 200-hour yoga teacher training with a minimum of 1,000 hours of direct yoga teaching experience

RYT500 = registered yoga teacher at the level of 500-hour yoga teacher training

E-RYT500 = experienced registered yoga teacher at the level of 500-hour yoga teacher training with a minimum of 2,000 hours of direct yoga teaching experience

RCYT = registered children's yoga teacher; a successful graduate of a 200-hour teacher training plus at least 85 hours of additional child-specific training, both from an RYS

RPCT = registered prenatal yoga teacher; a successful graduate of a 200-hour teacher training plus at least 95 hours of additional pregnancy-specific training, both from an RYS

YACEP = Yoga Alliance Continuing Education Provider; must be an E-RYT

Yoga Therapy

IAYT = International Association of Yoga Therapists, the regulating body for yoga therapy programs in the US and worldwide

C-IAYT = Certified yoga therapist by the IAYT; requires successful graduation from an accredited yoga therapy program; the program must require a minimum of 800 hours of yoga teacher/therapist training – i.e., at least 300 beyond a CYT500 or RTY500; the movement currently is to augment this requirement to 1,000 of training as the minimum requirement; maintenance of certification requires a minimum of 24 CEs every three years as well as successful completion of an ethics exam

APD = approved professional development – preferred CE for C-IAYTs; also the abbreviation for yoga therapists approved to provide APD

Summary and Definition of Relevant Acronyms Related to Yoga Services
IJYT = *International Journal of Yoga Therapy*, the PubMed-indexed research journal operated by IAYT; a free subscription comes with IAYT membership YTT = *Yoga Therapy Today*, the IAYT quarterly newsletter; a free subscription comes with IAYT membership SYTAR = Symposium on Yoga Therapy and Research – offered annually by IAYT SYR = Symposium on Yoga Research – offered annually by IAYT
Therapeutic Yoga
IAYT = International Association of Yoga Therapists, the regulating body for yoga therapy programs in the US and worldwide IAYT-Q = Qualified health professional with training in Foundations of Therapeutic Yoga, certified by the IAYT; requires successful graduation from an accredited therapeutic yoga program; the program must require a minimum of 300 hours of therapeutic yoga principles and practices training and evidence of a health profession or matriculation in a health professions program; maintenance of certification requires a minimum of 10 CEs every three years

Concluding Thoughts

The time has come to honor yoga's long tradition as a healing art and lifestyle practice. Therapeutically, yoga can be applied as a primary, secondary, and tertiary prevention strategy. It can be used to support human beings in a journey toward thriving, moving beyond healing and coping. As discussed in one of my blogs, yoga is a lifestyle as well as a means of practicing lifestyle medicine. It has much to offer to healthcare settings – for patients and providers alike. Integration of yoga into healthcare settings presents an innovative and multifaceted opportunity to revolutionize at least some of the challenges within current healthcare systems. Yoga's core principles are uniquely aligned with a commitment to comprehensive, coordinated, and integrated person-centered preventive and supportive care while enhancing provider wellbeing. The integration of yoga's ancient wisdom into modern healthcare can create a more resilient healthcare ecosystem that places emphasis on integrated and holistic wellbeing and lifestyles for patients and care providers alike.

For yoga to take its proper place in life and healthcare, we must create clarity about what yoga is and how a scope of practice can vary from yoga service provider to yoga service provider. In this book, I have simply offered my current ideas and recent thinking. A larger, nationwide effort is needed to establish clear guidelines for yoga service professionals to ensure ethical practice, guided by the ethical (*yama*) and lifestyle (*niyama*) practices and principles of the ancient yoga tradition, and aligned with professional practice codes in modern healthcare.

Bibliography and Citations

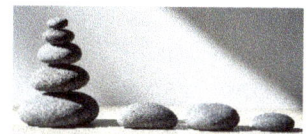

Abel, A. N., Lloyd, L. K., & Williams, J. S. (2013). The effects of regular yoga practice on pulmonary function in healthy individuals: A literature review. *The Journal of Alternative and Complementary Medicine, 19*(3), 185–190. 10.1089/acm.2011.0516

Addis, D. R., Wong, A. T., & Schacter, D. L. (2007). Remembering the past and imagining the future: Common and distinct neural substrates during event construction and elaboration. *Neuropsychologia, 45*(7), 1363–1377. 10.1016/j.neuropsychologia.2006.10.016

Altevogt, B. M., & Colten, H. R. (2006). *Sleep disorders and sleep deprivation*. National Academies Press. 10.17226/11617

Amen, M. D. (2017). *Memory rescue*. Tyndale House.

Badenoch, B. (2011a). *Being a brain-wise therapist: A practical guide to interpersonal neurobiology*. W.W. Norton and Company.

Badenoch, B. (2011b). *The brain-savvy therapist's workbook*. Norton.

Badenoch, B. (2018). *The heart of trauma: Healing the embodied brain in the context of relationship*. Norton.

Barkataki, S. (2020). *Embrace yoga's roots: Courageous ways to deepen your yoga practice*. Ignite Yoga and Wellness Institute.

Barnes, P. M., Bloom, B., & Nahin, R. L. (2007). Complementary and alternative medicine use among adults and children: United States. *National Health Statistics Report, 12*, 1–23. PMID: 19361005

Barnett, J. E., Shale, A. J., Elkins, G., & Fisher, W. (2014). *Complementary and alternative medicine for psychologists: An essential resource*. American Psychological Association. 10.1037/14435-000

Beaty, R. E., Thakral, P. P., Madore, K. P., Benedek, M., & Schacter, D. L. (2018). Core network contributions to remembering the past, imagining the future, and thinking creatively. *Journal of Cognitive Neuroscience, 30*(12), 1939–1951. 10.1162/jocn_a_01327

Birdee, G. S., Legedza, A. T., Saper, R. B., Bertisch, S. M., Eisenberg, D. M., & Phillips, R. S. (2008). Characteristics of yoga users: Results of a national survey. *Journal of General Internal Medicine, 23*(10), 1653–1658. 10.1007/s11606-008-0735-5

Boccio, F. J. (1993). *Mindfulness yoga: The awakened union of breath, body, and mind*. Wisdom Publications.

Bondy, D. (2020). *Yoga where you are*. Shambhala.

Borghardt, T. (2016). *Buddhistische psychologie*. Arkana.

Brems, C. (1999). *Psychotherapy: Processes and techniques*. Allyn & Bacon.

Brems, C. (2001). *Basic skills in psychotherapy and counseling*. Brooks/Cole.

Brems, C. (2015). A yoga stress reduction intervention for university faculty, staff, and graduate students. *International Journal of Yoga Therapy, 25*, 61–77. 10.17761/1531-2054-25.1.61.

Brems, C. (2020). Yoga as a mind-body practice. In J. Uribarri, & J. A. Vassalotti (Eds.), *Nutrition, fitness, and mindfulness: An evidence-based guide for clinicians.* (pp. 137–155). Springer Nature.

Brems, C. (2022). *Ancient wisdoms and science of yoga: A companion for 200-hour yoga teacher training for healthcare and allied healthcare settings.* Unpublished manuscript.

Brems, C. (2023). Finding truth, doing no harm, and being curious – the yoga of research and becoming a practitioner-scholar. *Yoga Therapy Today,* (Winter), 18–22.

Brems, C. (2024a). *Ancient wisdom and modern science of yoga: A companion for 200-hour yoga teacher training for healthcare and allied healthcare settings.* Self-Published.

Brems, C. (2024b). *Therapeutic breathwork.* Springer. 10.1007/978-3-031-66683-4

Brems, C., Colgan, D., Freeman, H., Freitas, J., Justice, L., Shean, M., & Sulenes, K. (2016). Elements of yogic practice: Perceptions of students in healthcare programs. *International Journal of Yoga, 9,* 121–129. 10.4103/0973-6131.183710

Brems, C., Justice, L., Sulenes, K., Girasa, L., Ray, J., Davis, M., Freitas, J., Shean, M., & Colgan, D. (2015). Improving access to yoga: Barriers to and motivators for practice among health professions students. *Advances in Mind-Body Medicine, 29*(3), 6–13. https://www.ncbi.nlm.nih.gov/pubmed/26026151

Brems, C., & Rasmussen, C. H. (2019). *A comprehensive guide to child psychotherapy and counseling* (4th ed.). Waveland.

Brown, K. W., & Ryan, R. M. (2003). The benefits of being present. *Journal of Personality and Social Psychology, 84*(4), 822–848. 10.1037/0022-3514.84.4.822

Brown, K. W., Ryan, R. M., & Creswell, J. D. (2007). Mindfulness: Theoretical foundations and evidence for its salutary effects. *Psychological Inquiry, 18*(4), 211–237. 10.1080/10478400701598298

Carroll, J. E., & Prather, A. A. (2021). Sleep and biological aging: A short review. *Current Opinion in Endocrine and Metabolic Research, 18,* 159–164. 10.1016/j.coemr.2021.03.021

Carter, J., Gerbarg, P. L., D'ambrosio, C., Anand, L., Dirlea, M., Vermani, M., & Katzman, M. A. (2013). Multi-component yoga breath program for Vietnam veteran post traumatic stress disorder: Randomized controlled trial. *Journal of Traumatic Stress Disorders & Treatment, 2*(3), 1–10. 10.4172/2324-8947.1000108

Chennaoui, M., Vanneau, T., Trignol, A. &., Arnal, P., Gomez-Merino, D., Baudot, C., Perez, J., Pochettino, S. &., & Eirale, C., & Chalabi, H.M. (2021). How does sleep help recovery from exercise-induced muscle injuries? *Journal of Science and Medicine in Sport, 24*(10), 982–987. 10.1016/j.jsams.2021.05.007

Clark, B. (2016). *Your body, your yoga.* Wild Strawberry Productions.

Cozolino, L. J. (2015). *Why therapy works: Using our minds to change our brains.* W.W. Norton and Company.

Cozolino, L. J. (2024). *The neuroscience of psychotherapy: Healing the social mind* (4th ed.). Norton.

Craig, A. D. (2014). *How do you feel? An interoceptive moment with your neurobiological self.* Princeton University Press.

Csikszentmihalyi, M. (2008). *Flow: The psychology of optimal experience.* HarperPerennial Modern Classics.

Damasio, A. R. (2012). *Self comes to mind: Constructing the conscious brain.* Vintage.

Datta, K., Tripathi, M., Verma, M., Masiwal, D., & Mallick, H. N. (2021). Yoga nidra practice shows improvement in sleep in patients with chronic insomnia: A randomized controlled trial. *National Medical Journal of India, 34*(3), 143–150. 10.25259/NMJI_63_19

De Michelis, E. (2004). *A history of modern yoga.* Continuum. 10.5040/9781472548436

Dittman, K. A., & Freedman, M. R. (2009). Body awareness, eating attitudes, and spiritual beliefs of women practicing yoga. *Eating Disorders, 17,* 273–292. 10.1080/10640260902991111

Easwaran, E. (2007). *The Bhagavad Gita.* Nilgiri Press.

Ekman, P., Davidson, R. J., Ricard, M., & Wallace, B. A. (2005). Buddhist and psychological perspectives on emotions and well-being. *Current Directions in Psychological Science, 14*(2), 59–63. 10.1111/j.0963-7214.2005.00335.x

Elwy, A. R., PhD, Groessl, E. J., PhD, Eisen, S. V., PhD, Riley, K. E., MA, Maiya, M., MA, Lee, J. P., MSW, Sarkin, A., PhD, & Park, C. L., PhD. (2014). A systematic scoping review of yoga intervention components and study quality. *American Journal of Preventive Medicine, 47*(2), 220–232. 10.1016/j.amepre.2014.03.012

Esteve-Gibert, N., & Prieto, P. (2014). Infants temporally coordinate gesture-speech combinations before they produce their first words. *Speech Communication, 57,* 301–316. 10.1016/j.specom.2013.06.006

Farb, N., Duabenmier, J., Price, C. J., Gard, T., Kerr, C., Dunn, B. D., Klein, A. C., Paulus, M. P., & Mehling, W. E. (2015). Interoception, contemplative practice, and health. *Frontiers in Psychology, 6,* 763. 10.3389/fpsyg.2015.00763

Farhi, D. (2005). *Bringing yoga to life.* HarperCollins.

Farhi, D. (2006). *Teaching yoga: Exploring the teacher-student relationship.* Shambhala.

Farhi, D. (2011). *Yoga mind, body & spirit: A return to wholeness.* Owl Books.

Ferrucci, P. (2007). *The power of kindness: The unexpected benefits of leading a compassionate life.* Jeremy P. Tarcher/Penguin.

Feuerstein, G. (2013). *The psychology of yoga: Integrating eastern and western approaches for understanding the mind.* Shambala.

Field, T. (2011). Yoga clinical research review. *Complementary Therapies in Clinical Practice, 17,* 1–8. 10.1016/j.ctcp.2010.09.007

Freeman, H., Brems, C., Michael, P., & Marsh, S. (2019). Empowering a community from the inside out: Evaluation of a yoga teacher training program for adults in custody. *International Journal of Yoga Therapy, 29*(1), 19–29. 10.17761/2019-00015

Freeman, H., Vladagina, N., Razmjou, E., & Brems, C. (2017). Yoga in print media: Missing the heart of the practice. *International Journal of Yoga, 10*(3), 160–166. 10.4103/ijoy.IJOY_1_17

Gard, T., Noggle, J. J., Park, C., Vago, D. R., & Wilson, A. (2014). Potential self-regulatory mechanisms of yoga for psychological health. *Frontiers in Human Neuroscience, 8,* 770. 10.3389/fnhum.2014.00770

Gard, T., Taquet, M., Dixit, R., Holzel, B., Dickerson, B., & Lazar, S. (2015). Greater widespread functional connectivity of the caudate in older adults who practice Kripalu yoga and vipassana meditation than in controls. *Frontiers in Human Neuroscience, 9,* 137. 10.3389/fnhum.2015.00137

Garland, E. L., Farb, N. A., R. Goldin, P., & Fredrickson, B. L. (2015). Mindfulness broadens awareness and builds eudaimonic meaning: A process model of mindful positive emotion regulation. *Psychological Inquiry, 26*(4), 293–314. 10.1080/1047840X.2015.1064294

Gerritsen, R., & Band, G. (2018). Breath of life: The respiratory vagal stimulation model of contemplative activity. *Frontiers in Neuroscience, 12,* 1–25. 10.3389/fnhum.2018.00397

Goleman, D., & Davidson, R. J. (2017). *Altered traits.* Avery.

Grant, A. (2021). *Think again.* WH Allen.

Grant, A. (2023). *Hidden potential: The science of achieving greater things*. Virgin Digital.

Gu, J., Strauss, C., Bond, R., & Cavanagh, K. (2015). How do mindfulness-based cognitive therapy and mindfulness-based stress reduction improve mental health and wellbeing? A systematic review and meta-analysis of meditation studies. *Clinical Psychology Review, 37*, 1–12. 10.1016/j.cpr.2015.01.006

Gupta, A., Kaur, J., Shukla, G., Bhullar, K. K., Lamo, P., KC, B., Agarwal, A., Srivastava, A. K., & Sharma, G. (2023). Effect of yoga-based lifestyle and dietary modification in overweight individuals with sleep apnea: A randomized controlled trial (ELISA). *Sleep Medicine, 107*, 149–156. 10.1016/j.sleep.2023.04.020

Hanh, T. N. (2011). *Anger: Buddhist wisdom for cooling the flames*. Ebury Digital.

Hartranft, C. (2003). *The yoga sutra of Patanjali: A new translation with commentary*. Shambala Classics.

Hayes, M., & Chase, S. (2010). Prescribing yoga. *Primary Care, 37*, 31–47. 10.1016/j.pop.2009.09.009

Hebb, D. O. (1949). *The organization of behavior: A neuropsychological theory*. Chapman & Hall.

Heyman, J. (2019). *Accessible yoga: Poses and practices for every body*. Shambhala.

Heyman, J. (2021). *Yoga revolution: Building a practice of courage and compassion*. Shambhala.

Heyman, J. (2024). *The teacher's guide to accessible yoga*. Rainbow Mind.

Hostetter, A. B., & Alibali, M. W. (2004). On the tip of the mind: Gesture as a key to conceptualization. https://escholarship.org/uc/item/0bq3923m

IPSOS Public Affairs. (2016). *2016 yoga in America study conducted by yoga journal and yoga alliance*. https://www.yogajournal.com/page/yogainamericastudy

Irving, W. (2019). *The stoic challenge: A philosopher's guide to becoming tougher, calmer, and more resilient*. Norton.

Iyengar, B. K. S. (2006). *Light on life*. Rodale.

Jessen, N., Munk, A., Finmann, L., Lundgaard, I., & Nedergaard, M. (2015). The glymphatic system: A beginner's guide. *Neurochemical Research, 40*(12), 2583–2599. 10.1007/s11064-015-1581-6

Jeter, P. E., Slutsky, J., Singh, N., & Khalsa, S. B. S. (2015). Yoga as a therapeutic intervention: A bibliometric analysis of published research studies from 1967 to 2013. *The Journal of Alternative and Complementary Medicine, 21*(10), 586–592. 10.1089/acm.2015.0057

Johnson, M. C. (2021). *Skill in action: Radicalizing your yoga practice to create a just world*. Shambhala.

Johnson, M. C. (2023). *We heal together: Rituals and practices for building community and connection*. Shambhala.

Jones, F. P. (1976). *Body awareness in action*. Schocken Books.

Justice, L., Brems, C., & Ehlers, K. (2018). Bridging body and mind: Considerations for trauma-informed yoga. *International Journal of Yoga Therapy, 28*, , 39–50.

Justice, L., Brems, C., & Ehlers, K. (2019). Bridging body and mind: Case series of a 10-week trauma-informed yoga protocol for veterans. *International Journal of Yoga Therapy, 29*(1), 65–79. 10.17761/D-17-2019-00029

Justice, L., Brems, C., & Jacova, C. (2016). Exploring strategies to enhance self-efficacy about starting a yoga practice. *Annals of Yoga and Physical Therapy, 1*(2), 1–7. https://austinpublishinggroup.com/yoga-physical-therapy/fulltext/aypt-v1-id1012.pdf

Kahan, D. M. (2017). Misconceptions, misinformation, and the logic of identity-protective cognition. *SSRN Electronic Journal,* , 1–9. 10.2139/ssrn.2973067

Kaminoff, L. (2021). *Yoga anatomy* (3rd ed.). Human Kinetics.

Khalsa, S. B., Cohen, L., McCall, T., & Telles, S. (2016). *Principles and practice of yoga in health care*. Handspring.

Kornfield, J. (2009). *A path with heart*. Random House Publishing Group.

Lasater, J. H. (2020). *Yoga myths*. Shambhala.

Lasater, J. H. (2021). *Teaching yoga with intention*. Shambhala.

Lorr, B. (2012). *Hell-bent: Obsession, pain, and the search for something like transcendence in competitive yoga*. St. Martin's Press.

McCall, M. C. (2013). How might yoga work? an overview of potential underlying mechanisms. *Journal of Yoga & Physical Therapy, 3*(1), 1. 10.4172/2157-7595.1000130

McCall, M. C. (2014). In search of yoga: Research trends in a western medical database. *International Journal of Yoga, 7*, 4–8. 10.4103/0973-6131.123470

Mingyur Rinpoche, Y., & Swanson, E. (2009). *Joyful wisdom*. Three Rivers Press.

Mitchell, J. (2019). *Yoga biomechanics*. Handspring.

Nivethitha, L., Mooventhan, A., & Manjunath, N. K. (2016). Effects of various prāṇāyāma on cardiovascular and autonomic variables. *Ancient Science of Life, 36*(2), 72–77. 10.4103/asl.ASL_178_16

Norman, A. (2021). *Mental immunity*. HarperCollins Publishers.

Panda, S. (2018). *The circadian code: Lose weight, supercharge your energy and sleep well every night*. Ebury Digital.

Panjwani, U., Dudani, S., & Wadhwa, M. (2021). Sleep, cognition, and yoga. *International Journal of Yoga, 14*(2), 100–108. 10.4103/ijoy.IJOY_110_20

Panksepp, J., & Biven, L. (2012). *The archaeology of mind*. Norton.

Park, C. L., Braun, T., & Siegel, T. (2015). Who practices yoga? A systematic review of demographic, health-related, and psychosocial factors associated with yoga practice. *Journal of Behavioral Medicine, 38*(3), 460–471. 10.1007/s10865-015-9618-5

Payne, L., Gold, T., & Goldman, E. (2014). *Yoga therapy & integrative medicine: Where ancient science meets modern medicine*. Turner Publishing.

Payne, P., & Crane-Godreau, M. A. (2015). The preparatory set: A novel approach to understanding stress, trauma, and the bodymind therapies. *Frontiers in Human Neuroscience, 9*, 178. 10.3389/fnhum.2015.00178

Porges, S. W. (2009). The polyvagal theory: New insights into adaptive reactions of the autonomic nervous system. *Cleveland Clinic Journal of Medicine, 76*(Suppl 2), S86–S90. 10.3949/ccjm.76.s2.17

Porges, S. W. (2011). *The polyvagal theory: Neurophysiological foundations of emotions, attachment communication, and self-regulation*. W.W. Norton & Company.

Porges, S. W. (2017). *The pocket guide to polyvagal theory: The transformative power of feeling safe*. W. W. Norton & Company.

Porges, S. W. (2022). Polyvagal theory: A science of safety. *Frontiers in Integrative Neuroscience, 16*, 871227. 10.3389/fnint.2022.871227

Porges, S. W., & Carter, S. C. (2017). Polyvagal theory and the social engagement system. *Complementary and integrative treatments in psychiatric practice* (pp. 221–240). American Psychiatric Association.

Porges, S. W., & Dana, D. (2018). *Clinical applications of the polyvagal theory: The emergence of polyvagal-informed therapies.* W.W. Norton.

Porter, K. (2013). *Natural posture for pain-free living.* Inner Traditions International.

Ranganath, C. (2024). *Why we remember.* Faber and Faber.

Razmjou, E., Freeman, H., Vladagina, N., Freitas, J., & Brems, C. (2017). Popular media images of yoga: Limiting perceived access to a beneficial practice. *Media Psychology Review, 11*, 2. http://mprcenter.org/review/popular-media-images-of-yoga-limiting-perceived-access-to-a-beneficial-practice/

Riley, K. E., & Park, C. L. (2015). How does yoga reduce stress? A systematic review of mechanisms of change and guide to future inquiry. *Health Psychology Review, 9*, 379–396. 10.1080/17437199.2014.981778

Ross, A., Friedmann, E., Bevans, M., & Thomas, S. (2013). National survey of yoga practitioners: Mental and physical health benefits. *Complementary Therapies in Medicine, 21*, 313–323. 10.1016/j.ctim.2013.04.001

Rountree, S. (2020). *The professional yoga teacher's handbook.* Bloomsbury.

Rountree, S., & DeSiato, A. (2019). *Teaching yoga beyond the poses.* North Atlantic Books.

Scaer, R. (2012). *8 keys to brain-body balance.* Norton.

Schacter, D. L., Addis, D. R., & Buckner, R. L. (2008). Episodic simulation of future events: Concepts, data, and applications. *Annals of the New York Academy of Sciences, 1124*(1), 39–60. 10.1196/annals.1440.001

Schacter, D. L., & Thakral, P. P. (2024). Constructive memory and conscious experience. *Journal of Cognitive Neuroscience, 36*(8), 1567–1577. 10.1162/jocn_a_02201

Schiffmann, E. (2013). *Yoga: The spirit and practice of moving into stillness.* Gallery Books.

Schmalzl, L., Crane-Godreau, M. A., & Payne, P. (2014). Movement-based embodied contemplative practices: Definitions and paradigms. *Frontiers in Human Neuroscience, 8*, 205. 10.3389/fnhum.2014.00205

Schmalzl, L., Powers, C., & Henje Blom, E. (2015). Neurophysiological and neurocognitive mechanisms underlying the effects of yoga-based practices: Towards a comprehensive theoretical framework. *Frontiers in Human Neuroscience, 9*, 235. 10.3389/fnhum.2015.00235

Schwartz, A. (2024). *Applied polyvagal theory in yoga: Therapeutic practices for emotional health.* Norton.

Sebanz, N., Bekkering, H., & Knoblich, G. (2006). Joint action: Bodies and minds moving together. *Trends in Cognitive Sciences, 10*(2), 70–76. 10.1016/j.tics.2005.12.009

Sengupta, P. (2012). Health impacts of yoga and pranayama: A state-of-the-art review. *International Journal of Preventive Medicine, 3*, 444–458. PMID: 22891145; PMCID: PMC3415184

Siegel, D. J., & Payne Bryson, T. (2012). *Whole-brain child: 12 revolutionary strategies to nurture your child's developing mind.* Scribe.

Singleton, M. (2010). *Yoga body: The origins of modern posture practice.* Oxford University Press. 10.1093/acprof:oso/9780195395358.001.0001

Smith, L. B., & Gasser, M. (2005). The development of embodied cognition: Six lessons from babies. *Artificial Life, 11*, 13–29. 10.1162/1064546053278973

Stephens, M. (2011). *Teaching yoga: Essential foundations and techniques.* North Atlantic.

Stern, D. (1985). *The interpersonal world of the infant.* Basic.

Stone, M. (2008). *The inner tradition of yoga.* Shambhala.

Sulenes, K., Freitas, J., Justice, L., Colgan, D. D., Shean, M., & Brems, C. (2015). Underuse of yoga as a referral resource by health professions students. *Journal of Alternative and Complementary Medicine, 21*(1), 53–59. 10.1089/acm.2014.0217

Sullivan, M. B., Erb, M., Schmalzl, L., Moonaz, S., Noggle Taylor, J., & Porges, S. W. (2018a). Yoga therapy and polyvagal theory: The convergence of traditional wisdom and contemporary neuroscience for self-regulation and resilience. *Frontiers in Human Neuroscience, 12*, 67–67. 10.3389/fnhum.2018.00067

Sullivan, M. B., Moonaz, S., Weber, K., Taylor, J. N., & Schmalzl, L. (2018b). Toward an explanatory framework for yoga therapy informed by philosophical and ethical perspectives. *Alternative Therapies in Health and Medicine, 24*(1), 38–46. https://www.ncbi.nlm.nih.gov/pubmed/29135457

Svatmarama, & Akers, B. D. (2002). *Hatha yoga pradipika (translated)*. YogaVidya.com.

Taylor, A. G., Goehler, L. E., Galper, D. I., Innes, K. E., & Bourguignon, C. (2010). Top-down and bottom-up mechanisms in mind-body medicine: Development of an integrative framework for psychophysiological research. *Explore: The Journal of Science and Healing, 6*, 29–41. 10.1016/j.explore.2009.10.004

Terracciano, A., Löckenhoff, C. E., Zonderman, A. B., Ferrucci, L., & Costa, J., Paul T. (2008). Personality predictors of longevity: Activity, emotional stability, and conscientiousness. *Psychosomatic Medicine, 70*(6), 621–627. 10.1097/psy.0b013e31817b9371

Thelen, E. (1995). Motor development: A new synthesis. *The Manchester School, 50*(2), 79–95. https://search.proquest.com/docview/38713200

Tsakiris, M., Jiménez, A. T., & Costantini, M. (2011). Just a heartbeat away from one's body: Interoceptive sensitivity predicts malleability of body-representations. *Proceedings of the Royal Society. B: Biological Sciences, 278*(1717), 2470–2476. 10.1098/rspb.2010.2547

Uithol, S., van Rooij, I., Bekkering, H., & Haselager, P. (2011a). Understanding motor resonance. *Social Neuroscience, 6*(4), 388–397. 10.1080/17470919.2011.559129

Uithol, S., van Rooij, I., Bekkering, H., & Haselager, P. (2011b). What do mirror neurons mirror? *Philosophical Psychology, 24*(5), 607–623. 10.1080/09515089.2011.562604

Vago, D. R., & Silbersweig, D. A. (2012). Self-awareness, self-regulation, and self-transcendence (S-ART): A framework for understanding the neurobiological mechanisms of mindfulness. *Frontiers in Human Neuroscience, 6*, 296. 10.3389/fnhum.2012.00296

Vladagina, N., Freeman, H., Razmjou, E., Freitas, J., Sulenes, K., Michael, P., & Brems, C. (2016). Media images of yoga poses: Increasing injury instead of access. Paper presented at the *144th Annual American Public Health Association Meeting and Exposition*,

von Allmen, F., & Seifarth, R. (2007). *Buddhismus*. Theseus-Verlag.

Vyasa. (2020). *The Bhagavad Gita*. Engage Classics.

Walker, M. (2018). *Why we sleep*. Scribner.

Ward, L., Stebbings, S., Sherman, K., Cherkin, D., & Baxter, G. D. (2014). Establishing key components of yoga interventions for musculoskeletal conditions: A Delphi survey. *BMC Complementary and Alternative Medicine, 14*(196), 1. 10.1186/1472-6882-14-196

White, G. (2007). *Yoga beyond belief*. North Atlantic Books.

Wilber, K. (2000). *Integral psychology*. Shambhala.

Wimbarti, S., & Self, P. A. (1992). Developmental psychology for the clinical child psychologist. In C. E. Walker, & M. C. Roberts (Eds.), *Handbook of clinical child psychology* (pp. 33–46). Wiley.

Witkiewitz, R., Roos, C. R., Colgan, D. D., & Bowen, S. (2017). *Advances in psychotherapy evidence-based practice*. Hogrefe.

Yang, T., Tang, Y., Liu, X., Gong, S., & Yao, E. (2024). Microglia synchronizes with the circadian rhythm of the glymphatic system and modulates glymphatic system function. *IUBMB Life, 76*(12), 1209–1222. 10.1002/iub.2903

Yeager, D. S., & Dweck, C. S. (2020). What can be learned from growth mindset controversies? *American Psychologist, 75*(9), 1269–1284. 10.1037/amp0000794

Żerek, M., & Sitarek, G. (2024). Sleep quality and immune function: Implications for overall health – A literature review. *Journal of Education, Health and Sport, 75*, 56048. 10.12775/JEHS.2024.75.56048

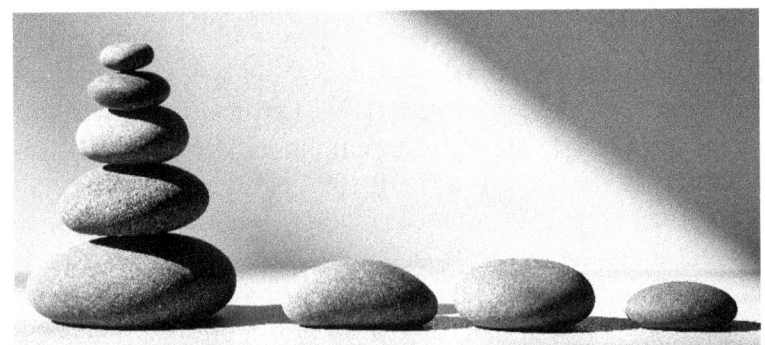

Index

Abhinivesha, 79, 113, 115, 116, 118, 119, 122, 128, 144, 273

Abhyasa, 30, 55, 217, 218, 222, 253, 255, 260, 261, 263, 264

Abundance, 15, 40, 41, 42, 60, 132, 164, 167, 171, 183, 186, 210, 263

Accessibility, 3, 4, 5, 8, 16, 18, 165, 172, 175, 177, 178, 182, 187, 188, 189, 191, 196, 200, 203, 241, 248, 250, 267, 268, 274, 277, 297, 298, 299

Adaptations, 17, 172, 173, 175, 181, 187, 196, 201, 204, 238, 240, 250, 252, 265, 267, 272, 274, 276, 277, 296, 302, 303

Adjusting, 24, 181, 196, 252, 276, 277

Affects, 4, 12, 13, 14, 15, 21, 22, 38, 45, 50, 51, 52, 56, 61, 65, 66, 71, 72, 76, 77, 78, 79, 81, 86, 89, 98, 105, 107, 110, 113, 114, 115, 120, 125, 127, 128, 129, 130, 136, 137, 140, 142, 143, 149, 150, 151, 154, 157, 158, 161, 162, 171, 173, 177, 182, 187, 194, 199, 205, 211, 218, 225, 226, 233, 243, 244, 251, 253, 254, 255, 257, 259, 267, 269, 279

Ahamkara, 81, 117, 154, 195, 231

Ahimsa, 32, 38, 39, 60, 190, 198, 267, 274

Alignment, 36, 46, 49, 65, 172, 176, 183, 186, 187, 191, 202, 203, 219, 223, 224, 225, 233, 234, 235, 242, 250, 251, 252, 253, 254, 256, 260, 262, 263, 268, 270, 272, 273, 276, 277, 278, 279, 281, 285, 286, 287, 288, 291

Allostasis, 24, 25, 51, 61, 74, 94, 95, 103, 108, 111, 223, 224, 264

Altruistic joy, 58, 88, 164, 166, 167, 210, 255, 256

Anandamaya kosha, 11, 63, 65, 70, 88, 97, 110, 155, 195, 213, 220, 222, 224, 255

Annamaya kosha, 11, 18, 47, 63, 65, 66, 69, 72, 73, 74, 75, 76, 78, 89, 92, 96, 97, 125, 150, 195, 199, 211, 212, 220, 222, 224, 231, 253, 254, 260, 262, 264, 272, 279

Apana, 76, 77, 219, 220, 227

Aparigraha, 42, 60, 267, 274

Appreciative joy, 4, 69, 87, 167

Arousal, 15, 21, 23, 24, 51, 56, 61, 65, 66, 74, 76, 77, 78, 79, 92, 93, 94, 104, 106, 107, 108, 109, 110, 111, 112, 113, 114, 117, 137, 140, 151, 154, 180, 199, 211, 224, 226, 227, 232, 236, 251, 253, 254, 255, 258, 259, 260, 262, 264, 267, 279, 282

Asana, 3, 5, 8, 15, 26, 27, 33, 36, 47, 48, 49, 50, 61, 125, 132, 176, 177, 186, 198, 202, 203, 209, 210, 211, 215, 217, 218, 228, 233, 235, 253, 254, 259, 272, 273, 281, 282, 288

Asmita, 71, 79, 113, 115, 116, 117, 121, 122, 128, 143, 226, 273

Assisting, 172, 173, 181, 200, 243, 252, 276, 277, 278

Asteya, 40, 41, 60, 267, 274

Attachment, 29, 30, 32, 55, 57, 76, 77, 79, 87, 112, 113, 114, 115, 116, 117, 119, 122, 123, 154, 155, 157, 163, 165, 166, 199, 207, 209, 217, 218, 226, 232, 242, 255, 259, 261, 263, 273

Attention, 7, 10, 18, 22, 23, 29, 44, 47, 49, 50, 52, 53, 54, 56, 57, 58, 61, 62, 66, 71, 80, 86, 87, 91, 99, 101, 106, 118, 121, 122, 127, 130, 134, 148, 153, 171, 172, 173, 185, 186, 187, 192, 193, 194, 196, 199, 200, 205, 206, 209, 210, 212, 215, 218, 220, 221, 223, 224, 228, 229, 230, 231, 232, 233, 235, 237, 238, 246, 248, 251, 253, 255, 263, 272, 273, 281, 288, 301, 302

Attunement, 15, 54, 55, 58, 61, 65, 87, 106, 149, 180, 196, 205, 206, 211, 212, 228, 231, 232, 234, 251, 276

Autonomic nervous system, 22, 23, 24, 50, 51, 53, 75, 79, 94, 95, 103, 104, 105, 108, 110, 125, 153, 212, 219, 226, 236, 258

Aversion, 18, 43, 77, 79, 80, 86, 89, 113, 114, 115, 116, 117, 119, 120, 121, 122, 123, 128, 129, 142, 143, 147, 151, 163, 164, 167, 199, 207, 209, 212, 215, 216, 226, 232, 254, 255, 257, 262, 273

Avidya, 68, 79, 91, 113, 115, 116, 118, 119, 120, 122, 123, 128, 143, 149, 152, 156, 157, 215, 226, 273

Awareness, 5, 11, 15, 17, 19, 22, 25, 26, 27, 28, 29, 32, 33, 34, 36, 41, 47, 49, 51, 52, 53, 54, 55, 56, 57, 58, 59, 61, 62, 64, 65, 66, 69, 70, 73, 74, 75, 76, 77, 78, 80, 82, 85, 86, 87, 91, 92, 93, 104, 110, 114, 119, 124, 125, 126, 130, 131, 136, 142, 147, 148, 149, 150, 155, 157, 158, 160, 161, 162, 164, 171, 173, 180, 182, 183, 184, 185, 186, 189, 191, 194, 196, 199, 200, 201, 202, 205, 206, 208, 209, 210, 211, 212, 213, 214, 215, 217, 219, 222, 223, 224, 225, 226, 227, 228, 229, 230, 231, 232, 233, 234, 235, 236, 237, 241, 243, 244, 245, 247, 250, 253, 259, 263, 277, 283, 285, 287, 296, 298, 299

Beneficence, 3, 4, 5, 8, 20, 175, 177, 178, 203, 250, 267

Bhagavad Gita, 5, 26, 31, 32, 33

Bias, 13, 14, 40, 53, 55, 80, 81, 82, 118, 127, 133, 150, 151, 154, 155, 156, 164, 165, 171, 182, 183, 184, 191, 199, 269

Biological imperative, 68, 75, 78, 83, 88, 152

Biopsychosociocultural factors, 4, 5, 8, 11, 12, 17, 36, 37, 41, 42, 43, 45, 47, 63, 64, 66, 67, 68, 71, 75, 78, 81, 83, 86, 87, 116, 123, 125, 126, 127, 131, 137, 150, 152, 156, 159, 164, 175, 177, 183, 193, 196, 203, 230, 244, 267, 300

Boundaries, 27, 102, 171, 173, 178, 179, 180, 184, 185, 197, 209, 211, 214, 237, 238, 247, 253, 258, 285, 293, 294, 295, 296, 298, 299
Bracing, 225, 226, 258, 259, 261, 262, 263, 265, 285
Brahma viharas, 59, 69, 87, 88, 115, 127, 144, 150, 154, 155, 157, 159, 161, 162, 163, 164, 167, 176, 177, 182, 183, 185, 197, 209, 210, 243, 293
   karuna, 163, 166, 167
   maitri, 62, 158, 163, 165, 166
   mudita, 163, 167
Brahmacharya, 41, 42, 45, 60, 267, 274
Brahmana, 227, 228
Brain waves
   alpha, 134, 137
   beta, 130, 134, 137
   gamma, 130, 134
   theta, 134, 136, 137, 139
Breathwork, 26, 50, 200, 201, 205, 212, 235
Buddhi, 82, 148, 155, 195
Buddhism, 19, 25, 26, 34, 37, 42, 59, 65, 72, 84, 88, 112, 113, 114, 115, 119, 128, 129, 130, 156, 166, 199, 210, 229, 242
Buddhist, 25, 26, 34, 59, 84, 88, 112, 113, 115, 119, 130, 156, 199, 210, 229
Collapsing, 102, 108, 225, 226, 258, 259, 260, 265
Compassion, 4, 5, 7, 15, 16, 18, 19, 31, 38, 39, 45, 58, 59, 62, 65, 69, 70, 73, 74, 86, 87, 88, 90, 91, 93, 96, 97, 100, 105, 123, 125, 133, 148, 155, 156, 157, 159, 160, 161, 163, 164, 166, 167, 171, 174, 176, 178, 179, 181, 182, 184, 190, 199, 203, 207, 209, 210, 213, 214, 216, 222, 223, 229, 230, 235, 236, 237, 239, 242, 243, 245, 252, 255, 263, 267, 268
Concentration, 3, 7, 18, 22, 28, 30, 36, 48, 53, 54, 56, 57, 58, 62, 65, 80, 86, 91, 116, 127, 148, 149, 153, 155, 161, 162, 196, 198, 201, 203, 207, 211, 213, 215, 223, 228, 229, 230, 255, 268
Confidentiality, 181, 185, 189, 203, 283, 296
Consistency, 98, 178, 179, 210, 237, 240, 298
Contentment, 4, 5, 15, 40, 43, 44, 60, 93, 143, 147, 207, 210
Credentialing, 295, 297, 298, 300, 304, 305, 306
Cuing, 37, 73, 77, 181, 196, 200, 201, 205, 210, 211, 212, 213, 215, 217, 219, 224, 228, 230, 232, 233, 236, 237, 239, 241, 242, 243, 244, 245, 246, 247, 248, 249, 251, 252, 253, 256, 258, 259, 265, 267, 276, 277, 278, 286, 288
Cultural skillfulness, 183
Default mode network, 57, 76, 82, 87, 89, 127, 137, 138, 224
Defense mechanisms, 123, 132
Demonstration, 172, 173, 175, 177, 212, 241, 242, 243, 244, 245, 250, 251, 253, 267, 276, 277, 278, 280, 285
Dharana, 3, 5, 8, 15, 36, 56, 57, 62, 176, 217, 235
Dharma, 31, 32, 34, 35, 116, 183, 199, 200, 205

Dhyana, 3, 5, 8, 15, 36, 58, 62, 176, 217, 235
Discernment, 19, 21, 22, 30, 33, 40, 44, 46, 56, 57, 59, 60, 70, 74, 79, 86, 87, 91, 93, 128, 129, 146, 153, 155, 158, 159, 160, 161, 162, 164, 185, 194, 199, 201, 210, 211, 231, 236, 237, 241, 242, 243, 245, 247, 251, 255, 258, 259, 268, 274, 277
Discipline, 7, 12, 28, 33, 34, 43, 45, 54, 60, 198, 210, 214, 217, 257, 295
Dorsal vagal
   collapse, 107, 108
   complex, 24, 107, 226, 233, 234
   state, 107, 108, 110, 117, 227
Drishti, 18, 91, 219, 220, 221
Dvesa, 79, 113, 117, 118, 122, 128, 142, 226, 273
Embodiment, 4, 11, 28, 47, 48, 59, 61, 63, 72, 73, 74, 89, 92, 94, 110, 111, 154, 165, 172, 215, 224, 225, 226, 235, 246, 259, 260, 262, 264, 276, 277, 280
Empowerment, 8, 37, 60, 61, 67, 175, 177, 180, 182, 187, 207, 226, 237, 238, 256, 258, 263, 268, 274, 283
Enlightenment, 9, 28, 29, 32, 54, 59, 115, 116, 152, 193, 198, 199, 214, 231
Environmental factors, 267
Equanimity, 4, 9, 16, 25, 31, 44, 65, 69, 86, 87, 88, 90, 91, 92, 97, 121, 122, 123, 133, 159, 163, 164, 165, 167, 180, 184, 193, 210, 213, 217, 218, 223, 224, 228, 235, 238, 254, 255, 263, 296
Equity, 5, 8, 14, 16, 18, 39, 41, 67, 172, 178, 184, 187, 188, 189, 190, 199, 267, 297, 298
Ethical commitments, 35, 157
Executive function, 13, 14, 21, 22
Exhalation, 51, 52, 53, 54, 71, 110, 205, 208, 218, 219, 223, 227, 264
Existential imperative, 20, 88, 144, 152, 167
Expansiveness, 219, 220, 221, 222, 226, 260, 261, 263, 281
Exteroception, 25, 49, 55, 61, 77, 104, 225, 229, 231, 233, 234, 244
Generosity, 40, 42, 58, 60, 65, 70, 86, 88, 96, 115, 154, 156, 163, 164, 165, 199, 209
Gunas, 4, 5, 32, 51, 53, 56, 57, 69, 74, 75, 76, 78, 79, 83, 92, 93, 96, 97, 98, 100, 101, 102, 103, 108, 110, 111, 112, 113, 115, 116, 117, 125, 126, 127, 128, 129, 130, 131, 136, 138, 140, 147, 148, 149, 150, 152, 153, 154, 157, 158, 159, 160, 161, 162, 165, 197, 212, 215, 226, 227, 231, 232, 251, 253, 254, 258, 272, 273
Habits, 3, 4, 8, 11, 15, 19, 20, 22, 30, 41, 45, 46, 48, 56, 57, 60, 61, 62, 70, 80, 81, 83, 84, 86, 89, 115, 121, 127, 133, 134, 136, 137, 138, 140, 141, 145, 149, 150, 151, 152, 153, 154, 155, 157, 159, 160, 161, 176, 212, 222, 225, 228, 231, 242, 253, 257, 258, 259, 260, 273
Hatha yoga, 26, 33, 186
Hatha Yoga Pradipika, 26, 33, 34, 71
Holism (see wholism), 9, 70, 193

Homeostasis, 3, 8, 21, 24, 25, 74, 94, 95, 103, 108, 111, 176, 223, 224, 228, 252
Humility, 93, 132, 136, 155, 165, 166, 183, 184, 187, 191, 238, 250, 251, 265, 302, 303
Hyperarousal, 74, 76, 78, 93, 94, 95, 96, 106, 111, 113, 130, 227, 237, 254
Immobilization, 24, 94, 95, 104, 107, 109, 111, 112
Impermanence, 25, 26, 79, 82, 116, 118, 119, 122, 144, 149
Implicit memory, 75, 78, 104, 107, 125, 126, 130, 136
Inclusion, 5, 7, 18, 172, 177, 178, 184, 188, 189, 190, 206, 238, 297, 298, 299
Informed consent, 189, 212, 279, 280, 294, 295, 297, 298, 299
   ongoing, 279, 280
Inhalation, 51, 52, 53, 54, 71, 205, 208, 227, 237
Integrated holistic yoga, 5, 7, 8, 9, 11, 12, 15, 20, 29, 35, 47, 50, 60, 63, 67, 91, 172, 175, 176, 177, 178, 186, 190, 193, 198, 200, 202, 205, 206, 209, 211, 250, 251, 280, 300, 301
   accessibility, 3, 4, 5, 8, 16, 18, 165, 172, 175, 177, 178, 182, 187, 188, 189, 191, 196, 200, 203, 241, 248, 250, 267, 268, 274, 277, 297, 298, 299
   beneficence, 3, 4, 5, 8, 20, 175, 177, 178, 203, 250, 267
   holism, 9, 70, 193
   integration, 3, 5, 8, 15, 16, 23, 24, 26, 28, 30, 36, 38, 49, 59, 60, 62, 66, 68, 69, 70, 74, 75, 81, 82, 85, 87, 96, 103, 134, 136, 163, 172, 175, 176, 177, 178, 194, 196, 197, 202, 205, 206, 207, 209, 210, 213, 215, 216, 217, 218, 226, 228, 260, 263, 308
   intentionality, 5, 8, 18, 22, 43, 60, 75, 79, 83, 88, 175, 178, 193, 194, 202, 203, 250, 256
   wholism, 9, 70, 193
Intentionality, 5, 8, 18, 22, 43, 60, 75, 79, 83, 88, 175, 178, 193, 194, 202, 203, 250, 256
Interconnection, 8, 12, 35, 59, 64, 71, 86, 91, 166, 167, 175, 177, 227
Interdependence, 7, 8, 10, 11, 12, 19, 26, 36, 38, 59, 63, 64, 65, 66, 67, 70, 71, 77, 81, 82, 83, 86, 88, 91, 105, 122, 123, 125, 137, 143, 151, 155, 158, 166, 175, 177, 209, 220, 229
Interior practices, 5, 7, 20, 22, 24, 146, 161, 198, 228, 239
International Association of Yoga Therapists (IAYT), 172, 303, 306, 307, 308
Interoception, 15, 23, 25, 49, 53, 54, 55, 61, 66, 69, 73, 76, 77, 78, 105, 153, 219, 225, 229, 231, 232, 233, 234, 235, 237, 240, 244, 245, 251, 276, 277
Interpersonal matrix, 4, 11, 12, 36, 43, 64, 66, 68, 78, 81, 83, 87, 105, 123, 131, 196, 301
Intervening, 277, 278, 296

Introspection, 7, 46, 60, 80, 84, 87, 137, 138, 152, 153, 158, 190, 198, 210, 227, 237, 268, 294, 295
Intuition, 56, 58, 68, 70, 137, 148, 150, 177, 197, 199, 201, 202, 205, 258, 276, 280
Ishvara pranidhana, 60
Karma, 5, 26, 29, 30, 31, 32, 33, 59, 149, 154, 158, 159, 160, 161, 162, 163, 197
   auspicious, 154, 159, 163
   inauspicious, 159, 160
   mixed, 159
Karuna, 163, 166, 167
Kleshas, 4, 5, 54, 55, 56, 57, 69, 76, 77, 78, 79, 83, 86, 113, 114, 115, 116, 117, 118, 119, 121, 122, 123, 125, 126, 127, 128, 129, 130, 131, 136, 142, 147, 148, 149, 150, 152, 153, 154, 155, 157, 158, 159, 160, 161, 162, 164, 165, 166, 197, 212, 215, 226, 227, 231, 232, 251, 254, 255, 258, 259, 261, 262, 273
   abhinivesa, 226
   asmita, 71, 79, 113, 115, 116, 117, 121, 122, 128, 143, 226, 273
   avidya, 68, 79, 91, 113, 115, 116, 118, 119, 120, 122, 123, 128, 143, 149, 152, 156, 157, 215, 226, 273
   dvesa, 79, 113, 117, 118, 122, 128, 142, 226, 273
   raga, 79, 113, 115, 116, 117, 118, 119, 122, 128, 142, 226, 273
Koshas, 4, 5, 9, 10, 11, 18, 20, 26, 35, 36, 38, 39, 40, 41, 42, 43, 44, 46, 47, 55, 56, 58, 63, 64, 65, 66, 67, 68, 69, 70, 71, 72, 73, 74, 75, 76, 77, 78, 79, 80, 81, 82, 83, 85, 86, 87, 88, 89, 90, 91, 92, 96, 97, 102, 110, 113, 116, 117, 125, 127, 143, 144, 145, 150, 151, 152, 154, 155, 163, 176, 177, 178, 182, 187, 193, 194, 195, 196, 197, 198, 199, 201, 202, 203, 204, 205, 206, 207, 208, 209, 211, 212, 213, 214, 215, 216, 217, 220, 222, 223, 224, 226, 228, 230, 231, 232, 235, 236, 241, 252, 253, 254, 255, 256, 258, 259, 260, 261, 262, 263, 264, 265, 272, 273, 279, 280
   anandamaya, 11, 63, 65, 70, 88, 97, 110, 155, 195, 213, 220, 222, 224, 255
   annamaya, 11, 18, 47, 63, 65, 66, 69, 72, 73, 74, 75, 76, 78, 89, 92, 96, 97, 125, 150, 195, 199, 211, 212, 220, 222, 224, 231, 253, 254, 260, 262, 264, 272, 279
   manomaya, 11, 18, 63, 65, 66, 69, 70, 79, 80, 81, 82, 83, 85, 89, 90, 97, 125, 150, 154, 195, 199, 212, 220, 222, 224, 231, 253, 255, 261, 262, 264, 273, 279
   pranamaya, 11, 18, 47, 63, 65, 66, 69, 75, 76, 77, 78, 79, 80, 85, 89, 92, 96, 97, 113, 125, 150, 195, 199, 212, 220, 222, 224, 231, 253, 254, 260, 262, 264, 273, 279
   vijnanamaya, 11, 18, 63, 65, 70, 81, 82, 83, 85, 86, 87, 88, 90, 97, 110, 127, 144, 150, 155, 163,

182, 195, 207, 213, 220, 222, 223, 224, 231, 255, 279
Langhana, 227, 228
Language considerations
connotations, 131, 244, 248, 250, 267, 269
language, 4, 5, 10, 13, 14, 17, 25, 27, 63, 69, 73, 79, 80, 81, 82, 86, 105, 125, 126, 127, 135, 136, 171, 173, 177, 178, 179, 180, 181, 182, 184, 185, 188, 190, 191, 200, 201, 236, 238, 240, 241, 243, 244, 246, 248, 249, 267, 277, 279, 282, 294, 296, 298
Layers of consciousness (also see koshas), 10, 58, 63, 64, 68, 230
Layers of experience (also see koshas), 11, 63, 64, 66, 71, 150, 158, 159, 176, 181, 197, 205, 206, 207, 209, 244
Layers of self (see also koshas), 12, 19, 20, 26, 28, 29, 47, 48, 49, 63, 64, 66, 67, 76, 155, 157, 158, 177, 197, 267
LET be, 235
Limbs of yoga, 3, 5, 8, 15, 24, 28, 35, 36, 37, 49, 59, 60, 131, 153, 176, 177, 194, 198, 203, 217
asana, 3, 5, 8, 15, 26, 27, 33, 36, 47, 48, 49, 50, 61, 125, 132, 176, 177, 186, 198, 202, 203, 209, 210, 211, 215, 217, 218, 228, 233, 235, 253, 254, 259, 272, 273, 281, 282, 288
dharana, 3, 5, 8, 15, 36, 56, 57, 62, 176, 217, 235
dhyana, 3, 5, 8, 15, 36, 58, 62, 176, 217, 235
niyamas, 3, 5, 8, 15, 33, 35, 36, 43, 44, 58, 115, 157, 161, 162, 171, 176, 177, 178, 183, 185, 187, 197, 209, 210, 293, 295, 298, 308
pranayama, 3, 5, 8, 15, 26, 33, 36, 50, 51, 52, 61, 125, 176, 198, 202, 203, 205, 210, 217, 228, 233, 235, 254, 270, 272
pratyahara, 3, 5, 8, 15, 36, 54, 55, 56, 57, 61, 153, 176, 207, 217, 233, 235
samadhi, 3, 5, 9, 16, 28, 30, 34, 36, 47, 59, 62, 193, 213, 228
yamas, 3, 5, 33, 35, 36, 37, 58, 60, 69, 115, 122, 154, 161, 162, 163, 164, 171, 176, 177, 178, 183, 185, 187, 197, 198, 209, 210, 293, 295, 297, 298
Lovingkindness, 4, 5, 16, 18, 31, 38, 39, 58, 62, 65, 69, 70, 86, 87, 88, 90, 105, 118, 123, 125, 133, 155, 156, 159, 164, 165, 166, 167, 179, 181, 184, 209, 210, 213, 214, 216, 217, 221, 230, 235, 242, 243, 252, 255, 263
Lucidity, 57, 86, 92, 130, 137, 148, 215, 217, 223, 255, 265
Maitri, 62, 158, 163, 165, 166
Manas, 81, 82, 154, 195, 231
Manomaya, 11, 18, 63, 65, 66, 69, 70, 79, 80, 81, 82, 83, 85, 89, 90, 97, 125, 150, 154, 195, 199, 212, 220, 222, 224, 231, 253, 255, 261, 262, 264, 273, 279

Manomaya kosha, 11, 18, 63, 65, 66, 69, 70, 79, 80, 81, 82, 83, 85, 89, 90, 97, 125, 150, 154, 195, 199, 212, 220, 222, 224, 231, 253, 255, 261, 262, 264, 273, 279
Meditation, 3, 7, 16, 17, 26, 28, 32, 34, 48, 50, 54, 58, 59, 62, 64, 65, 80, 86, 108, 109, 130, 137, 139, 153, 155, 161, 179, 191, 198, 199, 201, 207, 210, 211, 229, 230, 241, 246, 267, 270, 273, 274
Memory, 4, 15, 21, 22, 53, 68, 73, 75, 76, 78, 79, 80, 81, 82, 83, 84, 85, 87, 104, 107, 114, 124, 125, 126, 127, 128, 130, 133, 134, 135, 136, 137, 138, 139, 140, 142, 143, 144, 149, 153, 157, 255, 273
Mind states, 4, 5, 57, 58, 62, 66, 69, 83, 85, 114, 121, 128, 139, 147, 148, 149, 197, 212, 215, 223, 227, 251, 255, 267
ekagra, 147, 148
kshipta, 147
mudha, 147
niruddha, 147, 148
vikshipta, 147, 148
Mindfulness, 7, 15, 16, 17, 19, 22, 24, 25, 26, 29, 30, 31, 37, 48, 51, 54, 57, 60, 61, 73, 80, 81, 85, 86, 87, 91, 133, 134, 148, 149, 153, 155, 156, 157, 158, 161, 162, 163, 171, 180, 182, 183, 186, 196, 199, 200, 205, 211, 212, 218, 222, 228, 231, 232, 233, 234, 235, 238, 244, 245, 263
Misidentification, 29, 116, 117, 118, 154, 155
Misperception, 4, 84, 119, 127, 128, 130, 131, 133, 136, 142, 146, 154, 255, 273
Mobilization, 94, 95, 103, 104, 109, 111, 112, 291
Mudita, 163, 167
Neuroception, 23, 25, 49, 54, 55, 61, 66, 69, 73, 75, 77, 78, 94, 104, 105, 106, 107, 110, 153, 225, 229, 231, 232, 233, 234, 235, 240, 244
Neuroplasticity, 15, 58, 87, 135, 150, 159, 161
Nidra, 85, 126, 138, 186, 273
Niruddha, 148
Niyamas, 3, 5, 8, 15, 33, 35, 36, 43, 44, 58, 60, 115, 157, 161, 162, 171, 176, 177, 178, 183, 185, 187, 197, 209, 210, 293, 295, 298, 308
ishvara pranidhana, 60
santosha, 44, 60
saucha, 43, 44, 60
svadhyaya, 46, 185
tapas, 45, 60
Opening centering, 202, 205, 210, 253
Optimal functional breathing, 51, 53, 61, 205, 212, 235
Pancha vayu (see prana vayu), 77
Pancha vayus, 77
Parasympathetic nervous system, 3, 8, 51, 61, 94, 95, 103, 104, 105, 109, 111, 112, 176, 237
Patanjali, 3, 6, 26, 27, 28, 29, 54, 119, 126, 213, 215
Pattern locks, 4, 83, 121, 138, 149, 150, 153, 154, 155, 225
Peak pose, 179, 200, 202, 204, 206

Peak shape, 204, 205, 206, 207
Pedagogy, 169, 171, 173, 174, 175, 176, 178, 192, 194, 198
Perceptions, 3, 4, 8, 10, 15, 22, 23, 25, 36, 48, 49, 50, 73, 77, 80, 81, 83, 84, 89, 104, 105, 106, 109, 115, 120, 121, 126, 127, 128, 129, 130, 131, 133, 136, 138, 142, 143, 146, 148, 149, 150, 152, 154, 157, 159, 160, 162, 176, 229, 231, 232, 233, 234, 241, 246, 257, 273
Physical practices, 3, 7, 15, 17, 20, 47, 48, 49, 61
Polyvagal states, 51, 56, 76, 108, 109, 110, 125, 129, 153, 225, 227, 229, 254
Polyvagal States
  fight-or-flight response, 103, 104, 106
    social connection, 58, 94, 95, 96, 105, 106, 108, 111, 176, 229
Polyvagal theory, 4, 6, 51, 53, 74, 75, 78, 103, 110, 197, 233, 236
Postural alignment, 225
Pramana, 84, 126, 129, 130, 142, 273
Prana vayu, 77
Prana vayus, 76, 77, 78, 219, 221, 226, 228
Pranamaya kosha, 11, 18, 47, 63, 65, 66, 69, 75, 76, 77, 78, 79, 80, 85, 89, 92, 96, 97, 113, 125, 150, 195, 199, 212, 220, 222, 224, 231, 253, 254, 260, 262, 264, 273, 279
Pranayama, 3, 5, 8, 15, 26, 33, 36, 50, 51, 52, 61, 125, 176, 198, 202, 203, 205, 210, 217, 228, 233, 235, 254, 270, 272
Pratyahara, 3, 5, 8, 15, 36, 54, 55, 56, 57, 61, 153, 176, 207, 217, 233, 235
Prefrontal cortex, 23, 80, 82, 87, 132, 137, 163, 223, 229
Projective identification, 132
Proprioception, 25, 49, 54, 55, 61, 66, 69, 73, 75, 225, 229, 231, 233, 234, 244, 251
Props, 16, 17, 47, 172, 173, 175, 177, 180, 182, 188, 189, 196, 200, 201, 204, 205, 211, 212, 225, 238, 243, 250, 251, 255, 264, 265, 267, 268, 269, 270, 272, 274, 276, 296, 302, 303
Props (see yoga props), 16, 17, 47, 172, 173, 175, 177, 180, 182, 188, 189, 196, 200, 201, 204, 205, 211, 212, 225, 238, 243, 250, 251, 255, 264, 265, 267, 268, 269, 270, 272, 274, 276, 296, 302, 303
Raga, 79, 113, 115, 116, 117, 118, 119, 122, 128, 142, 226, 273
RAIN, 157, 164
Rajas, 5, 26, 27, 28, 32, 74, 76, 92, 93, 94, 95, 96, 97, 98, 100, 101, 102, 110, 111, 112, 115, 117, 128, 138, 147, 148, 165, 186, 226, 254, 262, 263, 272
Reactivity, 3, 4, 8, 15, 21, 22, 23, 24, 29, 30, 47, 51, 55, 56, 59, 61, 62, 75, 77, 79, 80, 87, 92, 106, 107, 110, 113, 125, 129, 130, 136, 138, 149, 150, 152, 153, 158, 164, 165, 176, 199, 206, 225, 229, 231, 232, 235, 238, 241, 263, 267, 269, 286
Reductionism, 10, 177, 193

Reflection, 15, 20, 46, 57, 60, 65, 82, 93, 96, 116, 131, 135, 152, 159, 199, 237, 239, 268
Relaxation, 21, 48, 54, 65, 73, 105, 108, 109, 137, 201, 214, 215, 226, 227, 255, 260
Resilience, 3, 7, 8, 13, 14, 15, 19, 20, 21, 24, 29, 36, 50, 59, 60, 62, 66, 67, 68, 74, 87, 92, 93, 94, 99, 106, 107, 111, 116, 140, 165, 167, 176, 182, 196, 198, 202, 206, 209, 210, 211, 213, 216, 218, 222, 223, 224, 227, 228, 237, 238, 241, 244, 252, 256, 258, 259, 260, 262, 263, 264, 265, 277
Responsiveness, 3, 4, 8, 15, 21, 23, 51, 59, 66, 79, 92, 138, 158, 164, 165, 176, 199, 207, 264, 272
Samadhi, 3, 5, 9, 16, 28, 30, 34, 36, 47, 59, 62, 193, 213, 228
Samana, 76, 77, 227, 228
Samskaras, 4, 30, 83, 89, 121, 136, 144, 149, 150, 152, 153, 154, 155, 156, 157, 158, 159, 160, 223, 231, 252, 258, 259, 262, 273
Sangha, 36, 219, 256
Sankalpa, 18, 91, 193, 194, 196, 200
SANKALPA
  Teaching with intention, 193, 194, 195
SANKALPA teaching with intention, 193, 194, 195
Santosha, 44, 60
Sattva, 53, 74, 76, 87, 92, 93, 95, 96, 97, 98, 100, 101, 102, 103, 110, 111, 112, 115, 128, 139, 141, 148, 165, 207, 226, 237, 254, 264, 265, 272, 273
Satya, 39, 40, 60, 190, 198, 267, 274
Saucha, 43, 44, 60
Self-regulation, 21, 22, 24, 25, 50, 53, 56, 62, 87, 172, 241
Sequencing, 23, 171, 173, 178, 179, 193, 197, 198, 200, 202, 203, 204, 205, 206, 207, 210, 237
Smriti, 84, 85, 134, 142, 228, 273
Social engagement, 23, 60, 73, 81, 87, 94, 104, 105, 106, 107, 108, 109, 110, 111, 112, 166, 206, 229
Sthira, 50, 213, 214, 215, 216, 226, 264
Sukha, 44, 50, 213, 214, 215, 216, 226, 264
Sutras, 3, 5, 6, 26, 27, 28, 29, 33, 34, 39, 40, 41, 42, 44, 45, 46, 47, 50, 54, 115, 116, 119, 126, 213, 215, 217, 218
Svadhyaya, 46, 185
Sympathetic nervous system, 22, 25, 53, 94, 103, 104, 106, 107, 108, 109, 110, 111, 112, 117, 186, 227, 233, 234, 236, 239, 240, 262
Tamas, 54, 74, 76, 92, 93, 95, 96, 97, 98, 101, 102, 110, 111, 112, 115, 117, 128, 138, 147, 148, 165, 219, 226, 254, 260, 261, 272
Tapas, 45, 60
Teacher qualities, 37
Therapeutic yoga, 68, 168, 175, 178, 186, 251, 300, 301, 302, 303, 305, 306, 308
Time management, 171, 173, 179
Transcendence, 5, 26, 34, 68, 69, 78, 115, 122, 156, 166

Trauma, 5, 13, 14, 21, 48, 71, 75, 76, 94, 95, 107, 111, 124, 132, 142, 152, 154, 180, 182, 183, 185, 197, 211, 232, 236, 237, 238, 239, 240, 241, 253, 258, 269, 296, 298
Truthfulness, 39, 40, 41, 42, 47, 60, 156, 165, 171, 210, 295
Upanishads, 25, 26, 31
Vagal brake, 104, 106, 227
Vagus nerve, 23, 75, 103, 104, 105, 106
   dorsal branch, 104
   ventral branch, 94, 104, 111
Vairagyam, 30, 55, 217, 218, 222, 253, 255, 261, 263, 264
Variations, 5, 20, 31, 47, 50, 173, 175, 181, 182, 187, 196, 201, 204, 211, 212, 238, 240, 250, 251, 257, 265, 267, 268, 272, 274, 276, 278, 302, 303
Vedana, 76, 78, 83, 113, 114, 115, 116, 125, 130, 140, 227, 231, 233, 251, 253, 254, 258
Vedanas, 83, 125, 130, 254
Ventral vagal complex, 23, 87, 104, 105, 106, 108, 109, 110, 233, 234
Ventral vagal state, 25, 105, 106, 107, 108, 110, 206
Vidya, 59, 68, 91, 113, 149, 215, 217
Vijnanamaya kosha, 11, 18, 63, 65, 70, 81, 82, 83, 85, 86, 87, 88, 90, 97, 110, 127, 144, 150, 155, 163, 182, 195, 207, 213, 220, 222, 223, 224, 231, 255, 279
Vikalpa, 84, 126, 137, 142, 273
Viparyaya, 84, 126, 130, 142, 273
Vrittis, 4, 5, 29, 54, 56, 57, 71, 83, 84, 85, 86, 113, 119, 126, 127, 128, 129, 130, 134, 136, 137, 138, 139, 142, 147, 148, 149, 150, 152, 153, 155, 157, 158, 159, 160, 161, 162, 163, 197, 212, 215, 217, 227, 231, 251, 255, 258, 273
   nidra, 85, 126, 138, 186, 273

pramana, 84, 126, 129, 130, 142, 273
smriti, 84, 85, 134, 142, 228, 273
vikalpa, 84, 126, 137, 142, 273
viparyaya, 84, 126, 130, 142, 273
VUCA, 12, 67
Warm-up, 179, 201, 205
Wholism, 3, 4, 5, 9, 10, 11, 60, 63, 70, 92, 95, 176, 177, 193, 194, 202, 209, 213, 215, 218
Withdrawal, 33, 48, 92, 95, 108, 109, 110, 112, 198, 233, 258, 260, 268, 271
Yamas, 3, 5, 8, 15, 33, 35, 36, 37, 50, 58, 60, 69, 115, 122, 154, 157, 161, 162, 163, 164, 171, 176, 177, 178, 183, 185, 187, 197, 198, 209, 210, 293, 295, 297, 298, 308
   ahimsa, 38, 39
   aparigraha, 42, 60, 267, 274
   asteya, 40, 41
   brahmacharya, 41, 42, 45, 60, 267, 274
   satya, 39, 40, 60, 190, 198, 267, 274
Yoga
   ethics, 54, 176, 178, 243
   props, 16, 17, 47, 172, 173, 175, 177, 180, 182, 188, 189, 196, 200, 201, 204, 205, 211, 212, 225, 238, 243, 250, 251, 255, 264, 265, 267, 268, 269, 270, 272, 274, 276, 296, 302, 303
   sutras, 3, 5, 28
   therapeutics, 68, 168, 172, 175, 178, 186, 191, 194, 202, 207, 212, 251, 300, 301, 302, 303, 305, 306, 308
   therapy, 68, 186, 300, 301, 303, 305, 306, 307, 308
Yoga Alliance (YA), 172, 173, 293, 297, 298, 302, 304, 305, 307
Yoga Sutras of Patanjali, 3, 6, 26, 28

www.ingramcontent.com/pod-product-compliance
Lightning Source LLC
Chambersburg PA
CBHW080517030426
42337CB00023B/4546